# Effective Medical Communication

Subhash Chandra Parija
Balachandra V. Adkoli
Editors

# Effective Medical Communication

## The A, B,C, D, E of it

Springer

*Editors*
Subhash Chandra Parija
Sri Balaji Vidyapeeth (Deemed-to-be University)
Pondicherry
India

Balachandra V. Adkoli
Sri Balaji Vidyapeeth (Deemed-to-be University)
Pondicherry
India

ISBN 978-981-15-3408-9 ISBN 978-981-15-3409-6 (eBook)
https://doi.org/10.1007/978-981-15-3409-6



This Springer imprint is published by the registered company Springer Nature Singapore Pte Ltd.
The registered company address is: 152 Beach Road, #21-01/04 Gateway East, Singapore 189721, Singapore

*Almighty God*

*To my wife Ms. Jyotirmayee Parija for self-less support and my mother Late Smt. Nishamani Parija and my father Late Shri Managovinda Parija for their blessings*

*Also to my Professional colleagues and mentors for their guidance*

*Subhash Chandra Parija*

*My wife Smt. Shyamala Adkoli for standing behind me; and my Gurus who have inspired me…*

*Balachandra V. Adkoli*

# Foreword

डॉ. विनोद कुमार पॉल
सदस्य
Dr. Vinod K. Paul
MEMBER

सत्यमेव जयते

भारत सरकार
नीति आयोग, संसद मार्ग
नई दिल्ली-110 001
Government of India
NATIONAL INSTITUTION FOR TRANSFORMING INDIA
NITI Aayog, Parliament Street
New Delhi-110 001
*Tele. : 23096809 Telefax : 23096810*
*E-mail : vinodk.paul@gov.in*

## Foreword

Communication is at the heart of medical profession's responsibility toward the society.

Stephen Covey, the author of "The 7 Habits of Highly Effective People" underlines communication as two distinct habits of leaders: Firstly, they 'Seek First to Understand, then to be Understood'. Secondly, they Synergize. Applying to medicine, communication is complete only when the message is understood by our patients. However, to make this happen, we need to understand not only our patients but also ourselves. By engaging in hearing, listening, feeling and finally, connecting, we would be shifting ourselves from defensive communication, to more respectful, genuine, sincere and empathic communication.

Sadly, communication skill is often found to be lacking among medical professionals. It is difficult to pin point one single factor for this lacuna.

The best strategy to overcome this gap in our profession is to start communication train medical students during early medical training and follow it throughout the career. In this background, finding a new book on communication is like a godsend. Indeed a paradigm shift is already taking place. Indian medical education is introducing modules on attitude, ethics and communication (AETCOM).

Though a number of books are available in the market, the present book edited by Prof Subhash Chandra Parija and Prof B.V. Adkoli is very special and different from the rest. This book addresses communication skills in a broader perspective, linked with the journey of a medical professional starting as undergraduate student, passing through the stages of post-graduation, faculty member and ending up as a leader in the profession. They have lined up twenty five chapters written by thirty one eminent leaders in health profession hailing from India, South East Asia, Middle East and U.K.

स्वच्छ भारत
एक कदम स्वच्छता की ओर

The topics range from patient doctor communication to mentoring, feedback, taking informed consent, writing prescription, making effective presentations, teaching, conducting workshops, managing conflicts and dealing with social media in a digital world.

The approach taken by the editors, viz., A, B, C, D, E approach is equally fascinating. It harmonizes the deliberations of authors coming from diverse background. The scenarios presented in each chapter are linked with a story a fictitious character 'Comini' a medico who passes through a journey from medical student to a senior faculty braving many odds and challenges. She is also the icon of woman empowerment taking place in India and elsewhere.

The editors pool together rich and diverse experience. Prof Subhash Chandra Parija, being a renowned medical microbiologist and a B.C. Roy Awardee of Medical Council of India brings rich experience of publication in national and international level. Prof B.V. Adkoli who is a leading medical educationist has long experience in faculty development and training of teachers in India and abroad. I am sure, this unique blend of experience and expertise, will immensely benefit the readers, thanks to the Publisher Springer Nature who have international presence in bringing high quality books.

In a nutshell, this book is for everyone, for those who wish to engage in serious reading or just glance through the stories and cartoons to capture the key messages. I hope this book will reach millions of doctors and students across the world to stimulate further work in medical communication.

VINOD K. PAUL
MD, PhD, FAMS, FNAsc, FASc, FNA
Member (Health) NITI Aayog
Government of India

# Preface

Communication in general is all about telling and selling. However, in medicine, it has a special significance. It is about empathic listening, connecting, and establishing bonds of trust with the patients. It is also about leading or working in a team to accomplish individual or collective tasks.

While the whole world of business, commerce, and industries is banking upon communication, the medical professionals have not fully explored the potentiality of communication in enhancing their effectiveness. They have emphasized the medical content rather than the psycho-social aspects of communication. Of late, the pendulum has been shifting. The popular slogan 'Content is the King' needs to be complemented with 'Communication is the Queen'! The science of medicine when delivered through the art of communication leads to a win-win situation for doctors, patients, and the society. The hard core medical science should embrace soft skills like leadership, motivation, and team building which rely mainly upon effective communication.

The felt need for strengthening communication skills among medical professionals prompted us to take up this project seriously. No doubt, a number of books in this field have hit the market, but still, we could not lay finger on any particular book that deals with the whole gamut of communication skills. We therefore decided to address communication skills in a broader perspective, as a journey of a medical professional starting as undergraduate student, passing through the stages of post-graduation, faculty member, and ending up as a leader in the profession.

This book has been designed to provide practical tips rather than extensive review of literature. The structure of the book, what we have termed as A, B, C, D, E approach is a novel attempt to harmonize the content and the style of chapters written by multiple authors. The scenarios depicted in each chapter through a fictitious character *Ms Comini* followed by one-minute exercise are an attempt to provoke thoughts in the mind of readers to ponder upon the issues. The cartoons are expected to convey the message loud and clear. In short, this book is not merely meant for reading, but to help the readers to think, apply, and create their own concept of communication.

We wholeheartedly thank all our contributors who have chipped in this project. Our publisher Springer Nature has shown a track record of executing the projects undertaken by the chief editor every time with a different flavour. We hope this book will also be received by the international reading community belonging to all ages and stages.

Pondicherry, India

Subhash Chandra Parija
Balachandra V. Adkoli

# About the Book

## The Genesis

Perhaps no other aspect in medicine has made so much of impact on the quality of patient care as communication. In fact, the heart of medicine lies in good patient–doctor relationship which is based on the art of communication. Sadly, with growing dependence on high end technology and diagnostics, the medical professionals have drifted away from the personal healing touch, resulting in strained doctor–patient relationship. The lack of communication skills has also hampered the interpersonal relationship among the health professionals which is a key factor for delivering quality care in a complex environment with various cadres of staff who are all interdependent. In order to bridge this *communication gap*, we decided to bring out a book which would serve as a guide for the teachers as well as students to develop communication skills. We were ably supported by 30 eminent faculty who willingly contributed chapters for this mammoth task.

## The Content Organization

We have adopted a different approach in organizing the content of this book. The topics chosen for the book are organized under five parts corresponding to five stages of development of a medical professional. They originate from the communication needs of a medico during various stages.

Part I 'Begin with a Bang' sets the stage for everyone to get sensitized to the overall landscape of communication.

Part II 'Catch them Young' addresses the communication needs of students and resident doctors to sensitize them about the modalities of verbal and non-verbal communication. Core topics such as patient–doctor communication, taking informed consent for research, skills related to prescribing medicine (using a novel 5-R framework), and how to make effective oral presentation in a seminar are discussed.

Part III 'Hold them Strong' addresses the needs of junior and mid-level faculty. The topics written in this part are teaching, learning, and assessing communication skills, communication in large class rooms, how to publish effectively, how to handle general public, media, press, and VIPs, social media, and medical education besides language skills.

Part IV is meant for the senior faculty and the leaders who 'Can't go Wrong'. This part covers skills for organizing workshops, communication skills for the leaders in health professions education, conflict management, and the future of communication in a digital world.

The final part, Part V, is all about 'Play Ping-pong' which means one has to consider the requirements of a specific situation. This part includes sensitive issues like palliative care, the role of medical humanities, communication skills perspectives from Middle East, Southeast Asian perspective, besides chapters on salutogenesis approach and the role of music in therapeutic communication which is an emerging area of interest. The final chapter gives the take home that communication skills can be learnt.

## The A, B, C, D, E Approach

The format of this book is entirely different. All the chapters have been organized in a uniform structure, what we describe as the A, B, C, D, E approach. This is based on the principles of adult learning besides the experience of editors.

A. *Assess the need* (This section states why this chapter is needed)
B. *Brief* (Lists the key objectives or issues to be discussed)
C. *Contextualize* (Presents one or two scenarios followed by one-minute exercise to ponder over the issue)
D. *Describe* (Describes the main body of the chapter, ending up in conclusion in the form of bullet points)
E. *Evaluate* (Raises a few questions or points to ponder)

We strongly suggest the readers to reflect on the scenario and take one-minute exercise as *set induction* for further in-depth reading of D-Describe section.

## The Value Addition

In the beginning of each chapter of the book, we have designed a cartoon around a fictitious character *Ms Comini*. Through *Ms Comini* we have given the key message of the chapter. The exercise given at the end of each scenario helps the reader to reflect and think about the content of the chapter. The evaluation at the end of the chapter is meant for self-assessment.

In summary, this book is designed in a flexible manner to cater to the diverse needs of readers. Those who wish to browse the book with an eye on key message can simply do so, bypassing the description. Those who wish to make serious reading can make use of the exercise and evaluation for a deep engagement with the book. It is therefore, a new experiment. We will be happy to receive comments, feedback, and suggestions from readers for improving this work. After all, we are talking about communication!

## Ms Comini

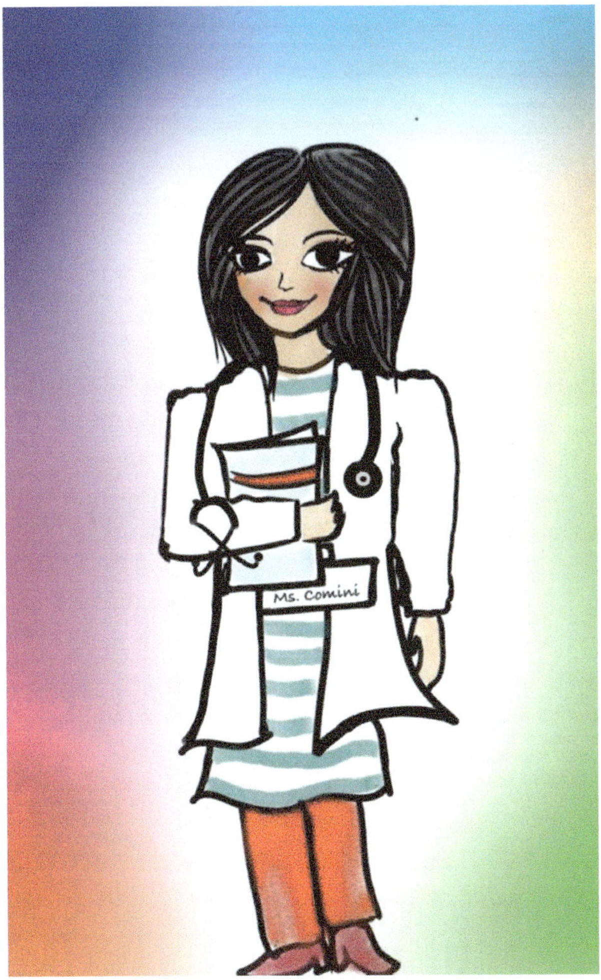


*Ms Comini* hails from a modest rural background. She starts her medical career in a premier medical institute. She is often subjected to a challenge of facing adverse situations during her training or while handling her job responsibility as a junior and then a senior faculty. However, with her positive thinking and innovative methods of handling situation, she comes out with flying colours. In fact, she converts problems into opportunities for learning and growth. Sometimes, she is an observer and at times she is a participant. *Ms Comini* represents a symbol of women empowerment which is taking place in India and many parts of the world.

# Acknowledgements

We wish to place on record our sincere thanks to all those who helped us in bringing out this book. The authors and co-authors of various chapters have done commendable job in submitting the manuscripts in time in spite of their preoccupation with multiple tasks.

Shri M.K. Rajagopalan, The Chancellor of Sri Balaji Vidyapeeth, has provided the academic ambience and support for us to venture this task of international publication.

The cartoons used in this book have been drawn by our second-year MBBS student Ms. Archana who has taken pains to draw all the cartoons amidst her studies, which is highly appreciated.

Several faculty and staff of Sri Balaji Vidyapeeth (Deemed-to-be University) have helped us at various stages. Dr. Ezhumalai has helped us in conducting plagiarism check. Dr. Richa Gupta has helped in grammar check. We also acknowledge with thanks the help received from Dr. Partha Nandi, Dr. M Shivasakthy, Dr. Suguna, Dr. Surekha, Dr. Vigneshvar Chandrasekaran, and Dr. Vinod Babu. Ms. Senbagame, Medical Education Unit has offered full secretarial assistance throughout this project. We thank them all.

We sincerely thank our publisher Springer Nature for extending wholehearted support to us in carrying out this project.

Pondicherry, India

Subhash Chandra Parija
Balachandra V. Adkoli

# Contents

# Contributors

**Balachandra V. Adkoli** Centre for Health Professions Education, Sri Balaji Vidyapeeth (Deemed-to-be University), Pondicherry, India

**Mona Hmoud Al-Sheikh** Medical Education Department, College of Medicine, Imam Abdulrahman Bin Faisal University, Dammam, Saudi Arabia

**N. Ananthakrishnan** Sri Balaji Vidyapeeth (Deemed-to-be University), Pondicherry, India

**Anshu** Department of Pathology, Mahatma Gandhi Institute of Medical Sciences, Wardha, Maharashtra, India

**B. Vishnu Bhat** Division of Medical Research, AVMC, Pondicherry, India

**Ananda Balayogi Bhavanani** Centre for Yoga Therapy Education and Research (CYTER), Sri Balaji Vidyapeeth (Deemed-to-be University), Pondicherry, India

**Gilly Burn** Care Response International and Cancer Relief India, Durham, UK

**Upreet Dhaliwal** Medical Humanities Group, University College of Medical Sciences, University of Delhi, New Delhi, India

**Amaya Ellawala** Faculty of Medicine, University of Sri Jayewardenepura, Nugegoda, Sri Lanka

**Muzaherul Huq** Formerly at WHO, SEARO, Dhaka, Bangladesh

**Muhammad Zafar Iqbal** Medical Education Department, College of Medicine, Imam Abdulrahman Bin Faisal University, Dammam, Saudi Arabia

**Tony George Jacob** Department of Anatomy, All India Institute of Medical Sciences, New Delhi, India

**Indika Karunathilake** Department of Medical Education, Faculty of Medicine, University of Colombo, Colombo, Sri Lanka

**Manoj Kumar Kingsley** Department of Neonatology, JIPMER, Pondicherry, India

**Rajiv Mahajan** Department of Pharmacology, Adesh Institute of Medical Sciences and Research, Bathinda, Punjab, India

**Nalin Mehta** Department of Physiology, All India Institute of Medical Sciences, New Delhi, India

**Shegufta Mohammad** Update Dental College and Hospital, Dhaka, Bangladesh

**Rasnayaka M. Mudiyanse** Department of Paediatrics, University of Peradeniya, Peradeniya, Sri Lanka

**Jyoti Nagmoti** Department of Microbiology, J.N Medical College, KLE Academy of Higher Education and Research (KAHER), Belagavi, Karnataka, India

**Subhash Chandra Parija** Sri Balaji Vidyapeeth (Deemed-to-be University), Pondicherry, India

**Swati Pawar** Mahatma Gandhi Medical College and Research Institute, Pondicherry, India

**Nirmala N. Rege** Department of Pharmacology and Therapeutics, Seth GS Medical College and KEM Hospital, Mumbai, India

**Peush Sahni** Department of Gastrointestinal Surgery and Liver Transplantation, All India Institute of Medical Sciences, New Delhi, India

**Santosh Salagre** Department of General Medicine, Seth G S Medical College and K E M Hospital, Mumbai, India

**Supten Sarbadhikari** FAIMER Regional Institute, Coimbatore, India

**Krishna Seshadri** Sri Balaji Vidyapeeth (Deemed-to-be University), Pondicherry, India

**Tejinder Singh** Departments of Pediatrics and Medical Education, Sri Guru Ram Das Institute of Medical Sciences and Research, Amritsar, Punjab, India

**Sumathy Sundar** Center for Music Therapy Education and Research, Sri Balaji Vidyapeeth (Deemed-to-be University), Pondicherry, India

**Avinash Supe** Formerly at Department of Surgical Gastroenterology, Seth GS Medical College and K E M Hospital, Mumbai, India

**Tashi Tenzin** Faculty of Postgraduate Medicine, Khesar Gyalpo University of Medical Sciences of Bhutan, Thimphu, Bhutan

**Raakhi K. Tripathi** Department of Pharmacology and Therapeutics, Seth GS Medical College and KEM Hospital, Mumbai, India

**Chamindri Witharana** Faculty of Medicine, University of Colombo, Colombo, Sri Lanka

# Last Page

Communication is a buzz word in medical profession. Developing effective communication skills among medicos should start early, reinforced regularly, and etched permanently in the behaviour, attitude, and practice of medical professionals across the board. This book on effective medical communication captures the essence of what communication skills are needed by a medico in his/her long journey starting as a medical student and ending up as leader in the profession. This is followed by practical tips on how to develop these skills. Another unique feature of this book is the approach taken by the editors in harmonizing the content under one common formula called A, B, C, D, E approach (A-Assess need; B-Brief; C-Contextualize; D-Describe; and E-Evaluate). All 25 chapters written by 32 leaders in the health profession hailing from India, Southeast Asia, Middle East, and the UK are based on scenarios followed by one-minute exercise.

The topics range from patient–doctor communication to mentoring, feedback, taking informed consent, writing prescription, making effective presentations, teaching, conducting workshops, managing conflicts, and dealing with social media in a digital world. In addition, specific issues like handling media and press, dealing with vulnerable groups, cultural sensitivities, role of medical humanities and salutogenesis approach using yoga and music therapy have also been covered.

The book is an effort to inform and engage a wide spectrum of audience, medical students, residents, faculty members, and administrators though its main focus is on faculty development which is instrumental for bringing about sustainable changes.

# About the Editors

**Subhash Chandra Parija** MBBS, MD, PhD, DSc, FRCPath, FAMS, FICAI, FABMS, FIMSA, FISCD, FIAVP, FIATP, FICPath is Vice Chancellor of Shri Balaji Vidyapeeth, Pondicherry. Prof. Parija, former Director at the Jawaharlal Institute of Postgraduate Medical Education & Research, Pondicherry, has nearly three-and-a-half decade of teaching and research experiences in Medical Microbiology.

Prof. Parija is a Food and Agriculture Organization (FAO) expert, being constituted to draft guidelines on food safety for parasites. Prof. Parija was awarded WHO fellowships for the study of DNA probes, PCR, and other molecular biological methods in the study of parasitic diseases at the University of Aberdeen, UK. Prof. Parija was a member of Research Advisory Board of BP Koirala Institute of Health Sciences, Dharan, Nepal, the member of Board of MD Examination in Parasitology, Colombo University, Sri Lanka, and the visiting Professor of the College of Medicine & Health Sciences, Sultan Qaboos University, Muscat, Oman, and Faculty of Medicine, University of Malaya, Malaysia. He is one of very few Medical Microbiologists of India to be conferred DSc, highest degree in research, for his contribution in the field of Medical Parasitology by Madras University.

Author of 15 books including *Textbook of Medical Parasitology*, *Textbook of Microbiology*, *Textbook of Microbiology and Immunology*, *Emerging and Re-emerging Infectious Diseases*, *Quick Review Series: Microbiology*, *Textbook of Practical Microbiology*, *Stool Microscopy* and *Sputum Microscopy: a Practical Manual*; editor of the book *Review of Parasitic Zoonoses* and two monographs *Immunizing Agents for Tropics: Success, Failure and Some Practical Issues* and *Kala-Azar: Epidemiology, Diagnosis and Control in Nepal*; Prof. Parija also has contributed several chapters mainly on parasitic diseases for the books, compendium of lectures and proceedings of scientific meetings. Prof. Parija has published more than 350 papers both in the national and international journals of repute. Some of his papers are quoted in textbooks and serial publications.

The development of simple, economical, and rapid diagnostic tests in serodiagnosis of parasitic diseases such as amoebiasis, cysticercosis, and hydatid disease and epidemiology of the parasitic diseases are his main fields of interest in research. Prof. Parija was the first to demonstrate that parasitic antigens are excreted in the urine in hydatid disease and cysticercosis, and urinary antigen could be detected for the diagnosis of these two diseases. He developed for the first time carbon immunoassay (CIA) and staphylococci adherence test (SAT) as two simple rapid diagnostic methods using a light microscope; rapid IHA, protein A IHA, and dot-ELISA for serum antibodies in the diagnosis of amoebic liver abscess, hydatid disease, cysticercosis, and lymphatic filariasis; and co-agglutination (Co-A), latex agglutination test, and CIEP for the detection of antigen in the serum and other body fluids in the patients with amoebic liver abscess, cysticercosis, and hydatid diseases.

Prof. Parija was first to report the use of LPCB, KOH, etc. in the wet mount preparation of stool for the detection of intestinal parasites including *Cryptosporidium*, *Cyclospora*, and *Isospora* by light microscopy; suggested thick smear of stool as a sensitive method for demonstration of intestinal parasites; suggested newer methods such as sucrose layer centrifugation method and formalin-acetone method for concentration of stool.

Prof. Parija was first to document and report the prevalence of *Entamoeba moshkovskii* from India, evaluate a multiplex PCR for simultaneous detection of *Entamoeba histolytica*, *Entamoeba dispar*, and *Entamoeba moshkovskii* in stool specimens for the diagnosis of intestinal amoebiasis, reported for the first time detection of *Entamoeba histolytica* DNA in the urine for the diagnosis of amoebic liver abscess; and reported *Arcanobacterium haemolyticum*-associated pneumothorax from India. He conducted for the first time the knowledge, attitude, and perceptions of rural people staying in two villages endemic for Kala-azar in Nepal and reported the cases of post-Kala-azar dermal leishmaniasis, cases of imported cutaneous leishmaniasis, a case of Kala-azar presenting with ulcers on the skin of the leg, a case of Kala-azar without hepatomegaly and LD bodies-negative cases of Kala-azar in Nepal, and cases of ocular rhinosporidiosis from Nepal. Prof. Parija for the first time documented the prevalence of hydatid diseases, prevalence of enterobiasis in children, prevalence of *Necator americanus* and *Ancylostoma duodenale* infections and *intracameral gnathostomiasis* from Pondicherry, India.

In recognition of his immense contributions in research of parasitic diseases, Prof. Parija has been honoured with several awards both international and national. The international awards include *BPKIHS Internal Oration Award 1997* conferred by BP Koirala Institute of Health Sciences, Dharan, Nepal, for overall contributions to the vision, mission, and goal of BPKIHS and contributions in the field of Microbiology and Parasitology.

The National awards include *Dr BC Roy National Award of the Medical Council of India 2003* for contribution to the development of Medical Microbiology, The *Indian Association of Biomedical Scientists Award 2015, Distinguished BHU Alumnus Award, 2012, DR PN Chuttani Oration Award 2007* of the National Academy of Medical Sciences, *Prof BK Aikat Oration Award 1998* of the Indian Council of Medical Research, *Major General Saheb Singh Sokhey Award 1992* of the Indian Council of Medical Research, *Dr SC Agarwal Oration Award 2001* of the Indian Association of Medical Microbiologists, *Dr BP Pandey Memorial Oration Award 1998* of the Indian Society for Parasitology, *Third Dr Datta Memorial Award 1999* by the Indian Association for the Advancement of Veterinary Parasitology, *Dr S.R.Memorial Award 2003* of the Bombay Veterinary College Alumni Association, *IAPM (Orissa chapter) Oration Award 1993* by the Indian Association of Pathologists & Microbiologists (Orissa Chapter), *Smt Kuntidevi Malhotra Award 1990* of the

Indian association of Pathologists & Microbiologists, *Dr S S Misra Memorial Award 1987* of the National Academy of Medical Sciences, *Young Scientist Award 1986* of the Indian Association of Medical Microbologists, and *Best Scientific Paper Award 1987* by the JIPMER Scientific Society. Professor Parija is the Editor-in-Chief of the journal, Tropical Parasitology published by the Indian Academy of *Tropical Parasitology*. He was also Editor of the Topical series on *Opportunistic infections and co-infections in HIV*, published by BMC, also Associate Editor of *BMC Infectious Diseases, BMC Journal of Case Reports, BMC Research Notes* and member of the Advisory board many on-line Journals, and reviews regularly for the international journals. He had served earlier as the member of the editorial boards of various journals both International (*Parasitology International, BMC Infectious Diseases, BMC Pathology, and Health Renaissance*) and National (*Journal of Veterinary Parasitology, Journal of Parasitic Diseases, Indian Journal of Medical Microbiology, Indian Journal of Pathology and Microbiology, and Journal of Biosciences*).

Prof. Parija has founded the Indian Academy of Tropical Parasitology, the only professional organization of Medical Parasitologists in India and propelled the Indian Academy of Tropical Parasitology as a President of this organization to its present admirable position. He has also initiated the *Tropical Parasitology*, a journal with a prime focus on the tropical diseases caused by parasites as the official journal of the IATP. With an effort towards harmonizing the laboratory practices, he has initiated the IATP to conduct external quality assurance programme throughout the country for the diagnosis of parasitic diseases.

He has been conferred with various fellowships such as FAMS Fellow, National Academy of Medical Sciences), FICAI (Fellow, Indian College of Allergy and Immunology), FABMS (Fellow, Indian Academy of Biomedical Scientists), FIMSA (Fellow, International Medical Science Academy), FISCD (Fellow, Indian Society for Malaria and Other Communicable Diseases), FIAVP (Fellow, Indian Association for Development of Veterinary Parasitology), FIATP (Fellow, Indian Academy of Tropical Parasitology), and FICPath (Fellow, Indian College of Pathologists) by professional bodies. Prof. Parija has visited many countries, delivered invited talks in parasitic diseases at universities, institutions, conferences, seminars, etc. and has chaired scientific sessions in the international as well as national conferences. He has guided both MD and PhD students and has been examiner for MBBS, MD, and PhD of various universities.

**Balachandra V. Adkoli** MSc, MEd, PhD, MMedEd, (Dundee) is presently working as the Director, Centre for Health Professions Education (CHPE), Sri Balaji Vidyapeeth. He started his career in general education as a Lecturer in a College of Education, Karwar, Karnataka, and Research Officer in Board of Education, Goa. Thereafter, he switched over to medical education and worked in two premier medical institutes in India, viz., Jawaharlal Institute of Postgraduate Medical Education & Research (JIPMER), Pondicherry (1985–1991) and All India Institute of Medical Sciences (AIIMS), New Delhi (1991–2012). He also had short stint at Medical Education Unit at the University of Dammam, Kingdom of Saudi Arabia (2008–2010) and Content Manager, National Health Portal, under Ministry of Health and Family Welfare, Government of India (2013–2015) before joining SBV.

During his tenure at AIIMS, New Delhi, he played key role in organizing Faculty development workshops, and running of a state-of-the-art media production facility, viz., KL Wig Centre for Medical Education & Technology (CMET). He served as a Resource Person for faculty development workshops organized by various medical colleges and specialty organizations in India and abroad. He has served as Short-Term Consultant to WHO-SEARO and World Bank-funded India Population Project.

Dr. Balachandra V. Adkoli has served as a Faculty of FAIMER Regional Institute, at CMC Ludhiana. FAIMER (Foundation for the Advancement of International Medical Education and Research), Philadelphia, USA, is a sister organization of ECFMG.

Other assignments held by Dr. Balachandra V. Adkoli include—Member, Steering Committee appointed by Ministry of Health and Family Welfare, Government of India, for starting National Health Portal, Member, National Curriculum Review Committee (NCRC) for the National Initiative for Allied Health Sciences (NIAHS) launched by the Ministry of Health and Family Welfare and Member of the Executive Committee, Academy for Health Professions Educators (India).

Currently, as the Director of CHPE he leads innovative programmes in Health Professions Education, including Certificate Courses, PG Diploma, MPhil, and PhD programmes, besides membership in several committees of SBV.

Dr. Adkoli is Accredited Educator for the Advanced Trauma Life Support (ATLS) Instructors course of ATLS India franchised by American College of Surgeons since 2010. He has authored or co-authored books (5), book chapters (23), and published more than 60 papers in medical education and allied topics. He is on the editorial board of three journals and peer reviewer for a number of journals.

# Part I

# Communication Skill for Everyone - Begin with a Bang!

# Communication Vocabulary and Landscape

# 1

Rasnayaka M. Mudiyanse and Amaya Ellawala

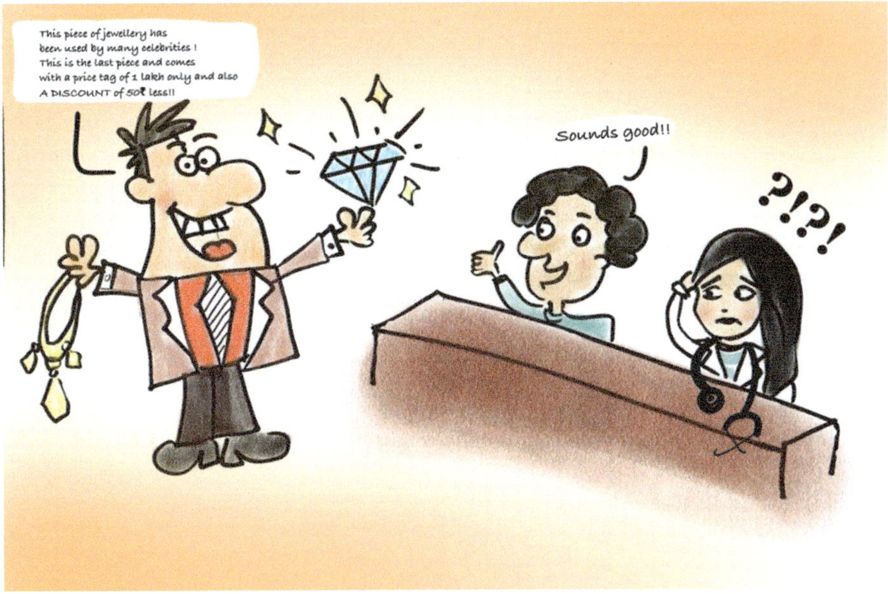


Effective communication is a trainable skill.—Mudiyanse and Ellawala.

R. M. Mudiyanse (✉)
Department of Paediatrics, University of Peradeniya, Peradeniya, Sri Lanka

A. Ellawala
Faculty of Medicine, University of Sri Jayewardenepura, Nugegoda, Sri Lanka



S. C. Parija, B. V. Adkoli (eds.), *Effective Medical Communication*,
https://doi.org/10.1007/978-981-15-3409-6_1

## 1.1 Assess Need

Communication is an integral part of life. One cannot refrain from communicating with others. In clinical practice, health care professionals communicate with patients to gather information to arrive at a diagnosis, plan management, execute a treatment, and monitor the progress of the illness. Communication is the tool that we use in the prevention, health promotion, advocacy, negotiations, and teaching.

Communication is intricately linked with the entire spectrum of competencies that health care professionals should possess. A good communicator invariably becomes an efficient learner, engaged and empathetic care provider, committed manager as well as an advocate in the society.

The value of communication in health care is highlighted repeatedly. However, issues linked to a communication failure are rampant. A vast majority of complaints about healthcare professionals, from patients and the public, stem from gaps in communication. Consequences such as poor patient satisfaction, poor health outcomes, and higher healthcare costs have resulted from such deficiencies. This has led to mounting dissatisfaction among the public regarding healthcare professionals.

In response, training programs for health care professionals have embraced communication skills as an integrated, spirally evolving, compulsory component of their curricula. In many settings, development of communication skills is emphasised during the undergraduate curriculum but is comparatively neglected during subsequent stages of training. As such, there is a need for the different training requirements along the continuum of learning to be objectively identified and documented.

## 1.2 Brief

In this chapter, an attempt has been made to:

- Define communication.
- Explain the interconnection of communication with patient-centredness, empathy, and competencies.
- Show how communication can be made efficient, effective, and supportive.
- Discuss the process, perception, and content in communication.
- Outline the evolution of models of communication.
- Discuss the process and skills of communication.

## 1.3 Contextualize

### 1.3.1 Scenario

Dr. Comini had no idea about the importance of communication skills or how to develop these skills. She decided to attend a training programme on communication skills, after hearing from a colleague that it had helped him immensely. Dr. Comini considered herself to be a good communicator and did not think she would learn anything new from the programme but decided to attend anyway. During the programme, she was introduced to many concepts of which she had previously been unaware. Most importantly, she learnt small changes that she could make to her current practice to make her communication more effective, sensitive, and patient-centered. By the end of the programme, she could feel a transformation within herself; from a doctor who talked to her patients, to one who talked, listened, and genuinely tried to understand their situation.

From that day forward, Dr. Comini applied her learning in her day-to-day practice, and began to see visible results. She developed better relationships with her patients, and began to witness improved treatment compliance and patient satisfaction. Communication with the rest of the health care team improved, and conflicts within the group reduced. As a result, over time, the health care unit to which Dr. Comini belonged documented better health outcomes, and became a popular choice for treatment, with patients travelling from around the country to seek the care of this skilled health care team.

***Exercise***: What was the turning point in Dr. Comini's journey as a faculty member? What benefits did she accrue from such exposure?

## 1.4 Describe

### 1.4.1 What Is Communication?

Communication has been defined as "*a process of sharing information, feelings, emotions, and values between two or more individuals*" [1]. This could be modified to suit communication in healthcare by adding "*efficiently resulting in a favourable change in behaviours of all the parties concerned*". In fact, communication could be recognised as a process of education that should achieve a favourable change in behaviour in practice.

Communication has a content, process, and perception. Traditionally, the content has been the prime focus in the teaching of medicine and includes information, ideas, feelings, or emotions that we share. However, the process—how you do it—and perceptions—intellectual interpretations that are intrinsically interwoven—become vital in meaningful conversations. The Shannon–Weaver Bi-directional Model of Communication is among the old, but still popular in the health care setting because of its simplicity [2] (Fig. 1.1).

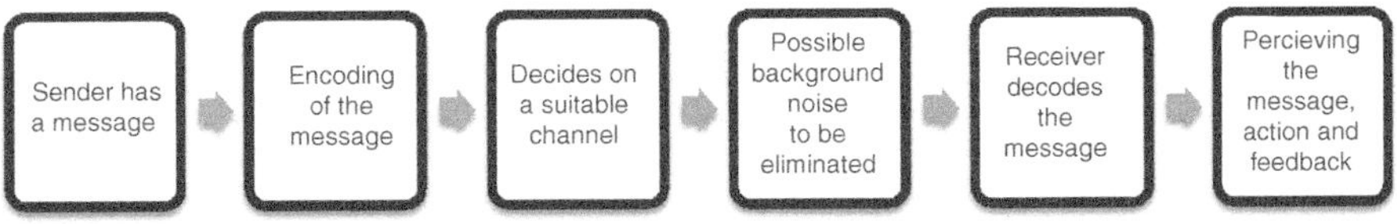


**Fig. 1.1** Shannon–Weaver Model adapted for health communication

The concept of communication has evolved greatly with time. Some of the models which were developed from time to time have been outlined in the Box 1.1.

**Box 1.1 Evolution of Models of Communication**

1. Aristotle model—One-way communication.
2. Linear models—Shannon–Weaver, SMCR model of Berlo [3].
3. Interactive models—Wilbur Schramm considered the impact of the message on the receiver and receiving feedback [4].
4. Transactional models—Barnlund [5], Newman and Summer recognise that individuals in reality simultaneously engage in sending and receiving messages [1].

#### 1.4.1.1 Patient Centredness

The traditional model or biomedical model of communication adopted data gathering and a factor analytic approach. It tended to marginalise the psychological and social aspects of individuals [3, 4]. George Engle highlighted the importance of psychosocial aspects of care, and proposed the biopsychosocial model of health care [5, 6]. This model, with its foundation of patient-centredness, the involvement of and collaboration with patients in decision making, ensures patient empowerment and treatment adherence, finally achieving a speedy recovery.

#### 1.4.1.2 Consumerism and Realistic Medicine

The exploitation of patients in a commercialised world could be curtailed by patient education and empowerment. However, the promotion of patient involvement in patient-centred care should not lead to consumerism, where the public considers health care as a consumer product, and demands services of their choice. The shifting emphasis in communication has been shown in Fig. 1.2.

#### 1.4.1.3 Empathy

Empathy is an essential attribute for a health care professional. Empathy drives a person to perceive, understand, and be attuned to the predicaments and emotions of another, communicate such feeling, and offer support. In fact, empathy occupies a central place in communication (Fig. 1.3).

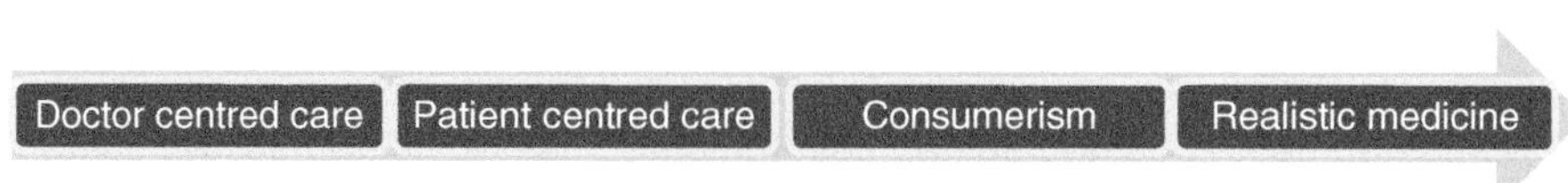


**Fig. 1.2** Shifting from doctor centred care to realistic care

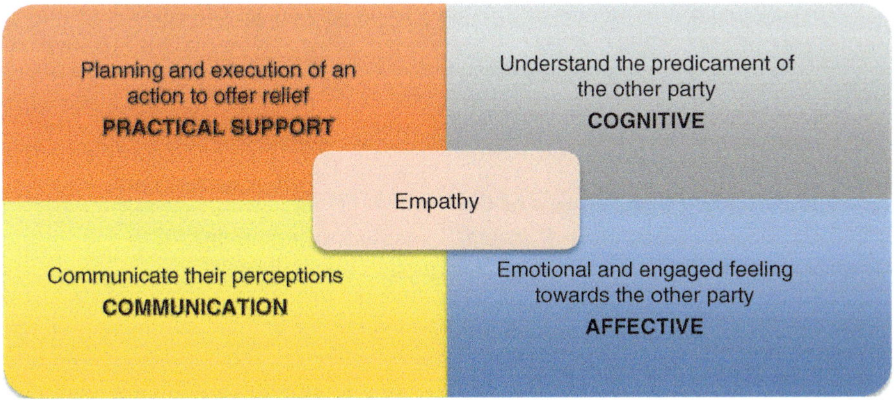


**Fig. 1.3** Elements of empathy

#### 1.4.1.4 Communication Skills and Competencies

Health care professionals are expected to embrace a wide spectrum of competencies in order to function as good doctors. Without communication skills, one cannot execute any of the other competencies in clinical practice.

The following are considered essential competencies for health care professionals (CanMEDS competencies):

- Expert: Possess and regularly update the required knowledge and skills.
- Communicator: Skilful communication with patients as well as all other collaborators in the discharge of duties.
- Collaborator: Work as partners in the process of delivery of services.
- Manager: Take the role of a leader appropriately and manage human and non-human resources wisely.
- Advocate: Promote behaviours conducive for better health in the society by education, practice, and role modelling.
- Scholar: Generate (by research and audit), assimilate (by learning), and disseminate (by teaching) knowledge.
- Professional: Conduct in a manner during as well as outside working hours as expected by regulatory bodies as well as the general public.

#### 1.4.1.5 Benefits of Developing Communication Skills

Communication should be effective, efficient, and supportive [7].

- An effective communication refers to accuracy, comprehensiveness, and relevance.
- The efficiency of communication indicates how quickly one could complete the process.

- Supportiveness of communication indicates psychosocial satisfaction offered to the patient.

The benefits of communication skills to patients, institutes, and the nation have been listed in the Table 1.1.

#### 1.4.1.6 Blocking Behaviours of Communication

At times, doctors tend to block patients' freedom of communication due to time constraints and enthusiasm to gather information relevant to them.

The following are blocking behaviours displayed by doctors:

- Asking closed-ended questions.
- Not dedicating adequate time for consultation and behaving as if they are busy.
- Looking away and not establishing eye contact.
- Giving explanations and solutions early even before the patient completes the story.
- Frequently checking the time.
- Responding or taking phone calls or texting.
- Demonstrating a lack of interest.
- Asking the patient to tell a short story.
- Taking notes or using a computer in a manner that the patient will be ignored.
- Engaging in other activities during the consultation.

**Table 1.1** Benefits of skilful communication to patients, health care professionals, institutions, and the nation

| *Benefits to patients* | *Benefits to professionals* |
|---|---|
| 1. Patient satisfaction | 1. Effective understanding of the patient problem |
| 2. Patient empowerment | 2. Capacity to develop effective and acceptable solutions to the problem |
| 3. Therapeutic adherence | 3. The satisfaction of health care workers (less vicarious trauma) |
| 4. Less expensive care | 4. Fewer conflicts with patients |
| 5. Improvement of holistic health | 5. Less likely to enter legal battles |
| 6. A good relationship with health care providers | 6. Higher popularity among the public |
| 7. Building trust in the health care system | |
| *Benefits to institution* | *Benefits to the nation* |
| 1. Institution becomes popular | 1. Empowered society |
| 2. Less hospital admission and minimise overcrowding | 2. Collaborative care makes health care less expensive |
| 3. Fewer investigations | 3. A trend towards health promotion |
| 4. Fewer conflicts with patient's or among stakeholders | 4. Reduced out of pocket spending |
| 5. Cost-effective care | 5. Reduced health care budget |
| 6. Patients become valuable stakeholders | |

### 1.4.2 Skills of Communication

Communication is a series of psychomotor skills supported by cognitive (intellectual) as well as affective (attitude) domains. Skills of communication contribute to effective conversations with patients in clinical practice as well as to successful motivational interviews, the development of teamwork, and leadership skills. Selected communication skills considered as essential have been listed in Table 1.2.

**Table 1.2** Essential skills to ensure effectiveness, efficacy, and supportiveness of communication; adopted from the Calgary Cambridge model

| | |
|---|---|
| ***Sequential skills*** | |
| Initiating the conversation | |
| 1. Attention to the environment | |
| 2. Mental preparation: leave ongoing work aside | |
| 3. Introductions: introduce self and try to know the client within his socioeconomic background | |
| 4. Building rapport: developing a trustworthy relationship | |
| 5. Effective opening question | |
| 6. Effective listening: attentive, reflective, and empathetic listening | |
| 7. Internal summaries | |
| 8. Screening questions | |
| 9. Developing an agenda to guide the conversation | |
| Gathering information | |
| 10. Effective questioning: a variety of questions and open to close cone | |
| 11. Summarising and checking understanding after each topic | |
| 12. Using transition and signposting | |
| 13. Evaluating patient perspectives: ideas, concerns, emotions, experiences, and expectations | |
| Collaborative planning and sharing information | |
| 14. Evaluation of patient's information need | |
| 15. Giving information using chunk and check closure | |
| 16. Closure with summaries and contract | |
| ***Longitudinal skills*** | |
| Building a relationship | Providing a framework for conversation |
| • Greeting | • Informing about time availability |
| • Respect and care | • Setting an agenda |
| • Body language | • Confirming the agenda |
| • Seating | • Signposting and transitions |
| • Eye contact | • Chunking the information to be given |
| • Attentive listening | • Checking for understanding |
| • Asking open-ended questions | • Summarising |
| • Giving explanations for your probing and clarifications | • Informing closure of the conversation |
| • Empathy | |
| • Sharing thoughts | |
| • Asking about perspectives | |
| • Collaborative planning | |
| • Developing a contract | |

#### 1.4.2.1 Sequential Skills

Attention to the environment and physical needs is vital. Noise, level of lighting, lack of privacy, room temperature, and even the mere arrangement of furniture can impede or support the process of communication. Physical needs like bladder and bowel movements, hunger, thirst, tiredness, and anxiety need due consideration.

Mental preparation: It is important for a professional to be mentally prepared, respectful, to stop other ongoing activities, and switch off the telephone so that complete attention could be offered to the client.

Introductions: Self-introduction and getting to know each other is civilised behaviour.

Building rapport: It is an essential pre-requisite for effective communication. The term rapport denotes something much stronger than mere friendliness.

The effective opening question is the first question that initiates the conversation. Commonly used phrases include: "*so tell me what brought you here today?*", "*Okay, tell me, what is the matter?*", "*why don't you tell me your story?*". This question should be phrased and timed skilfully, after building rapport, while indicating that you are ready to listen to the story respectfully. After the initial disclosure by the patient, the health care professional should summarise what was said and ask whether there is anything else. This is called the screening question. The screening question could be repeated until the patient has said all that he/she needs to say.

Effective listening is the most difficult, nevertheless the most valuable skill to develop. There are six levels of listening which have been highlighted in the Box 1.2.

**Box 1.2 Six Levels of Listening**

1. Ignoring.
2. Pretending to listen.
3. Selective listening.
4. Attentive listening.
5. Reflective listening.
6. Empathetic listening.

Developing an agenda: After the opening question, effective listening, and screening question, an agenda for the conversation should be proposed and confirmed with the patient.

Effective questioning: The conversation should follow the topics on the agenda. Following the opening question, clarification questions, probing questions, verification questions, close-ended questions or leading questions may have to be posed. Examples are provided in Box 1.3.

**Box 1.3 Types of Questions with Examples**

1. Opening question—the question asked at the beginning of the conversation after building rapport; *"so tell me what brought you here today?"*
2. Screening question—asking whether there is anything else after summarising the response to the opening question. *"Okay, I understand that you have a headache and vomiting. Is there anything else?"*
3. Clarifications questions—asking to clarify a point; *"you said you are suffering. What do you mean?"*
4. Probing questions—trying to probe on some information; *"are you sure that your child has had a fever for 2 weeks? Have you checked the temperature?"*
5. Verification questions—trying to verify the meaning; *"you said your child never eats, you mean he is a fussy eater?"*
6. Close-ended questions—asking questions expecting 1–2 words or short phrases. This is the commonest type of question used in conversations. *"Does he have a fever? For how many days?"*
7. Leading questions—the question guides the patients towards the response. *"You seem to be getting angry during feeding time. What do you do when you get angry?"*

The following items provide a guide to exploring sensitive and personal information (e.g., sexual life):

- Be empathetic.
- Use professional language.
- Provide explanations for asking specific questions.
- Ask close-ended questions.
- Address privacy as well as the availability of a chaperone.
- Ensure and assure confidentiality.

Responding to the patient: it is vital to respond to patients sensitively in a skilful manner. Types of responses with examples are provided below:

- Listening—highlighted earlier.
- Silence—Silence should be attentive. Merely being quiet is not sufficient.
- Facilitating.
- Empathising—Expression of empathy is an essential and integral part of good communication.

- Paraphrasing—Paraphrasing is repeating what was said using different words or a different order of words while retaining the same meaning.
- Echoing.
- Restatement—Restatement is similar to paraphrasing but using the same words and tone in order to add emphasis and promote further thinking.
- Clarifying.
- Probing—Some parts of the conversation may need further probing.

Summarising and checking understanding after each topic: Summarising the conversation at the end of each topic is a good practice to confirm as well as to demonstrate understanding.

Using transition and signposting: Using transitions and signposting is a valuable skill in any conversation.

Evaluating patient's perspectives: It is always worth exploring Ideas, Concerns, Emotions, Expectations, and Experiences (ICEEE) (Box 1.4).

**Box 1.4 Patients Perspectives (ICEEE)**

1. Ideas—patients have unique ideas about their problem.
2. Concerns—patient's concern may differ from that of the doctor.
3. Experiences—what do they experience, what is their plight?
4. Emotions—their feelings and emotions.
5. Expectations—expectations from their doctors, relatives, and society.

Giving information: Should follow an agenda based on patient's information need and information should be provided in manageable chunks. Understanding should be checked periodically.

Closure with summaries, contract, and greeting: Summarising the conversation and allowing the last chance for questions before suggesting a contract, should precede greeting, and closure of any conversation.

#### 1.4.2.2 Longitudinal Skills

These skills are helpful throughout the conversation. Only a list of items is presented as almost all skills have been described earlier in this chapter.

### 1.4.3 Building Relationships

- Greeting.
- Respect and care.
- Body language.
- Seating.

- Eye contact.
- Attentive listening.
- Asking open-ended questions.
- Giving explanations for your probing and clarifications.
- Empathy.
- Sharing thoughts.
- Asking about perspectives.
- Collaborative planning.
- Developing a contact.

### 1.4.4 Providing a Structure

- Informing about time availability.
- Setting an agenda.
- Confirming the agenda.
- Signposting and transitions.
- Chunking the information to be given.
- Checking for understanding.
- Summarising.
- Informing closure of the conversation.

#### 1.4.4.1 The Models of Communication in Healthcare

The models of communication in healthcare have been outlined (Table 1.3).

#### 1.4.4.2 Calgary Cambridge Model of Communication

The Calgary Cambridge model of communication is one of the most popular models of communication among medical as well as allied health science professionals.

**Table 1.3** Models of communication in health care

| | |
|---|---|
| • Physical, psychological, and social | • AACH-The three-function approach to the medical interview |
| • Stott and Davis | • The Calgary Cambridge approach to communication skills teaching |
| • Byrne and Long | • SAGUE framework for teaching and assessing communication skills |
| • Six category intervention analysis | • The Enhanced Calgary Cambridge Guides |
| • Helman's "*folk model*" | • Kalamazoo consensus |
| • Transactional analysis | |
| • Pendleton, Schofield, Tate, and Havelock | |
| • Neighbour | |
| • The disease and illness model | |

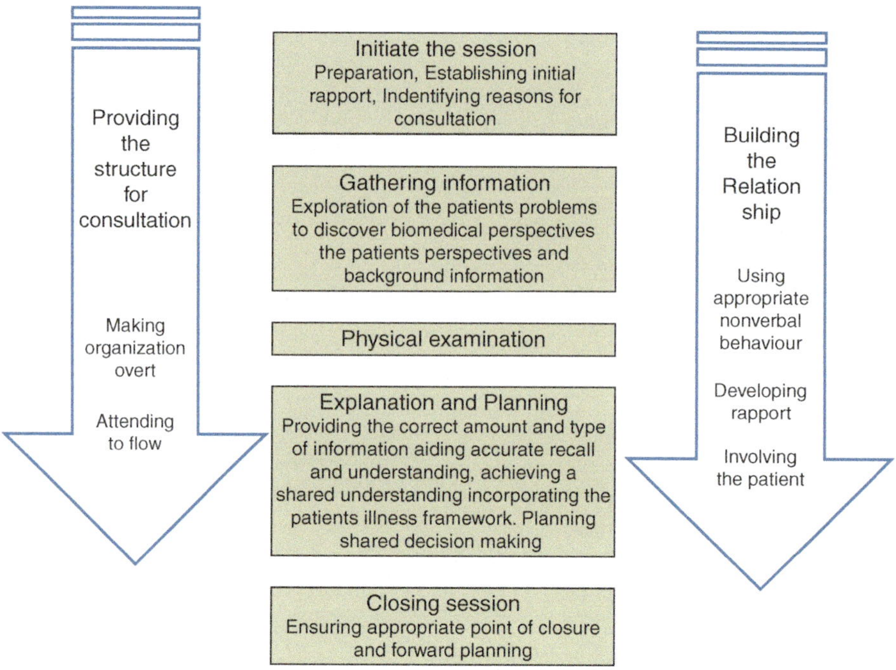


**Fig. 1.4** Calgary Cambridge model of communication

#### 1.4.4.3 Process of Communication in the Calgary Cambridge Model

Learning communication is not only a matter of learning about communication. It should inculcate a practice and change of attitudes so that the learner becomes a good communicator. It is a matter of changing people (Fig. 1.4).

The domains of learning involved in developing communication skills are as follows:

1. Knowledge—by lectures, discussion, reading material, watching videos.
2. Skills—by practice with actual patients or with actors who act like real patients.
3. Attitudes—by reflective learning and feedback from patients, teachers, and colleagues.
4. Relationship—developing relationships at the level of rapport is a separate skill that health professionals should focus on.

Active involvement of the learner is an essential ingredient in inculcating communication skills.

### 1.4.5 Conclusion

- Communication in healthcare should result in a favourable change in behaviours of all parties concerned.
- Communication should be effective, efficient, and supportive.
- Attention must be paid to the content, process, and perceptions of communication, in order to become an effective communicator.
- Effective communication requires both sequential and longitudinal skills.
- Patient centredness and empathy are two key principles of good communication with the patient.
- Effective communication results in numerous benefits to the patient, healthcare professional, institution, and community.

## 1.5 Evaluation

After reading this chapter, workout a flowchart which connects all the content and the message given in this chapter.

## References

1. Moss D, Newman A, De Santo B. What do communication managers do? Defining and refining the Core elements of management in a public relations/corporate communication context. J Mass Commun Quart. 2005;82(4):873–90. https://doi.org/10.1177/107769900508200408.
2. Weaver W. In: Shannon CE, Weaver W, editors. Recent contributions to mathematical theory of communication in the mathematical theory of communication. Urbana: University of Illinois Press; 1949.
3. Kurtz S, Silverman J, Benson J, Draper J. Marrying content and process in clinical method teaching; enhancing the Calgary – Cambridge guide. Acad Med. 2003;78(8):802–9.
4. Kurtz S, Silverman J, Draper J. Teaching and learning communication skills in medicine. 2nd ed. Oxford: Radcliffe Publishing Ltd; 2008.
5. Engle GL. The clinical application of the biopsychosocial model. Am J Psychiatr. 1980;137(5):535–44.
6. Balint E. The possibilities of patient-centred medicine. J R Coll Gen Pract. 1969;17(82):269–76.
7. Silverman J, Kurtz S, Draper J. Skills for communicating with patients. 3rd ed. London: CRC Press; 2013.

# Role of Mentoring in Developing Communication Skills

# 2

Subhash Chandra Parija and Balachandra V. Adkoli

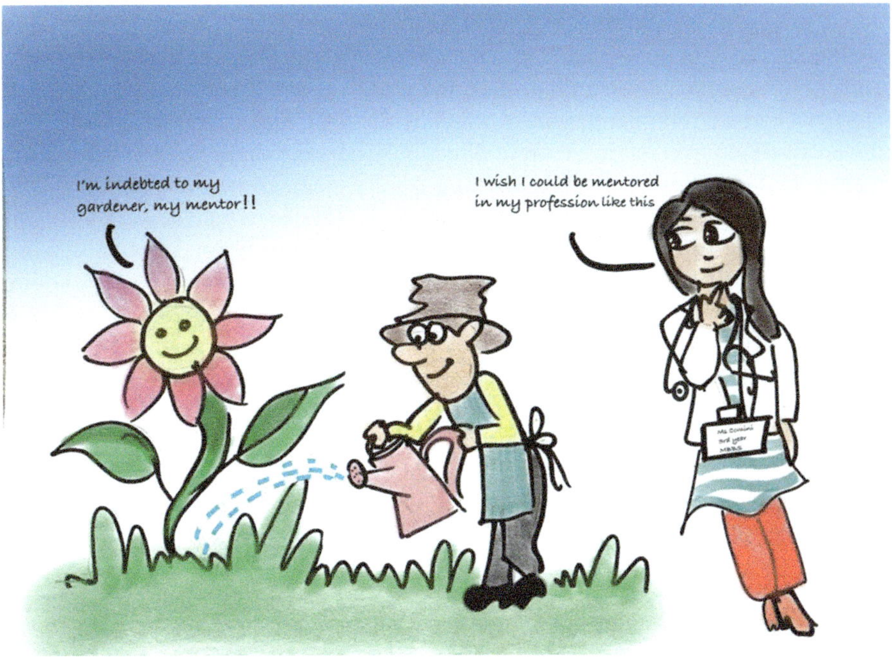


Mentoring is the most enriching experience for both mentor and mentee, for a professional career, lifetime—Parija and Adkoli

S. C. Parija (✉)
Sri Balaji Vidyapeeth (Deemed-to-be University), Pondicherry, India

B. V. Adkoli
Centre for Health Professions Education, Sri Balaji Vidyapeeth (Deemed-to-be University), Pondicherry, India



S. C. Parija, B. V. Adkoli (eds.), *Effective Medical Communication*,
https://doi.org/10.1007/978-981-15-3409-6_2

## 2.1 Assess Need

Achieving a successful career in medicine is a long and tedious journey. It means passing through several milestones, from under-graduation to post-graduation, and specialisation as a practitioner, consultant, researcher, or administrator. Any journey becomes smooth and enjoyable if one is lucky to find a suitable guide and a companion. Similarly, mentoring in medical career comes as a lifetime experience. It contributes to both professional achievement and personal development. Unfortunately, the value of mentoring is not explored in most of the medical colleges either because of lack of awareness or lack of motivation on the part of the mentor, mentee, or both.

The 'starting trouble' in the journey of a medico is quite but natural. The student is immersed totally in a different environment, new school, new friends, new faculty, and a new curriculum with a huge burden of biomedical information. Tests and exams roll out and become a nightmare.

When a medico passes through the grills of post-graduation, there are even more challenges. How to pursue speciality training, how to present a seminar or a journal club, how to pursue a research project and write a dissertation? Again, one has to depend a lot on a senior colleague or a faculty member who can guide and handhold the postgraduate student in the right direction. The story does not stop here. When the resident moves on to the position of a faculty member, new challenges appear. How to become an effective teacher, a competent clinician, or a research supervisor to excel amidst stiff competition?

The trick of the trade lies in following someone as a 'role model'. By entering into long term 'mentor–mentee relationship', it is possible to attain a high level of professionalism in a competitive world. Unfortunately, medical schools in the present context are neither prepared nor equipped to address the issue of mentorship in all its dimensions to come out with some practical tips. The need for mentoring has been keenly felt in medical education [1]. Its implications in enhancing research skills have also been advocated by the research community [2, 3].

## 2.2 Brief

The purpose of this chapter is to sensitise the students, teachers, and the administrators in medical education to appreciate the role of mentoring for effective communication. We propose to:

- Recognise the importance of mentoring in medical education.
- Identify the various qualities and attributes of an effective mentor, mentee and the role to be played by medical schools to foster a successful mentor–mentee system.
- Explain the mentoring needs of undergraduates, postgraduates, and faculty members.
- Offer practical tips for designing a sound mentorship program in medical schools.

## 2.3 Contextualize

### 2.3.1 Scenario 1

Ms. Comini, a somewhat shy and modest girl, hailing from a remote village, suffered a cultural shock when she got admission in a metropolitan medical college which is a premier medical institute in the country. This medical institute which was reputed for its 'high standards of the curriculum' started with anatomy dissection hall, welcoming the freshers, with cadavers and specimens. Her classmates gave a strange look. Her food habit, clothing, and the life style were totally different. For the first time in her life she had migrated to a new place and subjected to hostel life with all strangers. At that point of time ragging by the seniors was also quite common and scary. Ms. Comini became home sick and almost felt like running away from the campus.

Soon there was an announcement from the Dean that every undergraduate would be allotted a mentor, who is a faculty member. The mentor was expected to spend some time with the mentee in helping the latter to cope up with the studies and address other issues.

This came as a blessing in disguise for Ms. Comini. One Dr. DM, an endocrinologist was allocated as the mentor to Ms. Comini. DM was initially reluctant to help Ms. Comini because he was busy with his research project related to the iron deficiency among the tribal community. However, looking at the Ms. Comini's background, he thought, one day, this girl might help him in collecting data, especially from the tribal community for his research.

Thus a mentoring process started and took off quickly. Dr. DM not only helped Ms. Comini in overcoming her 'inferiority complex' but encouraged her to submit a student research project, which was approved by the funding agency in the first attempt itself. After that, there was no looking back for Ms. Comini. She finished her graduation with a gold medal, got a postgraduate seat in the same institute, and ultimately appointed as a faculty member in the same college.

### 2.3.2 Scenario 2

When Dr. Comini joined the premier medical institute as a faculty member in Medicine, she was allotted lectures to be delivered to a large class. This was a nightmare for Dr. Comini who had no experience in teaching. The last benchers made a huge noise, and she lost control though she was a gold medallist.

At this point of time, Prof GD, who was the chairman of the Medical Education Unit (MEU), came as a guiding star. He was looking for a junior faculty who would be willing to join MEU to launch some curriculum reforms. Dr. Comini responded to Prof GD with humility and respect, which led to a mentoring relationship knowingly or unknowingly. Prof GD not only gave her practical tips to handle large class but also persuaded her to take up a course in medical education from a reputed centre. She got the opportunity to practise microteaching, which helped her to improve her teaching skills. She was inducted as a member of the faculty of MEU.

Prof GD encouraged Comini to pursue PhD in medical education, which she did putting up a lot of hard work. At times her colleagues and seniors tried to put obstacles in between. However, Dr. Comini received constant encouragement from her mentor. Not only she completed her PhD but also published papers in journals with high impact. Prof GD also motivated her to apply for copyright for the research tools which she had developed as a part of her PhD. She succeeded in securing copyrights. Based on her expertise and experience, she bagged the faculty award for excellence.

***Exercise***: Now think of the above scenarios and reflect on the factors that led to the success of a girl from a remote part of the country!

## 2.4 Describe

### 2.4.1 What Is Mentoring?

The word mentor originated from Greek mythology, wherein a person named *Mentor* was entrusted with the responsibility of 'caretaker' for his colleague's son [2]. The ancient Indian version of mentorship is called *Gurukul* in which the disciple (*Shishya)* lived in the *ashram* (hermitage) of Guru, served him, and religiously learnt sixty four *vidyas* (skills) needed for future career. The *Guru—Shishya* relationship was the epitome of mentorship. However, this system was faded out with time, when formal schooling took away the responsibility of Guru.

#### 2.4.1.1 Key Features of Mentoring

- Mentoring is a two-way process in which the mentor and the mentee enter into a reciprocal relationship for a long term career enhancement and personal development of both [3].
- Mentoring relationship is marked by mutual trust, respect, and shared vision of objectives.
- The mentor is more than a teacher or a coach. He is a guide, confidante, counsellor who contributes to mentee's professional as well as personal growth.
- Mentoring can be formally arranged by an institution to support its academic program. It gives ample scope for catering to the needs of diverse learners, especially the high performers and the low performers.
- Mentoring can take place informally in the corridor, canteen, or home, when the mentor agrees to offer guidance, counselling, and support as and when needed by the mentee. Informal mentoring can result in a long-lasting and rewarding experience for both. This is because of the autonomy and flexibility involved in the process. Again there is no 'control' exercised by an authority to monitor the progress.

### 2.4.2 Importance of Mentoring

Fields of knowledge, such as engineering and art or crafts, are based on the apprenticeship model. The medical education, however, followed formal training mostly in western medicine or the modern system of medicine since its inception. Looking retrospectively, medical education in India and neighbouring countries like Sri Lanka, Nepal, Bangladesh, etc. witnessed a steep increase in the establishment of medical schools as well as the enrolment of students. This resulted in a shortage of teachers affecting the quality of teaching-learning [4]. With the explosion of knowledge, there is a further need to cope up with the heavy curriculum by adopting strategies such as self-directed learning. This requires an efficient system of mentoring.

In fact, the competency-based medical education, which is the current trend in medical education relies heavily on self-directed learning as well as reflective practice by the learner by maintaining a portfolio or e-portfolio [5–6]. However, this process has to be aided by the mentor.

The new millennial medicos who are borne after the 2000 A.D. are drastically different from an earlier generation of learners. They are tech-savvy, multitasking, digitally connected, and adaptable. If they are mentored with senior faculty who have been trained in the pre-IT era, both will be benefitted mutually.

With the system of education becoming more cost-intensive and accountable, educators need to design new ways of cutting the cost and making the system more efficient. Mentoring may be a cost-effective and feasible solution.

### 2.4.3 Attributes of a Good Mentor and Mentee

Mentoring is not an ad hoc and aimless process. It is based on the sound principles of adult learning propounded by many educationists. These underline the importance of motivation, self-directed learning, contextual learning, feedback, reinforcement, and reflective practice as the key elements [7–10]. Each of these principles has a bearing on the practice of mentoring (Table 2.1).

**Table 2.1** Principles of adult learning and implications for mentoring

| Adult learning principles | Implications for mentoring |
|---|---|
| Adult learners are self-directed learners | Mentor them to set their own goals, pursue learning at their own pace, in their style |
| Adults bring a wealth of information and previous experience | While mentoring, facilitate *construction*<br>Do not impart *instruction* |
| Adults are motivated by 'value attached' to the task and their perceived self-efficacy | Demonstrate the relevance of the task<br>Help them build self-confidence |
| Adult learning is facilitated by feedback from the peers and self-reflection | Provide feedback and obtain feedback. Promote reflection and practice all the time |
| Adults are sensitive about their ego and self-pride | Provide a non-threatening and respectful environment. Make learning an enjoyable task rather than a workload |

**Table 2.2** Qualities and attributes of mentor and mentee

| Mentor's attributes | Mentee's attributes |
|---|---|
| Encourages, supports, and motivates the mentee | Respects and appreciates the kind gesture |
| Listens to the mentee patiently before giving suggestions or hints | Acts on the suggestions given by the mentor sincerely |
| Handles the problems of the mentee in a responsible and ethical manner | Confides problems to the mentor without any inhibition |
| Takes the initiative in serving as a role model by setting an example, practising what he/she is preaching | Takes the initiative in seeking necessary help from the mentor, for example, maintaining punctuality in attendance, attending to logistics |

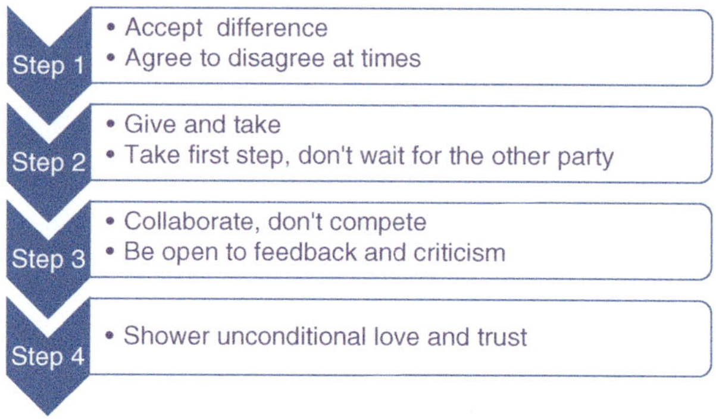


**Fig. 2.1** The magic formula for a successful mentor–mentee journey

For successful mentoring, both mentor and mentee should contribute their best (Table 2.2). The partnership, in the beginning, looks like mentor dominated. However, the relationship becomes reciprocal in a long term partnership.

Should the mentor be a subject expert? Not really. He should be a facilitator. He should have the skill to lead the mentee to acquire such expertise.

The mentor should be a friend, guide, and a philosopher. Friend, because he has to respond to the needs of the mentee. Guide, because he has to guide the mentee towards reaching the greater heights. Philosopher, because he should lead the mentee to discover the truth.

Successful mentoring requires understanding, adjustment, and at times, sacrifice on the part of both. For example, mentor and mentee may come from a different culture and may have a different lifestyle altogether. If they can accept these differences, nothing can stop them from coming closer. An attitude of 'giving and taking' will quicken the process of mentoring. A spirit of collaboration rather than competition will pave the further way towards better progress (Fig. 2.1).

### 2.4.4 Problems and Pitfalls in Mentoring

All is not well with the current practice of mentoring across the medical schools in the developing countries.

- Most of the mentoring happens on paper, not in practice! Often the Dean notifies the list of mentors and mentees according to a routine, practically feasible way.
- Mentor–Mentees are notified without consulting the preference of either.
- Nothing moves till the previous day of the exam when mentor and mentee meet for the first and last time since mentor's signature is a mandatory requirement for writing the exam.
- Mentors are too busy with their multiple tasks assigned to them. For them, it is an additional 'burden'.
- Mentees do not think that the mentor would be helpful. They resort to their senior friends who give them useful tips on how to study and 'finish' the course!
- Deans issue circulars and claim that mentoring is being 'practised strictly'.

### 2.4.5 Mentoring Needs at Various Stages

Mentoring is a lifelong process. It is a continuous journey. However, the specific need at each stage varies from stage to stage, which determines the roles played by the mentor and the mentee (Fig. 2.2).

#### 2.4.5.1 Before Admission

Mentoring is needed even before entering medical schools. It is necessary to organise a sensitization program for all the aspirants of medical colleges as a prelude to their admission. Such a program can help the aspirants about what to expect from medical schools, and what preparations are required for entering into a medical career.

#### 2.4.5.2 During Undergraduate Training

As soon as students are admitted to a medical school, they are lost in the new environment. The challenges before them are how to cope up with a new curriculum and how to get adjusted to a new environment. Sometimes there could be food issue, hostel accommodation issue, language issue, or cultural issue or even homesickness after leaving their sweet homes.

**Fig. 2.2** Mentoring needs vary at different levels

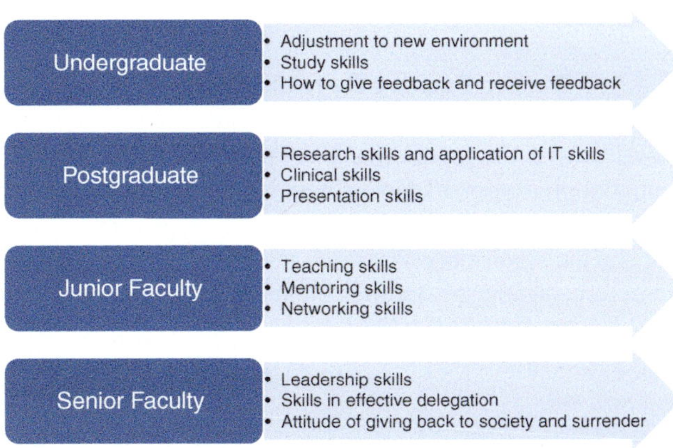
Undergraduate
• Adjustment to new environment
• Study skills
• How to give feedback and receive feedback
Postgraduate
• Research skills and application of IT skills
• Clinical skills
• Presentation skills
Junior Faculty
• Teaching skills
• Mentoring skills
• Networking skills
Senior Faculty
• Leadership skills
• Skills in effective delegation
• Attitude of giving back to society and surrender

The institutional response should be to establish mentoring arrangements with mutual agreement. Criteria such as sharing the same geographical background, language, and culture may be considered while fixing mentor–mentee pairs. Organising a foundation course can help acquire IT skills, language skills, and study skills which are important for laying a sound foundation.

A well-designed test for identifying the learner's style of learning, ability, and aptitude will go a long way in identifying mentee's needs. Many hidden talents come to the surface with proper assessment. Some medical schools also administer a questionnaire called Visual, Aural, Reading, and Kinaesthetic (VARK) Questionnaire to identify the preferred learning style of the learner, viz., Visual, Aural, Reading, and Kinaesthetic. This will help the mentor to guide the mentee to deploy a preferred style for better learning. Undergraduate mentoring can be considered as a foundation stage for building a long term 'mentor–mentee relationship'.

#### 2.4.5.3 During Postgraduate Training

The problems faced by postgraduate students are how to develop clinical skills, acquire research skills such as writing a research protocol, review of literature, research design, tool development, data collection, analysis, and reporting in the form of a dissertation. Skills pertaining to the journal clubs, seminars, presenting posters or papers during national and international conferences should also form the part of mentoring.

Mentoring for research follows the same rules applicable to education. However, a certain degree of research experience and expertise will add value for mentoring a research fellow [1].

Many of the medical schools are now shifting to competency-based medical education (CBME) [5–6]. One of the key features of this approach is a day-to-day interaction with the supervisor by means of an e-portfolio. The essential skills needed here are a willingness to share personal experiences, including success and failure stories. The desirable skills are research and publication skills, IT skills, web-surfing, information retrieval, application of biostatistics, and ethical norms. Awareness of new trends such as genomics, imaging techniques, nanotechnology, robotics, Artificial Intelligence, Internet of Things (IoT), etc., will be a great asset for a mentor.

#### 2.4.5.4 During Faculty Development

Mentoring is not a luxury but a necessity even for a faculty member who aspires to be a leader in the profession. The faculty members who have access to mentoring by eminent professionals have a better chance of success in their professional development. The mentoring relationship at this stage will be somewhat different. The mentor and the mentee become more of collaborators or partners in progress. Mentoring, therefore, leads to mutual benefit. Entering into collaborative projects and networking with various departments, institutes, and professions will be a part of the mentoring process at this level.

The senior faculty who are expected to mentor the juniors are caught in a peculiar dilemma. With the obsolescence of knowledge and stiff competition for survival, senior mentors need young mentees to assist them in adopting new technologies. Hence mentor–mentee is a win–win situation, and it is not 'one-way traffic'.

### 2.4.6 Practical Tips to Start Mentoring in Medical Schools

Medical schools should promote mentoring either through formal arrangement, informal approach, or both. Formal approach needs a deliberate attempt to train the mentors by means of Faculty Development Programs (FDP) [11]. While most of the FDPs are limited to developing pedagogical skills of teachers, a time a come to address soft skills such as mentoring skills, feedback skills, and motivational techniques which can make difference to the lives of their students. How to train the faculty members in these aspects is a challenge for the educators. Because such skills not only require role models who can make an impact, but also internalisation of these practices in the institute's culture. Only one or two mentors however competent they are cannot make an impact unless the entire medical fraternity shares such a practice. The following steps are needed for effective implementation of mentoring in medical institutions:

- Allocation of mentor–mentee based on mutual preference (not coercion!).
- Leaving enough flexibility and autonomy to the mentor–mentees.
- Providing proper ambience and logistics support for mentoring.
- Monitoring, removing hurdles, and facilitating long term mentorship.
- Recognising and rewarding every mentor–mentee pair in a unique manner.
- Fostering a culture of mentoring and feedback.

The future of mentoring will be enabled by the availability of smart devices and technologies which make virtual mentoring a reality. However, the core issues of mentoring viz., offering a helping hand combined with head and heart will continue forever irrespective of the changing time and expanding space.

### 2.4.7 Conclusion

- Mentoring is a practical and effective solution to bring transformative learning.
- Mentors are not borne. They are made. Mentoring can be learnt.
- While formal approaches are much needed to lay a foundation, the informal approaches can contribute to a long enduring relationship.

- Mentoring should be stage-specific rather than department-specific.
- A culture of mentoring and feedback go together.

## 2.5 Evaluate

- Who is the mentor to whom you want to give due credit for your success in life? What did you learn from him/her? What did you contribute to his/her growth?
- Based on the attributes of a good mentor–mentee relationship, what steps will you take to strengthen your mentoring strategy?

## References


1. Modi JN, Singh T. Mentoring in medical colleges: bringing out the best in people. Int J User-Driven Healthc. 2013;3(3):106–15. https://doi.org/10.4018/ijudh.2013070108.
2. Joshi P. Choosing a suitable research area and supervisor. In: Parija SC, Kate V, editors. Thesis writing for Master's and Ph.D. program. Singapore: Springer; 2019. p. 19–26.
3. Keyser DJ, Lakosi JM, Lara-Cinisomo S, Schultz DJ, Williams VL, Zellers DF, et al. Advancing institutional efforts to support research mentorship: a conceptual framework and self assessment tool. Acad Med. 2008;83(3):217–25.
4. Sood R, Adkoli BV. Editorial medical education in India – problems and prospects. J Ind Acad of Clin Med. 2000;1(3):210–2.
5. Ten Cate O. Competency-based postgraduate medical education: past, present and future. GMS J Med Educ. 2017;34(5):Doc69. https://doi.org/10.3205/zma001146. Published online 2017 Nov 15. http://www.naac.gov.in/images/docs/Manuals/HSM-University-22Feb19.pdf
6. Medical Council of India. Competency based undergraduate curriculum for the Indian medical graduate. New Delhi: Medical Council of India; 2018. Available at www.mciindia.org/CMS/information-desk/for-colleges/ug-curriculum.
7. Knowles MS and Associates. Andragogy in action: applying modern principles of adult learning. San Francisco: Jossey Bass; 1984.
8. Kolb DA. Experiential learning: experience as the source of learning and development. Englewood Cliffs: Prentice Hall; 1984.
9. Gibbs G. Learning by doing: a guide to teaching and learning methods. London: Further Education Unit; 1988.
10. Schon DA. Educating the reflective practitioner: toward a new design for teaching and learning in the professions. San Francisco: Jossey Bass; 1987.
11. Srinivas DK, Adkoli BV. Faculty development in medical education in India: the need of the day. Al Ameen J Med Sci. 2009;2(1):6–13.

# Feedback: How to Give and Take?

3

Balachandra V. Adkoli and Subhash Chandra Parija

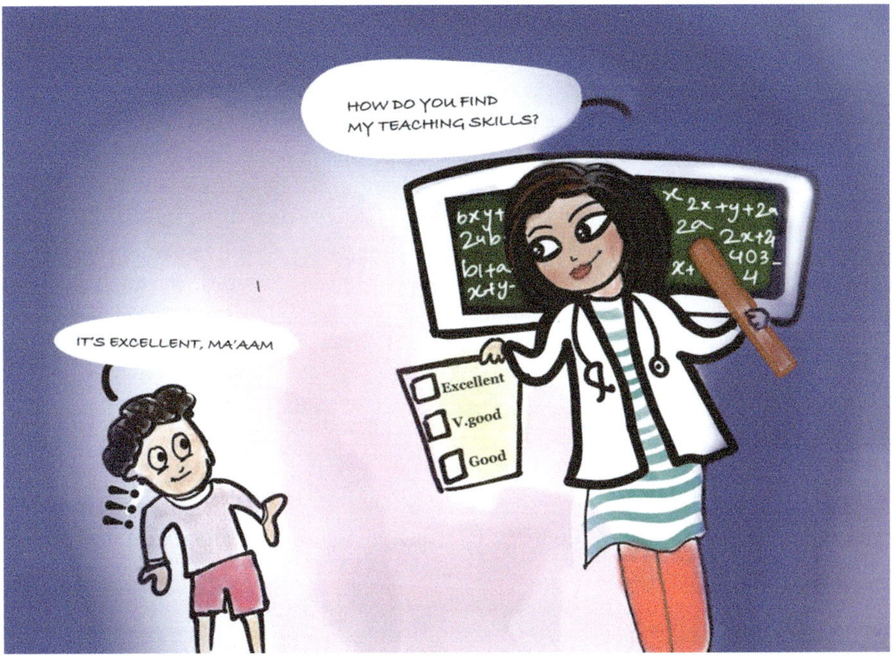


Feedback is the official receipt issued for successful communication—Adkoli and Parija

B. V. Adkoli (✉)
Centre for Health Professions Education, Sri Balaji Vidyapeeth (Deemed-to-be University), Pondicherry, India

S. C. Parija
Sri Balaji Vidyapeeth (Deemed-to-be University), Pondicherry, India



S. C. Parija, B. V. Adkoli (eds.), *Effective Medical Communication*,
https://doi.org/10.1007/978-981-15-3409-6_3

## 3.1 Assess Need

Feedback holds the key to successful communication. In fact, without feedback, communication is incomplete, ineffective, and can be even dangerous. While feedback can bridge many communication gaps in human interaction, it can also cause communication gaps resulting in a strained relationship between health professional and the patient or between two competent professionals.

Feedback is perhaps, most important in all communications, whether it involves patients, community, or day-to-day interpersonal communications with peers, seniors, and members of the health team. All the time, we need to check whether the message has been conveyed to others in the manner it is meant for. Only through feedback, we can find out the strengths and deficiencies in the system. Feedback, therefore, is a powerful instrument for improving communication, to enhance competency and deliver a better quality of care.

While feedback from patients is vital for improving patient care, feedback in teaching-learning activities is vital for the growth of learner and the effectiveness of the teacher. Feedback is essential at all stages of instruction: before instruction, in assessing learners' previous knowledge; during instruction, in monitoring the progress; after the instruction, in assessing the learning outcome.

Unfortunately, the medical training dominated from a paternalistic approach has hampered the practice and the power of listening to the patients. On a similar note, the absence of feedback in teaching-learning has affected the quality of training. The competency-based approach to medical education which is the current trend in medical education relies heavily on feedback [1]. Feedback does not happen by chance. There are deliberate techniques and models of giving and receiving feedback. Deliberating on the role of feedback is, therefore, not a luxury but a necessity.

## 3.2 Brief

The purpose of this chapter is to sensitize the students, teachers, and the administrators regarding the power of feedback in effective medical communication. Towards this end we:

- Discuss the role played by feedback in strengthening effective communication and learning—What? Where? When? and How?
- Discuss various models of giving feedback.
- Offer a few tips for giving feedback, receiving feedback, and responding to the feedback.
- Highlight the need for promoting a culture of feedback.

## 3.3 Contextualize

### 3.3.1 Scenario 1

Ms. Comini a girl from rural background having admitted to the premier institute was subjected to the grill of first semester exam against all odds: a shift in the medium of instruction from local language to English; problems of adjustment to the new environment; poor attendance because of episodes of illness caused by a change in the food habit. Somehow she wrote the exam, and waited for the report card to see how she has performed.

One Dr. FB was faculty in-charge of conveying the students' performance in a proper manner. Dr. FB was a taskmaster, authoritative, and short-tempered too. He thought he should parade the students, one by one in the whole class to see that everyone takes him seriously. When it was Ms. Comini's turn, Dr. FB was even more furious and started blasting her with a sarcastic remark, to begin with: 'Madam I am totally disappointed with your performance, you scored 5 in physiology, 3 in biochemistry and a big zero in anatomy! MBBS course is not your cup of tea. You better quit..or else….' At this point of time, Ms. Comini burst into tears.

***Exercise***: Reflect for a minute on the comments made by Dr. FB. What is your feedback on Dr. FB's feedback?

### 3.3.2 Scenario 2

Dr. Comini is now a faculty member in the Department of Medicine. She is given the responsibility of mentoring a fresher Mr. DR who is the son of a wealthy businessman, who had joined medicine because of parental pressure. He was not serious with studies but spent time with sophisticated gadgets, friends circle, and partying late nights. Dr. Comini, having accepted his mentoring, noticed his behaviour and started her first interaction by welcoming him to a street play at a rural health centre. Mr. DR took pictures and selfies with the actors and audience, which was appreciated by Dr. Comini. Thus a bond of affection was formed between the mentor and the mentee. Dr. Comini suggested Mr. DR to make use of his photography skills to capture practical experiments in physiology, dissection skills in anatomy, and complex concepts in biochemistry for complementing the classroom teaching. At every step, Dr. Comini would only help Mr. DR in setting *his* own goals, finding out *his* method of achieving that goal, and just appreciating him about *his* achievement.

***Exercise***: Reflect for a minute on the mentoring style of Dr. Comini. Make your assessment.

## 3.4 Describe

### 3.4.1 What Is 'Feedback'?

The word feedback has a long list of synonyms: criticism, advice, pointer, reaction, comment, response, opinion, and view! Though feedback may take all these '*avatars*', what is central to the concept of feedback is that it is an honest opinion about the '*act*' and not a '*person*' given in a palatable manner to improve the performance of an individual. Feedback is based on the observed behaviour of an individual. Feedback is a two-way process. Its focus is on *improving* the learner and not *proving*. Feedback is a potential tool that can make or mar the quality of patient care, teaching, or assessment.

The origin of feedback and the importance attached to this crucial concept dates back to ancient times. The ancient Indian dictum *(Manusmriti)* emphasizes that feedback should be given in a palatable manner (Box 3.1).

**Box 3.1 The Ancient Indian Dictum on how to Give Feedback**

Feedback is not a creation of educators of modern times. It is embedded in the history and civilization of mankind. One of the earliest quotes on how to give feedback comes from the following verse of *Manusmriti* an ancient Indian masterpiece stating—'*Sathyam bruyaat, priyambruyaat, nabruyaat, sathyapriyam*' (Manusmriti 4-138), which means 'Speak the truth, speak in a pleasant manner, do not speak bitter truth'.

Unfortunately, academia is neither informed about its potential benefits nor the dangers of its absence in the system of education. Applied to education, feedback plays a significant role in learning. Feedback is an essential component of communication which is an integral part of competency, in addition to knowledge, skills, and attitudes [1]. The journey of a medical student begins with mostly receiving feedback from peers, seniors, and sometimes, from other health team members. Receiving positive feedback from a teacher is every student's dream! On the other hand, receiving negative feedback from students is a nightmare for every teacher! Unfortunately, neither the teachers nor the students are formally trained to give or receive feedback. Nevertheless, the literature in this field has started coming up [2–6].

The current scenario of feedback in many countries, including India, offers a grim picture. Consider the journey of a medical professional starting from medical student, and then a faculty member and ultimately as a Head of the Department or Institute. The medical student is a passive 'recipient' of feedback, and a senior professional is often the 'giver'. In between these two ends, we have midlevel faculty who give and take feedback in a small measure. Hence, there is a need for giving and taking honest feedback at all levels.

**Table 3.1** The meaning and scope of Feedback

| What feedback is about? | What feedback is not about? |
|---|---|
| Guiding the learner to correct his/her mistakes | Finding fault with the learner |
| Listening and directing what is right and what is wrong | Telling and judging who is right or who is wrong |
| Monitoring the progress of the learner | Sitting on the judgement about learner's competence |
| Encouraging and motivating the learner | De-motivating or threatening the learner with the probable consequences |
| Briefly specifying the strength and limitations | Making an elaborate list of deficiencies |
| Informing the learner's strengths and weaknesses privately | Exposing the learner's weakness to the whole class |
| Telling the points immediately | Lodging a complaint later |
| Planning a future strategy | Digging about the past |

The term feedback is often misunderstood as an exercise to find fault, criticize, or judge a person (Table 3.1).

### 3.4.2 When to Give Feedback?

Feedback should be given immediately after the event. Otherwise, it will lose its seriousness. For instance, if the feedback of a test performance has to be effective, it should be given as quickly as possible. There is a saying that 'justice delayed is justice denied'. This is highly applicable for giving feedback. However, the tricky thing is that feedback is well taken only when the other party is receptive to feedback! If the receiver has a fixed mindset or a defensive attitude to negative feedback, no amount of feedback will work.

### 3.4.3 Where to Give Feedback?

While formal feedback is given in a classroom, there is no restriction of place for giving informal feedback. It can be given in the corridor, canteen, outpatient settings, bedside, wards, community, or even market place. The informal setting works better for receiving honest feedback. Based on our experience of obtaining feedback as a part of program evaluation, we found that the participants have a tendency to tick mark the rating scale, and somehow finish the evaluation rating scale. However, when we meet them informally over a cup of coffee, they tell the real story!

Preparing the recipient for the feedback is very important. There is a need to create a receptive ambience to establish rapport before giving feedback. It has to be a non-threatening environment. Positive feedback may be given in public, but negative feedback should be given privately on one-to-one basis after taking the person into confidence.

### 3.4.4 How to Give Feedback?

Giving feedback is art and science put together. While logic helps in convincing the person about the performance, emotional touch contributes to building trust. We offer some tips for giving effective feedback (Fig. 3.1).

- Be specific and non-judgmental in giving your feedback. Instead of telling 'Overall, you did very well', you may tell what did you find well, and how can you improve further. For example, you can say 'you have answered correctly, but you could have used bullet points instead of a continuous paragraph'.
- Be truthful and honest in your comment. If the truth is bitter, make it palatable like 'sweet coated pills'. For example, in counselling an obese patient, instead of telling 'You are obese or overweight, stop eating too much' you may politely say 'You look healthy, but with some diet control, you will be great!'
- Always give a constructive suggestion as to how to improve. Still, better is to help the *student* in finding a solution. Mere pointing out the deficiency is no feedback at all. For example, instead of telling 'Your handwriting is very poor', you may say that 'Do you think you could improve your handwriting? Why don't you practise one hour per day? Would you like to try writing in capital letters?'
- Show a genuine passion and concern for the improvement of the learner while giving feedback. For example, you may promise to throw a party to your mentee when he achieves A-Grade.
- Offer only one or few points during each encounter. Too many points will be forgotten or not taken seriously. If there are many lacunae, point out one or two at a time and then help learner in overcoming those deficiencies.

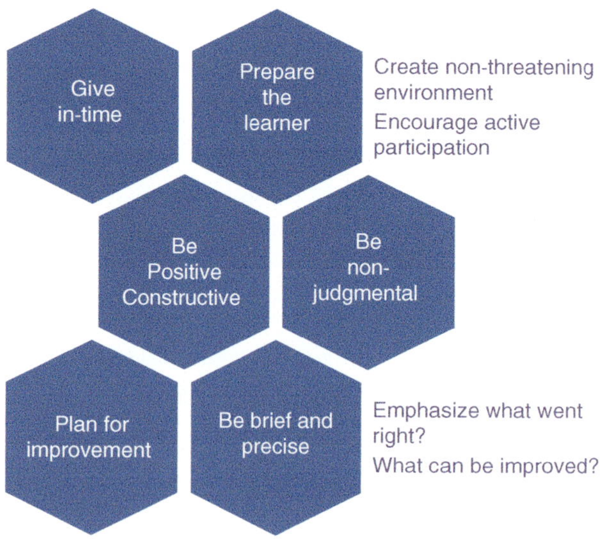


**Fig. 3.1** Tips for giving effective feedback

### 3.4.5 How to Receive Feedback?

Receiving feedback requires courage, tolerance, and a receptive mind. When we queried a large number of teachers as to how often they take feedback from their students, we were surprised to see very few responses. This may be due to the 'fear of getting negative feedback' or their perception that the respondents are not mature enough to give feedback. Many people take a defensive stand when someone gives negative feedback. This is like insulting the person who has given feedback after a request has been made. We offer the following tips for handling feedback effectively.

- Be attentive and keen to listen to ALL feedback (even if you think it is 'rubbish') with rapt attention and interest!
- Acknowledge all feedback with thanks.
- Do not be defensive. If you have solicited feedback from someone, ignoring means disrespect to the giver.
- You may not accept all feedback, but 'keep it in your pocket', reflect later, and see its worth.
- Encourage feedback from multiple sources over a period of time before taking major decisions.
- An isolated episode of extreme positive or negative feedback needs to be checked by taking a second opinion.
- Guard yourself against extreme feedback, liberal appreciation, or ruthless criticism.
- The one who gives critical remark is more helpful than a person who praises you lavishly. You need to assess the credibility of the person, his motive, and conflict of interest if any.

### 3.4.6 Models of Giving Feedback

The literature on feedback includes several models of giving feedback [2]. We discuss three models which are useful for a day-to-day interaction between a learner and teacher.

#### 3.4.6.1 Sandwich Model

As the name suggests, this model involves feedback sandwiched between plus points and minus points.

- The teacher appreciates what learner did well.
- Points out the deficiencies.
- Reinforces the strengths again giving a few tips.
- The learner listens to comments offered.

This model is flawed because it is dominated by the teacher, hence, one-way traffic. The only good thing about it is the fact that both strengths and deficiencies are pointed out in a balanced manner.

#### 3.4.6.2 Pendleton Rules

Here the learner becomes a part of the feedback process.

- The learner describes what he/she did well—positive aspects or strengths.
- The teacher amplifies and adds to what learner confessed—negative aspects or deficiencies.
- The learner describes what did not go well.
- The teacher amplifies and adds to what learner confessed.
- The learner sums up major highlights.
- The teacher adds and complements.

This model is an improvement over the sandwich model. It involves both the teacher and the learner. Moreover, it covers both strengths and deficiencies. An agreed plan for action is also initiated here.

#### 3.4.6.3 Learning Conversation

This involves feedback exchange between teacher and learner in the form of regular encounters.

- The teacher initiates a conversation with a learner looking back to latter's performance in a particular event individually or in class.
- The learner describes his/her experience, strengths, and weaknesses which he/she felt.
- The learner identifies the key issues.
- The teacher explores these issues with the whole class, and receives inputs.
- A plan of action is decided and informed to the learner to try next time.
- The learner tries out the action plan in his/her routine practice.
- The learner reports his/her experience this time… the conversation continues…

This is perhaps the best model considering that it ensures continuous development of the learner. Since the learner is responsible for taking a decision, this model conforms with the principle of self-directed learning.

### 3.4.7 The Role of Faculty Development

In the end, the role of faculty development should be highlighted more than anything else to support feedback. Faculty Development Programs have generated much interest among medical teachers. The practice of microteaching is a wonderful example of developing feedback skills in addition to other teaching skills. The Competency-Based Medical Education (CBME) requires the collection of evidence from multiple sources [1]. Multi-Source Feedback (MSF) is gaining much

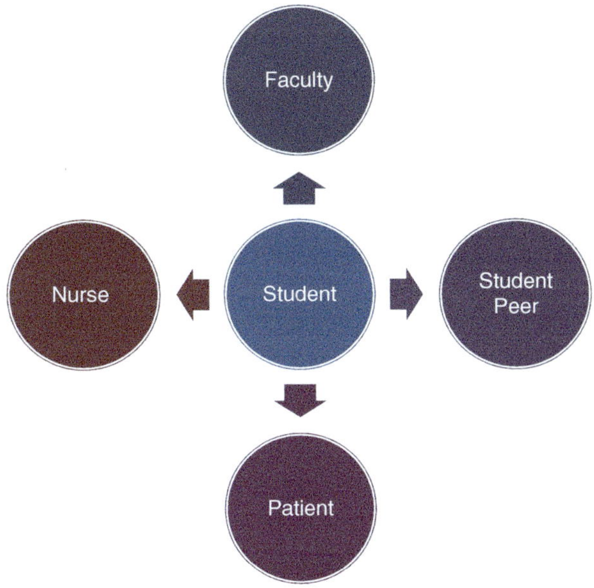


**Fig. 3.2** Multiple source feedback

momentum not only at the internship and postgraduate level but also in designing strategies for assessment of health personnel functioning at various levels (Fig. 3.2).

The task of promoting a culture of feedback is a long drawn agenda which needs to be addressed collectively by all stakeholders. In countries like India, where professional hierarchy dominates all walks of life, it is difficult to change the mindset of seniors overnight. Once the top leadership is convinced about it, the battle is half won. A beginning should be made to bring this culture by way of encouraging questions, criticisms, and comments by the young minds in classrooms, and beyond. Even 'best critique' awards can be instituted. However, changes will take time. It is worthwhile waiting.

### 3.4.8 Conclusion

- Feedback is a potential tool for determining whether communication has occurred.
- It is a two-way interaction with the goal of improving the performance of the learner, participant, process, or a program.
- Good feedback should be brief, timely, honest, non-judgmental, given in a non-threatening environment, along with a constructive suggestion.
- Feedback should be given only after preparing the person to receive feedback.
- Receiving feedback is as important as giving feedback.
- A culture of giving and taking feedback is essential for effective communication.

## 3.5 Evaluation

After reading this chapter, prepare a list of the strengths and deficiencies of this chapter. The next step is to post your comments to the authors, with or without mentioning your identity. Let us join together and work to create a culture of feedback!

## References


1. Epstein RM, Hundert EM. Defining and assessing professional competence. JAMA. 2002;287(2):226–35.
2. Anshu. Effective feedback in medical education. In: Bhuiyan PS, Rege NN, Supe A, editors. The art of teaching medical students. 3rd ed. New Delhi: Elsevier; 2015. p. 248–60.
3. Cantillon P, Sargeant J. Giving feedback in clinical settings. BMJ. 2008;337:a1961.
4. Krackov SK. Giving feedback. In: Dent JA, Harden RM, editors. A practical guide for medical teachers. 3rd ed. London: Churchill Living Stone; Elsevier; 2009.
5. Ende J. Feedback in clinical medical education. JAMA. 1983;250:777–81.
6. Adkoli BV. The role of feedback and reflection in medical education. SBV J Basic Clin Appl Health Sci. 2018;2(1):34–40.

# Part II

# For Students and Residents: Catch Them Young!

# 4 Effective Non-verbal Communication

B. Vishnu Bhat and Manoj Kumar Kingsley

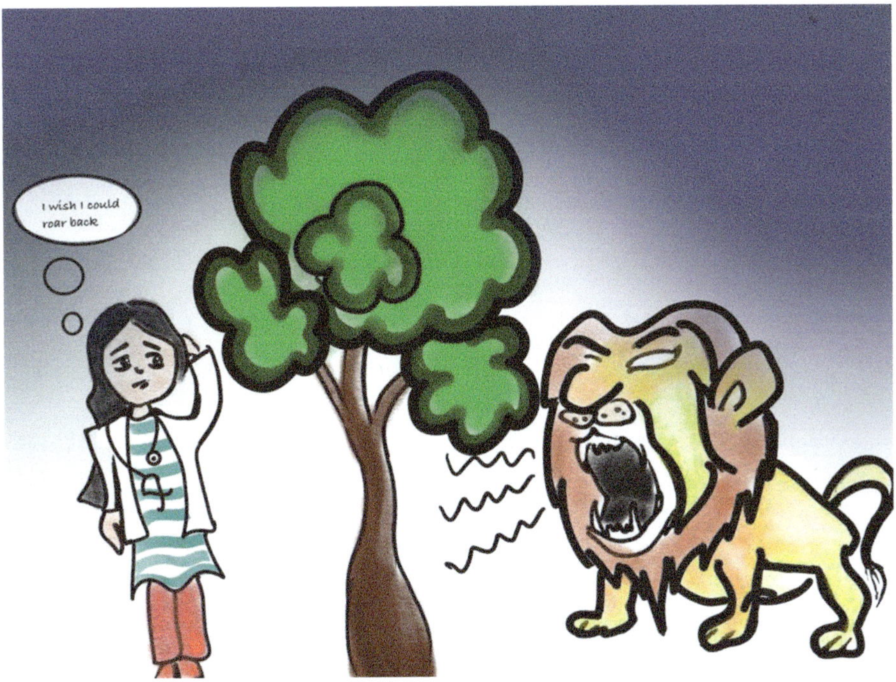


Better use of non-verbal tools of communication can make a big difference in the doctor-patient relationship than what we currently assume—Bhat and Kingsley

B. V. Bhat (✉)
Division of Medical Research, AVMC, Pondicherry, India

M. K. Kingsley
Department of Neonatology, JIPMER, Pondicherry, India


S. C. Parija, B. V. Adkoli (eds.), *Effective Medical Communication*,
https://doi.org/10.1007/978-981-15-3409-6_4

## 4.1 Assess Need

Any individual needs to communicate with others in daily life, and many daily activities can not be accomplished without communication. Effective and smooth communication is mandatory for the success of any organization or individual. It can be accomplished when the cyclic process of message transmission is smooth between the sender and the receiver (Fig. 4.1).

Non-verbal communication can be defined as communication without using words of speech, using voluntary or involuntary non-verbal signals. Unfortunately, in the clinical setting, more importance has been given to verbal communication though non-verbal behavior depicts more accurately the patient's attitude and emotional state of mind. Developing one's communication skills is an art that has to be developed throughout ones career. In the healthcare profession, any miscommunication or misunderstanding can be very costly. Physicians need to reassess their communication skills as there is an increase in malpractice litigations in recent times. It has been found that effective patient–doctor communication has shown to improve health outcome [1]. Despite all the technological advancements, patients still look for loving, caring, and compassionate doctors who are their first and best medicine.

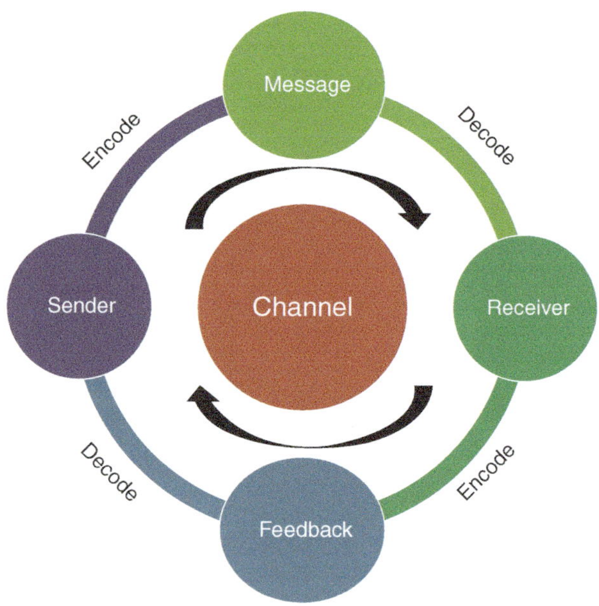


**Fig. 4.1** Communication cycle

## 4.2 Brief

The purpose of this chapter is to reveal the importance of non-verbal communication among the students, teachers, and physicians in medical education. The power of non-verbal communication and the change it can make in the student or patients' mentality has been discussed. In essence, in this chapter, we shall discuss:

- Importance of non-verbal communication in medical education.
- Classification of non-verbal communication.
- Different types of non-verbal communication.
- How to improve non-verbal communication?
- Obstacles to effective non-verbal communication.

## 4.3 Contextualize

### 4.3.1 Scenario 1

Dr. Comini is working as a doctor in a premier medical institution. One of her patients has been diagnosed with cancer. The tests have confirmed the diagnosis, and she has to inform the news to the patient and his family. It is a typical situation which arises in the life of most doctors. Now instead of showing a tense face with a hopeless look, Dr. Comini chooses to keep a calm face with a normal confident look. She decides to convey the message to the family first. With a gentle look and calm voice, she reveals the results of the diagnosis to the patient's family first. She gives them the confidence through her non-verbal actions such as an encouraging voice tone, a pat on the shoulders, leaning forward in her chair which reveals her care and interest in them. She tells them how to face the situation. She assures them of her full support. She cites the example of several other patients she has dealt with who have recovered from similar situations. This turned the grim situation of the patient and his family into a one of hope and confidence.

Now, after 6 months of radiation therapy and other medicines which were administered to the patient, there was a significant improvement in the condition. The patient is far better now, and the whole family is happy and thankful to Dr. Comini for her kind and positive way of handling things.

***Exercise***: Think of the consequences if Dr. Comini had not resorted to the manner in which she handled the situation.

### 4.3.2 Scenario 2

Dr. JY is a pediatrician in a hospital. This incident occurred when he was treating a 5-year-old child with pneumonia. He had given a slight overdose of the medicine by mistake. The next day he found out the medicine was more for a 5-year-old child, and it had caused increased side effects like vomiting and abdominal pain. Now the parents of the child were worried and angry that Dr. JY had given more medicine than required. Dr. JY understood his mistake and with a subtle look and smile started explaining the situation to the family. With proper use of non-verbal skills, he explained that he had not given the wrong medicine, but the dose was little extra. He reassured touching the father's hand that the situation is entirely under control, and he has now reduced the dosage of medicine. The family was satisfied with the gentle behavior combined with the proper explanation given by Dr. JY and decided to continue the treatment under him.

***Exercise***: Discuss the effect of non-verbal communication during medical error disclosures to improve the patients satisfaction.

## 4.4 Describe

### 4.4.1 What Is Non-verbal Communication?

Non-verbal communication is the process of sending and receiving messages without using either spoken or written words. It is the non-linguistic transmission of information through visual, auditory, tactile, and kinesthetic channels. It is also called as sign language or silent language, comprising of all behaviors performed in the presence of others or perceived either consciously or unconsciously [2]. Existing data shows that most of the clinical communication skill teaching focuses on verbal communication [3]. However, it has been found that non-verbal communication accounts for 80% of essential communication between individuals [4]. Studies have found that in a conversation, <15–20% of the concepts are expressed through spoken words.

Non-verbal communication is often more subtle and effective than verbal communication as it can deliver the message without words. For example, a pleasant smile from the doctor could mean a lot to the patient despite his condition or current situation. Thus body language, facial expressions, and the way we present ourselves before others are more powerful than our words.

### 4.4.2 Importance of Non-verbal Communication

Non-verbal communication is one of the crucial aspects of communication having various functions:

- It is used to reinforce the verbal message. For instance, while showing directions, we tend to point our hands or fingers towards the needed direction.
- It can complement or contradict the verbal message. For example, a "*wink*" contradicts a message, whereas a "*nod*" reinstates a positive message.

- It can even substitute verbal messages. For instance, when a teacher wants a student to keep quiet, the teacher may use gestures using finger on lips to signify the message.
- It can be used to regulate interactions. For example, non-verbal signals can be used to convey whether the other person should speak or not.
- Appropriate and timely use of verbal and non-verbal actions by teacher correlate well with students' progress and good behavior.
- Better non-verbal communication skills are associated with significantly greater patient satisfaction in different types of clinical encounters with standardized patients [5].

### 4.4.3 Classification of Non-verbal Communication

There are two basic categories of non-verbal communications—non-verbal signals conveyed by the body and non-verbal messages produced by the broad setting (time, space, and silence) [6]. It can be intentional or unintentional as well. From our handshakes to our hairstyles, our body language decides how we relate with other people.

Broadly, non-verbal communication can be classified into four different categories [7]:

1. Kinesics: head and body movements (smile, leaning postures, etc.).
2. Vocalics: non-linguistic vocal cues (sound pitch, silence time, etc.).
3. Haptics: body contact (touch, pat, handshakes, etc.).
4. Proxemics: spatial cues (distance between doctor and patient, etc.).

### 4.4.4 Types of Non-verbal Communications

1. *Facial expressions*

   A major proportion of non-verbal communication involves facial expression. It is the most studied non-verbal behavior to identify and interpret. While talking with someone, the changes in facial expression are noted vividly, and convey your mindset to other person. Smiling, nodding, raising eyebrows, rolling eyes, yawning, and sneering are some of them. Though non-verbal communication can vary across cultures, the meaning for classic facial expressions such as happiness, fear, disgust, surprise, anger, or sadness remains the same across cultures [6].
2. *Gestures*

   Gesturing is a robust phenomenon found across ages and cultures. Gestures include the deliberate movement of head, hands, arms, and legs. Some of the frequent gestures include waving, pointing, and using fingers. For instance, raising thumb means to show "*OK*."
   (a) Gesturing can act as a tool which displays the speaker's unspoken thoughts.
   (b) An encouraging gesture can change the way how students or patients think or visualize things which might alter the course of therapy or learning.

(c) When asking a question to a particular student it is important that the teacher does not point his finger towards him/her as this may cause anxiousness.

(d) Gestures are the crucial components which can be used to create language especially in the case of children who do not already have a language. They know something which they cannot say and use gestures.

3. *Eye contact*

Our eye movements reveal what is going on inside our mind. A person's emotions can be read through the eyes, and in many instances it is not the same as the words that are spoken. It can signify different emotions such as hostility, interest, and attraction [6]. Eye contact with audience increases the speakers' credibility. A teacher who is able to comfortably look into the eyes of all the students shows his confidence and passion. It does not mean that you have to stare intensely into a person's eyes continuously which may make him/her very uncomfortable.

4. *Body posture*

Body posture is an effective means of non-verbal communication. For instance, slouching, folding arms, crossing legs, or sitting erect, all can reveal different messages. With hunched shoulders, face supported by the hands or elbows in table signifies that the person is not much interested in what the other person is saying. Leaning too far back on the chair with mouth covered by hands implies that you are expressing hostility towards the other person's opinion, and you are restricting your views by covering your mouth [8].

While talking to a person, it is important to stand with feet approximately 18 inches apart. This implies a comfortable distance. Feet too close to one another imply that one is not comfortable and is nervous. Feet too far signify that we are ready to attack someone or fight or you are over cautious. Maintaining a feet distance of 18 inches while standing gives the audience the impression that you are comfortable and relaxed. Similarly arms folded against chest especially while standing and talking signify resistance. Juggling with the fingers and nails while talking or listening to someone implies that you are not interested in listening. Likewise criss-crossing of legs, tapping of toes implies that either you are nervous or you are ready to leave.

Movements which are not purposeful, putting hands inside pocket, or clasped them behind the back are not advisable. These hand positions reveal that either you are bored or hiding something.

5. *Paralanguage or voice signals*

Speech related non-verbal behaviors include pitch, tone of voice, rhythm, prosody, volume, and speed of speaking. Paralinguistics comprise of several factors such as the tone of voice, loudness, inflection, and pitch [6]. A statement expressed in a strong tone of voice may draw the interest and approval of the listeners. On the other hand, a hesitant tone may create discontent and lack of interest.

The speaking time, gap, or pause is one of the dominance related behaviors. In a doctor–patient communication such type of behaviors were found to be complementary in action [9].

**Table 4.1** Types of non-verbal communication

| Non-verbal skill | Expressions |
|---|---|
| Facial expressions | Smiling, frowning, sneering, yawning |
| Gestures | Waving, pointing, and using fingers |
| Eye contact | Comfortably looking at eyes, staring, blinking, raising eyebrows, rolling eyes |
| Body postures | Sitting erect, slouching, arm crossing, folding arms, legs crossing |
| Paralanguage | Rate, rhythm, prosody, volume, tone, and pitch of voice |
| Distance | Personal space between two people while communicating |
| Touch | Pat on the back/shoulders, hugging, pushing, hand shake |
| Appearance | Color, clothing, hairstyle |

6. *Distance*

   It is very important to maintain proper distance when communicating with others. The amount of distance between two persons can be interpreted differently depending on various cultures. For instance, it can either signify attraction or can signify intensity. Language of space can be classified as intimate space (within 45 cm), personal space (45 cm–1.2 m), social space (1.2–3.6 m), and public space (3.7–4.5 m). People are very protective of their personal or intimate space which is approximately from 6 to 18 in. This personal space is generally reserved for their spouse, family, or close friends. When you talk to another person ideally the distance must not be too close but yet not too far (30 in) [8].
7. *Touch*

   Any actual touching may signify attraction or a level of intimacy. Touch may take different forms and can have various meanings. Some examples include shaking hands, patting the back, and hugging. Touch can be used to convey various emotions such as affection, sympathy, or familiarity. It varies depending on the intimacy, gender, age, status, and cultural background of the persons. A hand shake which is firm, warm, and not overpowering signifies sincerity and genuineness [8].
8. *Appearance*

   The choice of dress, color of clothing, hairstyle, and personal appearance is considered as important tools of non-verbal communication. Appearance can alter the physiological reactions, judgments, and interpretations [6]. Different colors can evoke different moods. Patients look up to doctors with great respect and it is very important to present oneself in a tidy and well groomed manner. Likewise students look up to teachers as role models. Table 4.1 shows the different types of non-verbal skills and the various expressions associated with them.

### 4.4.5 How to Improve Non-verbal Communication?

- Maintain eye contact while speaking.
- Use pleasant facial expressions like a gentle smile.
- Use proper gestures to complement your speech.
- Do not point fingers while talking.

- Mind your posture.
- Be conscious of personal space.
- Beware of your voice tones and sound.
- Be neatly dressed and well groomed.

### 4.4.6 Obstacles to Effective Non-verbal Communication

Different factors such as culture, gender, generation, context, collegiality, cooperation, self-disclosure, and reciprocity affect the outcome of effective communication. No single gesture or behavior means the same in every culture, context, or situation. All non-verbal behavior must be interpreted within context. Different contexts can convey different meaning of the same non-verbal signal. Likewise, the same gesture or use of non-verbal skills in different kind of scenarios can mean different things in different cultures. Physicians must be trained to the situation.

There have not been many studies on how physicians and older patients interact with one another. Old people in nursing homes tend to less frequently communicate with hands or trunk movements than with facial expressions, head movements, speaking variations, and paralinguistic signs [6]. Identifying and improving non-verbal communication may actually improve the verbal exchange between physician and older patients and thus may improve medical care of older patients [10].

### 4.4.7 Conclusion

- Non-verbal communication is a crucial component of effective communication.
- Verbal communication is complete and effective only when it is accompanied with proper use of non-verbal skills.
- Effective use of non-verbal expressions like - smile, eye contact, forward lean, tone of voice, and gesture can improve the doctor–patient relationship and patient satisfaction.
- Medical students and budding doctors must be trained appropriately for effectively using non-verbal tools in their profession.
- Though research has focused on the effect of non-verbal behavior of the doctor on the patient satisfaction there has been not much information on the non-verbal behavior of the patients.

## 4.5 Evaluate

1. What was your impression about importance of non-verbal communication? What are the changes you will employ from now to improve your non-verbal skills?

2. Have you come across someone (your professor, HOD, or your mentor) who make good use of non-verbal skills? What are the things you can learn from their behavior? Do you think by employing those skills in your life from now it can make a change in the people/patients associated with your life?

## References


1. Stewart MA. Effective physician-patient communication and health outcomes: a review. CMAJ. 1995;152(9):1423–33.
2. Bambaeeroo F, Shokrpour N. The impact of the teachers' non-verbal communication on success in teaching. J Adv Med Educ Prof. 2017;5(2):51–9.
3. Mast MS, Hall JA, Köckner C, Choi E. Physician gender affects how physician nonverbal behavior is related to patient satisfaction. Med Care. 2008;46(12):1212–8.
4. Gorawara-Bhat R, Cook MA, Sachs GA. Nonverbal communication in doctor-elderly patient transactions (NDEPT): development of a tool. Patient Educ Couns. 2007;66(2):223–34.
5. Griffith CH 3rd, Wilson JF, Langer S, Haist SA. House staff nonverbal communication skills and standardized patient satisfaction. J Gen Intern Med. 2003;18(3):170–4.
6. Ben-Nun L. Non-verbal communication skills. B.N. Publication House, Israel; 2014.
7. Liu C, Calvo RA, Lim R. Improving medical students' awareness of their non-verbal communication through automated non-verbal behavior feedback. Front ICT. 2016;3:11.
8. Hull RH. The art of nonverbal communication in practice. Hear J. 2016;69(5):22–4.
9. Mast MS. On the importance of nonverbal communication in the physician-patient interaction. Patient Educ Couns. 2007;67(3):315–8.
10. Irish JT. Deciphering the physician-older patient interaction. Int J Psychiatry Med. 1997;27(3):251–67.

# 5 Doctor–Patient Communication

Krishna Seshadri

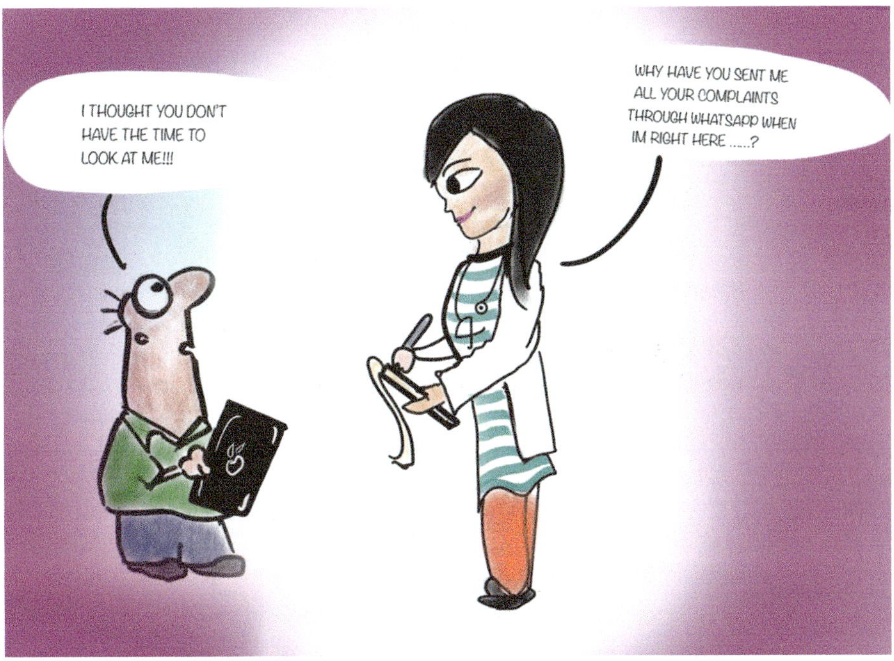


Communication is the sheet anchor of the doctor-patient relationship—Krishna Seshadri

K. Seshadri (✉)
Sri Balaji Vidyapeeth (Deemed-to-be University), Pondicherry, India



S. C. Parija, B. V. Adkoli (eds.), *Effective Medical Communication*,
https://doi.org/10.1007/978-981-15-3409-6_5

## 5.1 Assess Need

The nature of doctor–patient communication is determined foremost by the nature of the physician–patient relationship. As the nature of the doctor–patient relationship (DPR) has evolved, so has the nature of and need for communication.

The DPR is defined by four key elements: (a) the values of the patient, (b) the obligation of the physician, (c) the concept of patient autonomy, and (d) the concept of the physician's role [1].

A paradigm shift has occurred in the DPR—from paternalism to increased involvement of the patient in the decision-making process. This evolution has essentially involved increasing the amount and quality of information shared with the patient, facilitating and ensuring a process of understanding that will allow the patient to participate in the decision-making process and make informed choices. It is quite obvious that the sheet anchor of this process is in the content, nature, and tone of communication involved. As a corollary, it can be stated that the nature of communication in many ways determines the nature of the DPR.

Several other factors have influenced the evolving nature of the DPR and thus the need for better and efficient communication. Foremost of these has been the ready availability of medical information primarily through the internet and social media. Unfortunately, the quanta of legitimate information available to the discerning patient have been swamped by mis- and often dis-information much to the patient's peril and the disenfranchisement of doctors. The knowledge of factors affecting patient–doctor communication is of vital importance (Table 5.1).

The corpus of medical knowledge and its complexity has changed enormously in the last five decades. State of the art in modern medicine is increasingly dependent on advances in molecular biology genetics, various "*omics*", etc. that is difficult to comprehend for many physicians. Many of these "*advances*" are often small increments over existing standards of care available at significantly enhanced cost. Their treatment by the public information process, viz. the news cycle, lay press, and social media provides an exaggerated and often distorted picture to the patient invariance to the perception of the physician.

The societal perception of physicians and the medical profession has evolved over the years. Advances of medicine with its cost escalation, ownership patterns, remuneration, and industry relationships have all resulted in straining DPR. When the doctor–patient relationship is deconstructed, trust emerges as its vital component. The most important determinant of trust is effective communication.

**Table 5.1** Factors affecting the doctor–patient communication

| |
|---|
| 1. Doctor–patient relationship |
| 2. Availability of information in the public domain |
| 3. Growth in the complexity of medicine |
| 4. The societal perception of physicians and the profession |

## 5.2 Brief

This chapter will highlight:

- The purpose of communication.
- Benefits of effective and appropriate communication.
- Barriers to effective communication.
- Common errors in communication.
- Elements of effective communication.
- Strategies for improvement.

## 5.3 Contextualize

### 5.3.1 Scenario

A note from the diary of an eminent specialist: "*It was humiliating. After so many years...to sit in front of a medical director and listening to how I need to be better. What does the man think he is? And that lady - patient experience officer tells me – 'Please listen to your patients some more. Look at your patients in the eye. Don't be distracted by your phone'. Where do they get these people from? Twenty-five years in the field. Over 20000 surgeries - trained so many students and I have to listen to these upstarts. One disgruntled patient and they react like this. No gratitude for what I have done for the institution*".

***Exercise***: How you would have reacted if you were in the position of the specialist?

## 5.4 Describe

### 5.4.1 The Purpose of Communication

Communication is a core clinical function. Effective communication: (a) facilitates the acquisition of adequate and appropriate data that will guide diagnosis and care, (b) promotes patient empowerment and participation in shared decision making, and (c) establishes an empathic and caring relationship with patients. It is clear that these constructs of communication are major determinants of patient behaviour outcomes and satisfaction and in-turn of effective health care delivery [2, 3] (Fig. 5.1).

The etymological meaning of communication emphasizes the shared process that forms the basis of the doctor–patient relationship. While data gathering and information transfer about diagnosis, prognosis, and therapy are its obvious constructs, communication forms the basis on which the therapeutic relationship is built and nurtured. Effective communication is believed to be a tool that positively influences patient outcomes. Above all, it is the means through which *trust* is infused to the partnership between the patient and physician.

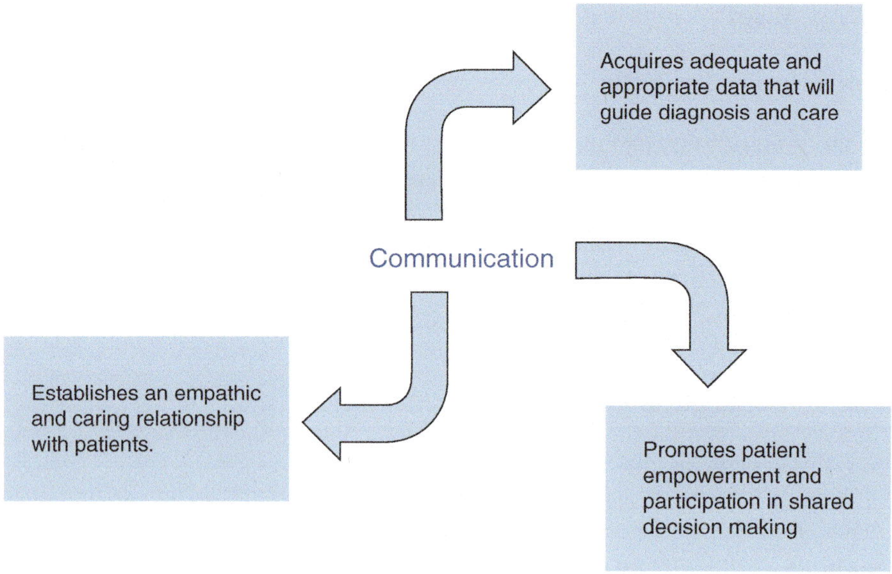


**Fig. 5.1** The purpose of communication

**Table 5.2** Barriers to effective doctor–patient communication

| |
|---|
| Anxiety, fear, and expectations |
| Practice environment |
| Inadequate training |
| Evolving patient constructs |

### 5.4.2 Benefits of Effective and Appropriate Communication

A doctor who communicates effectively is perceived by patients as competent [4]. Undoubtedly, effective doctor–patient communication allows a better assessment of the patient's clinical and emotional state. It is associated with greater satisfaction, agreement with the proposed plan, greater treatment adherence, and recovery [5]. Other reported benefits include improvements in pain tolerance, better mental health, shorter hospital stays, and fewer referrals [6].

Patient satisfaction scores significantly correlate with physician communication skills, and this, in turn, is associated with fewer malpractice complaints, greater physician satisfaction, and less burnout [7].

### 5.4.3 Barriers to Effective Communication

The barriers to effective communication are listed in Table 5.2.

#### 5.4.3.1 Anxiety, Fear, and Expectations

Several barriers spoil effective communication between patients and doctors. Patient's anxiety, fear, and unrealistic expectations contribute to this phenomenon. The attitude of physicians, their values, skills, and misperception of their own communication skills are important contributors to ineffective communication. It is well known that physicians overestimate their ability to effectively and appropriately communicate with patients.

#### 5.4.3.2 Practice Environment

Constraints of time and inability to manage time effectively contribute to poor communication skills among doctors. Fear of litigation promotes defensive behaviours in clinical care. In the age of social media, physicians are worried continuously about increased scrutiny, loss of reputation, mental and physical assault. Breakdown of traditional family support, changing family norms, unrealistic patient expectations lead to new barriers to effective communication.

#### 5.4.3.3 Inadequate Training

Some aspects of poor doctor–patient communication can be explained by the lack of training. Communication is often deemed to be learnt automatically. It is also considered part of the hidden curriculum. Skills, myths, and mistakes are observed, acquired, adopted, practised, and transmitted passively from one generation of doctors to the next without the opportunity to be learnt formally, assessed, honed, and improved.

One of the consequences is inflated self-importance among physician trainees—leading to paternalism, inappropriate understanding of what constitutes adequate and appropriate information, and a reduced perception of the patient as the most important participant in the decision-making process.

Long working hours, the demands of medicine, and the numbing exposure to human suffering, especially during an internship where supervised learning is minimal often leads to a reduction in compassion and empathy [8]—which reflect in poor communication skills.

The traditional clinical encounter in a medical school rarely addresses the psychosocial and emotional aspects of patient care. The consequence is "*avoidance*" in clinical care—doctors tend to ignore rush or skip over emotional or coping issues of patients, often leading to an increase in patient distress [8] and dissatisfaction. "*Avoidance*" by the physician, in addition, leads to inadequate disclosure of information by patients resulting in poor outcomes.

Training programs seldom provide opportunities for trainees to examine and reflect on their emotional reactions to human suffering. The lack of an opportunity to safely reflect, explore, and discuss their reactions to suffering and lack of guidance in helping patients and families cope with illness lead to untested ill-formed reactions and defences that seriously endanger communication and the doctor–patient relationship.

The absence of formalized training in communication skills in summary (pitched at a clinical and empathetic level appropriate for patient-centered care) is a serious flaw in the education system that leaves young physicians unprepared for a changing world.

#### 5.4.3.4 Evolving Patient Constructs

As medicine and society evolve, so have patient's values perceptions and needs. Patients actively seek involvement in their own care and have begun to assert their own knowledge, beliefs, and values in the care equation. Often there is resistance to the position of authority that the physician occupies in the doctor–patient relationship. This, at times, is taken to an extreme that leads to a breakdown in communication. Evidence and guideline-based medicine often lead to boiler plating of health care that ignores inequality, social equations, and structural constraints which are critical influencers of health care [9]. The demanding "*educated*" patient empowered by social media, who perceives the doctor as a privileged money-grubber erects a miscommunication wall that can seldom be breached easily.

### 5.4.4 Common Errors in Communication

The physician–patient relationship is intensely intimate. While the physician has many patients—the patient usually has one doctor. Every word said and unsaid, and every expression is latched on by the patient. From patient interviews, several themes of communication errors made by physicians emerge [10] (Table 5.3).

#### 5.4.4.1 Non-verbal

Most of us infer more from what is unsaid than what is said. Eye contact, facial expressions, hand gestures all tell a story that is more compelling than the verbal narrative provided by physicians. The addition of the computer EMR and phone screen in the clinic or bedside has further diverted physician attention from the patient. Eye contact is strongly related to the perception of truth and trust in communications. Patients frequently interpret lack of eye contact as lack of interest in their problems or as frank disrespect.

#### 5.4.4.2 Tone

How words are said is as important as what is being said. Volume, rhythm, pitch, intonation, and speed of delivery are perceived, analysed, and inferred by patients. A flat tone often conveys lack of interest. Raise in volume is often equated with

**Table 5.3** Common errors in doctor–patient communication

| | |
|---|---|
| Non-verbal | Lack of eye contact<br>Inappropriate facial expressions or hand gestures |
| Tone | Inappropriate volume pitch, rhythm, speed |
| Listening | Interrupting too soon |
| Choice of words | Defensive and accusatory words |
| Information | Too little or too technical |
| Attitude | Lack of empathy and respect |

"*shouting*". Slow delivery is equated with maturity and wisdom. Lack of pauses is construed as not interested in ascertaining the understanding of the patient or of not providing an opportunity for the patient to ask questions.

#### 5.4.4.3 Listening

Not listening is probably the most common complaint that patients express against physicians. The "*His - Story*" as a patient narratives is one of the oldest themes in clinical medicine. Physicians, however, interrupt patients commonly and all too soon (median of 18–23 s) [11]. Listening by physicians is seldom "*active*" leading to discontentment among patients.

#### 5.4.4.4 Choice of Words

Inappropriate choice of words translates into a perception of a lack of sensitivity and tact. Words that are threatening or defensive lead to judgements by patients on the lack of professionalism and attitude of physicians.

#### 5.4.4.5 Information

Often information provided by physicians is perceived as inadequate. This includes an explanation of results of investigations, the disease, its prognosis, lifestyle, and dietary changes required options of care and side effects of therapies. Lack of updates in admitted patients is a common grouse amongst families. Of note, the quality of the information provided also leaves much to be desired. A judgement on the physician's part that this is "*sufficient*", without thought to the patient's needs, expectations, and values are in part responsible for break down in communication.

#### 5.4.4.6 Attitude

Lack of empathy and respect are often cited as major drawbacks amongst physicians. Failure to demonstrate an understanding of the patient's situation and being judgmental is often deciphered from the way a physician communicates. The physician's communication skills also tell the patient the quantum of respect that the physician has for the patient. Not introducing oneself or not obtaining permission prior to examination or using respectful and polite language are common examples that reflect the attitude of the physician, and affect the tone and demeanour of the DPR.

### 5.4.5 Elements of Effective Communication

The best strategy for effective communication is a matter of debate. Individual physician styles matter and indeed, the physician must not lose his personality and individuality while communicating. However, there is a need for acquiring some minimal common skills in communication. Many professional bodies have defined the key elements of communication that physicians must acquire (Table 5.4).

#### 5.4.5.1 Setting the Stage

A culturally appropriate greeting that conveys respect and self-introduction (for new patients) is a good start. Enquire which language of communication that the

**Table 5.4** Elements of effective communication

| | |
|---|---|
| Setting the stage | Appropriate greeting, language, explain the use of EMR or mobile devices |
| Eliciting information | Open-ended, active listening, summarizing to convey an understanding |
| Sharing information | Assess what is known, what needs to be conveyed, prioritize, de-jargonize; allow questions; ask the patient to summarize understanding; provide access to more information |
| Decision making | Shared decision making. Help the patient take the decision—but do not make it for him or her |
| Support | Empathy and respect; be available |

patient would prefer. Establishing eye contact early and maintaining them periodically convey interest. Writing or filling up the EMR should ideally be postponed until the end of the interview. If this is not feasible—stating to the patient that you will periodically be entering or writing the data gathered reassures them that break in engagement is not necessarily because of a lack of respect. Use of a large screen that is visible to the patient, and that allows them to view the data entered is a further reassurance that you are not viewing the screen for any other reason. If a mobile phone has to be present in the examination room, then it should ideally be "*face down*".

#### 5.4.5.2 Eliciting Information

An open-ended starting question such as "*what brings you here today*"—allowing to state the concern without interruption establishes caring. Listening actively includes attention, acknowledgement of the information provided through verbal and non-verbal cues, and clarifying information that is provided. A simple way of reassuring the patient that you have indeed listened to him or her is to summarize your understanding of the narrative—"*As I understand*". It also allows the patient to restate incorrect information or correct misunderstanding [7]. Allow and actively explore the social and psychological impact of the illness and the coping mechanisms employed by the patient and the family. Asking "*Is there anything else that you would like to tell me?*" is a good way to reassure the patient that you have and are willing to provide the time required to help sort out the issue.

#### 5.4.5.3 Sharing Information

Before sharing information, it is useful to start by assessing what the patient already knows [12]—"*Can you tell me what you know about your condition*". Patients often bring in prior (right or wrong) impressions of their illness from previous clinical encounters and other sources of information. Assessing and understanding what the patient knows or has misunderstood about his or her illness allows the physician to prepare for the task at hand.

Also, assess what the patient wants to know [12]. Patients are in a continuum wanting to know very little to every detail that a physician has to offer [13]. Finding and providing what the patient expects to be told are the key to the right communication. Slowing down the delivery and providing adequate pauses allow better comprehension. Prioritize information that needs to be provided, especially if time is a constraint. Between each category of information, it is wise not only to summarize but also elicit the degree of understanding [7]—"*Can you tell me what you have understood so far?*" This allows us to decide the level at which the information should be provided. In crucial areas such as when administering informed consent before surgery/procedures a suggested approach would be to present the risks and benefits of the procedure and then allow the patient to decide how much additional information that they require [14]. It goes without saying there is a pressing need to *Keep it Simple* and de-jargonize language. There is also a need to de-statistics (sic) the narrative.

Paying attention to the questions posed by the patient is crucial. If the questions reflect that the patient has comprehended the information provided, then further detail is warranted. If they reflect confusion or misunderstanding, return to more basic information is desirable. Silence must be assessed by observing non-verbal cues—does it reflect quiet understanding? Does it reflect a lack of comprehension or discomfort?

It is good to provide more information through other resources—"*We have some reading material available. Would you like to review them*". It is important to add—"*After you review them you can ask me further questions (at the same or subsequent visit)*".

It is useful to decide on what can wait for a subsequent meeting and obtain the patient's acquiescence. This is useful in chronic care conditions where many factors have to be addressed, and lack of time and increased quantum of information will reduce the effectiveness of communication. It is good to ask an open-ended question at the end of the information sharing process—"*Is there anything else that you would like to know?*" This gives the patient the impression that the time that they deserve and desire has been provided. It leads to a nod and smile from many patients that is quite gratifying.

#### 5.4.5.4 Decision Making

Supporting and facilitating patients to make an informed decision is a key component of doctor–patient communication. At one extreme point, patients would like to independently assess the information provided, seek further information elsewhere, and make their own choices. At the other, patients would like to outsource the decision making to the physician. Despite giving detailed information, patients often undergo significant conflict in the decision-making process. One approach is to provide basic information tailored to the level of understanding, and then provide further information on demand that will help narrow down the options and choose the best.

Patients may sometime choose the lesser of the choices offered or refuse to consider any of them. The exercise of value judgement by the patient must be respected. The clinician brings in his or her knowledge, experience, and wisdom into the decision making. The patient and family bring in their experiences and values into decision making. A refusal to consider any of the choices must not be dismissed—it must be respected. However, that should not in itself be considered final. Exploring the reasons for refusal would be worthwhile. A good therapeutic choice is made when the clinical judgement of the patient seamlessly aligns with the value system of the patient.

#### 5.4.5.5 Support

The support that a clinician provides to patients is a key component of the healing process. Empathy and respect are key components of the support process. Illness often destroys the sense of infallibility and immortality. It precipitates a wide range of behaviour, from anger to defensiveness, diffidence, or depression, which need support. Exploring the need for support without being unduly intrusive is a skill that requires practice. "*Being available for*" is a trait that is respected by patients and families. Often physicians lose interest in patients when further therapy is not possible or futile. Patients and families highly value the comfort that the doctor provides, especially when an illness is terminal. Failure to cure is seldom viewed as failing on the part of the physician. However, *failure to provide support is viewed seriously*.

### 5.4.6 How to Improve?

Recognition of the need to inculcate communication skills into the curriculum is a heartening trend in medical educations. Recently, the regulatory authority for medical education in India made three substantial additions to the curriculum that will allow learners to emerge with a well-honed set of communication skills. These include (a) recognition of communication as a domain of learning, (b) a shift to outcome-based learning with an increased focus on acquisition and assessment of skills (including communication skills), and (c) introduction of a longitudinal program in communication skills as part of the AETCOM (attitude ethics and communication) module.

While the need for next-generation is being addressed by educators and regulators, it is incumbent on physicians to constantly improve their communication skills. A willingness to assess correctly improve and excel is key to keeping up with the demands of the changing patient–doctor relationship.

#### 5.4.6.1 Assess Ourselves

The first step in improvement is to find out what we are good at, what we are not, what needs strengthening, and what needs change. Informal ways can be a start with moving to formal improvement methods over time.

Introspection is clearly the first step. In most instances, external help is desirable and useful. Colleagues, including office staff and nurses, are good sources of feedback. Patients often express their displeasure or discontent to them. They also pick up comments of patients in hallways. Asking a trusted colleague to observe and give feedback is worthwhile to consider. One should not get defensive but listen to the feedback carefully and try to work upon them.

As a more formal exercise is to go to a communications skills lab and to work with a standardized patient and receiving multisource feedback (MSF) which combines self-review, feedback from an expert and the patients themselves. MSF provides a clear idea of where we are and what needs to be done. This can be supplemented by attending formal workshops or learning sessions (Fig. 5.2).

#### 5.4.6.2 Make a Plan and Improve

It is possible to learn new tricks as long as there are a will and commitment. Some sacrifices may be required. For example—lengthening the time of appointments and seeing fewer patients, removing distracters such as phones. Marking some patient encounters to "*try out*" some of the changes and following it up with feedback and reflection is one way to implement change. The reflections should include—what went well? What did not? What could be done better? If this were to happen again—what should be done differently? This should lead to a further action plan. The results of such intervention may not be seen instantly, but seen over a period of time in the form of a smile on the face and the twinkle in the eyes of the patient.

*After some angst and diffidence, the doctor in the scenario called his nurse Ms. K and told her. "Ms. K, you have been working with me for the last 25 years. Tell me what should I change about the way I talk to patients?" Ms. K smiled and began.*

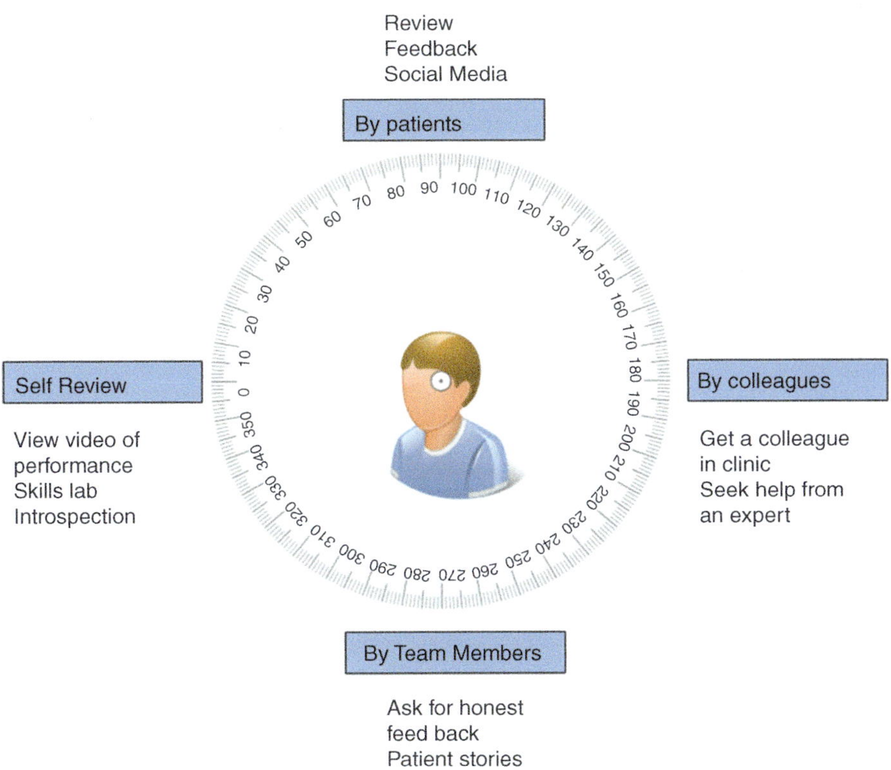


**Fig. 5.2** Assessment for improving communication—A 360° approach

### 5.4.7 Conclusions

1. Communication is the sheet anchor of the doctor–patient relationship.
2. Effective communication is associated with positive medical outcomes.
3. Doctors who communicate well are considered competent by patients.
4. Changing expectations, practice environment, and inadequate training in communication are the major challenges in acquiring effective communication.
5. Common errors in communication include lack of eye contact, use of inappropriate gestures, use of the wrong tone pitch beside the incorrect choice of words.
6. Lack of empathetic listening, frequent interruptions, and being judgmental are perceived as major barriers to effective communication.
7. Assessing the patient's requirement of information, ensuring understanding, encouraging questions, and assessing ones' own strengths and weakness through introspection and eliciting feedback from colleagues will go a long way in improving communication.

## 5.5 Evaluate

1. What would you do to avoid the situation mentioned in the scenario outlined in section C - Contextualize?
2. Have you been at the receiving end of a bad evaluation by patients? What was your reaction? What did you do?
3. What is the one thing that you have learnt from this chapter? What is the one thing about yourself that you will commit to change?

## References


1. Emanuel EJ, Emanuel LL. Four models of the physician-patient relationship. JAMA. 1992;267(16):2221–6.
2. Tongue JR, Howard R, Forese LL. Communication skills for patient-centered care. J Bone Joint Surg. 2005;87A(3):652–8.
3. Stewart MA. Effective physician-patient communication and he1alth outcomes: a review. CMAJ. 1995;152(9):1423–33.
4. Hall JA, Roter DL, Rand CS. Communication of affect between patient and physician. J Health Soc Behav. 1981;22(1):18–30.
5. Stewart M, Brown JB, Donner A, et al. The impact of patient-centered care on outcomes. J Fam Pract. 2000;49(9):796–804.
6. Ha JF, Longnecker N. Doctor-patient communication: a review. Ochsner J. 2010;10(1):38–43.
7. Maguire P, Pitceathly C. Key communication skills and how to acquire them. BMJ. 2002;325(7366):697–700.
8. DiMatteo MR. The role of the physician in the emerging health care environment. West J Med. 1998;168(5):328–33.
9. Lee RG, Garvin T. Moving from information transfer to information exchange in health and health care. Soc Sci Med. 2003;56(3):449–64.

10. Kee JWY, Khoo HS, Lim I, Koh MYH. Communication skills in patient-doctor interactions: learning from patient complaints. Health Prof Educ. 2018;4(2):97–106.
11. Phillips KA, Ospina NS. Physicians interrupting patients. JAMA. 2017;318(1):93–4.
12. Travaline JM, Ruchinskas R, D'Alonzo GE, Jr. Patient-physician communication: why and how. J Am Osteopath Assoc. 2005;105(1):13–8.
13. Miller SM. The interacting effects of coping styles and situational variables in gynecologic settings: implications for research and treatment. J Psychosom Obstet Gynaecol. 1988;9(1):23–34.
14. Lankton JW, Batchelder BM, Ominsky AJ. Emotional responses to detailed risk disclosure for anesthesia, a prospective, randomized study. Anesthesiology. 1977;46(4):294–6.

# Communication Training for Obtaining Informed Consent for Medical Research

# 6

N. Ananthakrishnan

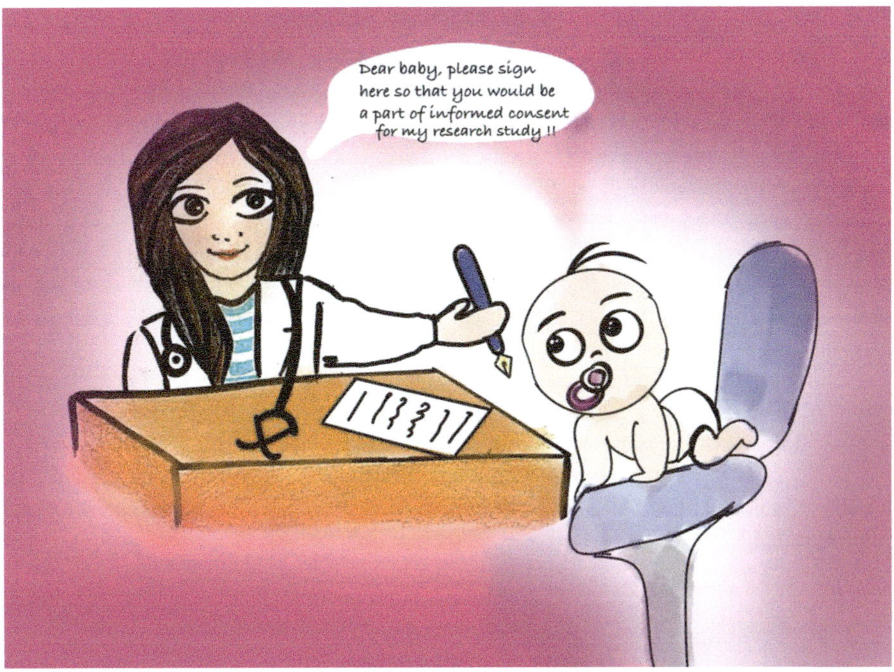


Obtaining informed consent from the patients or participants in research is a mandatory requirement for the researcher—N. Ananthakrishnan

N. Ananthakrishnan (✉)
Sri Balaji Vidyapeeth (Deemed-to-be University), Pondicherry, India



S. C. Parija, B. V. Adkoli (eds.), *Effective Medical Communication*,
https://doi.org/10.1007/978-981-15-3409-6_6

## 6.1 Assess Need

Medical practice requires constant interaction between health care providers and those who seek care at these facilities. In addition, modern medicine also requires a strong focus on continued research for the benefit of mankind. It is estimated that the doubling time of medical knowledge in 1950 was 50 years; in 1980, 7 years; and in 2010, 3.5 years. In 2020, it is projected to be 0.2 years—just 73 days [1]. According to an estimate, students who join medicine in 2010 would experience three doublings before they complete the course, and those who join in 2020 would experience four doublings [1]. Medical research on either patients or other subjects/ volunteers has, therefore, become an undeniable existential fact of medical practice.

In addition to the health care provider and the patient or the researcher and the participant, there are additional individuals who are involved in this interaction. The caregivers are engaged in constant interaction with patients, relatives, members of the community, or other interested parties. This situation makes communication even more demanding. The need for effective communication, both verbal and written in both these scenarios, viz. obtaining proper informed consent either in providing health care or organizing, planning, and carrying out medical research, cannot be over emphasized [2, 3]. Communication is one area which is vital to the practice of medicine but receives little attention during the training of future doctors. The guiding principles of medical ethics, beneficence and non-malfeasance, justice and equality, and autonomy mandate such training. Increasing awareness in the general population of their rights and privileges and lack of proper training among the health care providers lead to potential conflict or worse, disaster scenarios in the form of adverse effects on the users of health care facilities or subjects of medical research and increasing litigation.

Communication handicaps are even more in developing countries, because of the poor socio-economic status of the participants, their lack of awareness of their rights, the perceived hierarchical superiority of the health care provider over the patients or subjects of research which inhibits their desire to raise questions, and finally the near-universal use of technical language by the researcher which is incomprehensible to the participants.

## 6.2 Brief

This chapter is not intended to be a definitive treatise on the ethical issues in medical research, and will address only those issues pertaining to the need for effective communication in this field and methods of ensuring such competence.

- What is informed consent?
- What are the issues to be considered in taking informed consent?
- How to write a good participant information sheet (PIS)?
- What is meant by vulnerable groups? What precautions should be taken while obtaining informed consent from a vulnerable group?

- How to deal with research on archived specimens?
- Can subjects be deceived in the process of obtaining informed consent?
- What are the requirements while using videography or audiography?
- How to organize the process of recording interaction between researcher and subject?
- How to train medical students in obtaining informed consent for research?

## 6.3 Contextualize

### 6.3.1 Informed Consent for Research in Health Care Settings

The poor quality of communication between the researcher and the participants has recently been emphasized in a publication on the "*Quality of informed consent in cancer trials in India*:" by Gota et al. [4]. Despite what was considered as an adequately obtained informed consent, at a major cancer treatment center in India, participants in the clinical trial had wrong perceptions of anticipated benefits. Nearly 60% thought they would benefit somehow by participation in the trial, one-third thought that their survival or outcome will improve and one-fourth thought their treatment would be better and faster if they agree to participate in the trial. All these could be interpreted as inducements for participation by the uninformed observer. This shows the relative failure of the informed consent process to convey the correct information to the participants.

### 6.3.2 Scenario 1

In 2010, death of four girls who were a part of a human papilloma virus vaccine trial had raised the alarm about the nature of research in India as well as the value attached by the State to the lives of its citizens. This trial was conducted in Andhra Pradesh and Gujarat by a Non-Governmental Agency, with support from the Indian Council of Medical Research (ICMR) and local health authorities, and was funded by the Bill and Melinda Gates Foundation [5]. When the government stopped the trials, three doses had already been administered to 30,000 participants, mostly tribal girls aged between 9 and 14. Subsequent investigation revealed several errors in communication and obtaining informed consent [6]. These were:

1. The subjects of the research were vulnerable, being from poor socio-economic and ill-informed backgrounds.
2. Many of the girls were residents of hostels and consent was obtained from the hostel authorities bypassing the parents.
3. Parents were not available to monitor side effects.
4. For non-residential children, the consent form was sent through the children to get parental signature without any prior contact between the researchers and the parents to provide the information required to obtain informed consent.

5. The children and through them, the parents were informed that it was a "*Government program, harmless, with no effect on fertility and would provide lifelong protection against cancer*".

***Exercise***: Even assuming that the deaths occurred were unrelated to the intervention, do you think this is a clear case of poor research communication?

### 6.3.3 Scenario 2

A trial conducted at a major Regional Cancer Centre in India, with a collaborator from a top university in the USA, had used an experimental drug on 25 patients with tongue cancer between 1999 and 2000. This was revealed by a whistleblower. The patients were not aware that it was an experimental drug, and their consent had been obtained without the proper information. An enquiry raised several questions:

1. Did the participants know that it was an experimental drug?
2. Did they know of the risk involved?
3. Did they know that they had a choice to refuse participation?
4. Were they explained that the drug trial might lead to commercialization by a major pharmaceutical company?
5. Were they apprised of possible adverse effects?

The answers were all in the negative [7].

***Exercise***: Think how lack of adequate procedure in obtaining informed consent can be a contentious issue forever.

## 6.4 Describe

The process of informing the subjects of research has always remained a rather unsatisfactory area. Frequently, this forms the subject of detailed discussions between the investigators and members of the Ethics Committee. The ICMR has recently updated its guidelines on research on human participants [8, 9]. Government of India as the regulatory authority has notified its own updated recommendations this year [10]. Though the source documents used would be the guidelines as they pertain to India, there is very little difference in the guidelines of various countries and what has been mentioned here would apply to most of them.

The informed consent process involves three essential components:

(a) Providing information to potential participants/subjects of research,
(b) Ensuring information is comprehended by them, and
(c) Assuring voluntariness of participation in the research.

Informed consent protects the individual's autonomy to freely choose whether or not to participate in the research, and the process of obtaining consent should explain medical terminology in simple terms which the average patient/participant, without a background of medical knowledge, can understand.

## 6.4.1 Participant Information Sheet (PIS)

### 6.4.1.1 Major Issues

Participant information sheet (PIS) is the written document which is provided to the patient or the participant of the research which lays down the essential elements which formed the basis of prior verbal communication in a language that the participant/patient would understand and be able to affix his signature as a sign of having read and understood the document. Some of the key features of PIS and tips for writing the same have been given in Box 6.1.

**Box 6.1 Tips for Writing a Good Patient Information Sheet (PIS)**

- Make PIS document available both in English and in the language of the patient.
- Avoid medical jargon; write in a simple language that a lay person can understand.
- Talk to the subject face to face before writing PIS in the patient's language. Record the proceedings and use it for back translation in to English. Writing it in English first always makes the language more technical.
- Make it clear that the study is part of research, and not routine patient care; state the purpose of the research.
- Explain that participation is entirely voluntary, and they may decline to participate or withdraw after initial concurrence without any adverse effect on the quality of care provided to them by the health care facility.
- Explain why the patient is being considered for inclusion in the study, how frequently he would have to return for contact with the health care facility or the researcher.
- Whether any sample he provides would be stored, and if so what would be its duration of storage and to what use it may be put to in future. Make it clear that the patient/subject retains the right to refuse retention of the sample beyond the study or its use for other purposes without his consent.
- Furnish the identity and details of the researcher.
- Explain all the benefits of participation to the patient, short term and long term.
- Some studies may not involve immediate benefit to the subject but may lead to future improvement in management of that particular problem. This has to be explained to the patient in situations where the benefit to the subject is nil.

- In case of study on volunteers, where there is no expectation of benefit, this fact should also be conveyed to them before entry.
- Explain all the risks to the patient, short term and long term.

In randomized trials, before randomization, the participant has to be told of the standard of care for his problem, the alternatives available for its management, the risk vs. benefit of the two or more arms and convinced of the equipoise. The decision to give consent or withhold it can be made only thereafter.

#### 6.4.1.2 Economic Issues

There are several economic issues pertaining to medical research.

- Whether the subject will be compensated for the loss of livelihood due to participation?
- Whether travel expenses for participation would be reimbursed?
- Whether there is insurance for trial-related risks or adverse consequences?
- Whether there is provision for compensation for research-related injury and/or harm?
- Will participation in research involve payment for the participation by the sponsor?
- If the study shows benefit, will the subject have access to continued treatment by the beneficial drug?
- In the case of commercialization after the study, does the subject have any right to be compensated further or share benefits of commercialization?

All these issues may vary from trial to trial. It is the responsibility of the researcher to convey the answers to these questions both verbally in lay terms and record them in the PIS and obtain written consent of the participant.

#### 6.4.1.3 Confidentiality and Privacy Issues

The trial subject's right to privacy and confidentiality must be protected with special care in sensitive, potentially stigmatizing, and socially vulnerable situations. All identifiers from the record should be anonymized before the data is put in the public domain. Plans for publication, future use of the biological specimen provided, and other issues mentioned earlier should be conveyed in advance of the trial and proper consent obtained.

#### 6.4.1.4 Vulnerability

Vulnerability is defined as "*a situation where subjects of research by virtue of their age, cognitive status, health status such as pregnancy or lactation, socio-economic status, hierarchical compulsion, lack of decision making powers, comprehension issues or other causes, perceive that they are not in a position to refuse consent or feel hesitant do so for fear of causing offence or for fear of being denied proper care.*"

Those who belong to the vulnerable groups [8] are shown in Box 6.2.

**Box 6.2 Vulnerable Groups**

- Economically and socially disadvantaged.
- LGBTQIA community.
- Children up to 18 years.
- Pregnant/lactating women.
- Women with poor decision making powers/poor access to health care.
- Tribals and marginalized communities.
- Refugees, migrants, homeless, residents of conflict zones, riot areas, or disaster situations.
- Cognitively impaired, differently abled.
- Terminally ill.
- Those suffering from stigmatizing diseases such as HIV, Hansen's disease, etc.
- Those with diminished autonomy due to dependency or hierarchical system, defense personnel, prisoners, institutionalized subjects, health care workers.

The onus lies on the researcher to ensure strong justification for including the vulnerable population in the study. The researcher should make extra efforts to explain to the subjects why they are being included, and take greater care to see whether the information provided has been understood by soliciting further questions. In vulnerable groups, a legally authorized representative may be required to give consent, where appropriate. Such subjects may require additional information to facilitate comprehension. By virtue of the social effects of some of the issues, additional measures may be needed to safeguard privacy and confidentiality of the vulnerable subjects because any violation of privacy or confidentiality of these subjects them to possible enhancement of risk of increased vulnerability.

#### 6.4.1.5 Research on Children

These have been summarized in the ICMR guidelines [9]. Research on children is permissible only when the topic of research cannot be carried out in adults, e.g. research on hyaline membrane disease, neo-natal hyper-bilirubinemia, etc. Any research on children is permissible only if there is benefit to the particular child or children in general. For purposes of informed consent, children are divisible in to three age groups, viz. those under 7 years of age, those between 7 and 11 years of age, and those between 12 and 18 years beyond which age they attain legal maturity. The guidelines for taking informed consent from these groups have been shown in Table 6.1.

#### 6.4.1.6 Deception in Research

There may be situations, particularly in public health research where an element of deception may be required since revealing the facts may lead to modification of behavior and defeat the purpose of the study, such as collecting information on

**Table 6.1** Tips for informed consent from children in conducting research

| Age group | Guidelines | Comments |
|---|---|---|
| For children below 7 years of age | Consent is required only from the parent/legally authorized guardian (LAR) | |
| For those between 7 and 11 years of age | The researcher, in the presence of parents should explain in simple terms what is going to be done and what is expected of the child | The child's concurrence to participate in verbal terms is mandatory; the same is to be documented and signed by the parents in the PIS |
| For those between 12 and 18 years of age | In addition to this oral assent, the assent should also be obtained in writing. The form should be countersigned by the parent/LAR | The assent form for these children is not a mere repetition of the PIS for the parents but be written in simple terms |
| Those above 18 years of age | Treat them as legal adults for all purposes | Use the same guidelines applicable for adults |
| For research in children with a potential for harm, consent from both parents is mandatory | | |

health seeking behavior of members of the community or their attitude to various illnesses or their attitude towards the girl child vis-a-vis the male child in providing health care or nutrition or education. Such information may be required for influencing policy or altering the perception of the population or for interventions for purposes of improving health care services. Prior intimation of the purpose in this case and detailed discussion may elicit wrong information. The ethical committee should take care in giving consent for such studies, make sure it is non-invasive, ensure extra care is taken in gathering data, and make sure the study has important outcomes of significant public interest which would be defeated by prior information. The piece of information which needs to be withheld should be informed to the Ethics Committee and approval obtained. However, the researcher should debrief the participants or communities after completion of the research [8].

#### 6.4.1.7 Informed Consent for Research on Archived Specimens

A common concept in researchers is that any further research on biological specimens obtained in the past for other purposes and kept in the archives can be re-used for fresh research without further consent of the providers of the original biological sample since they are no longer current patients or the specimens have been anonymized.

Researchers applied to the Institute Ethics Committee at a medical college to use archived specimens of thyroid cancers for restudy and classification as per current knowledge as part of postgraduate training. The study was given a certificate of waiver of consent by the concerned Ethics Committee. The specimens were anonymized and could not be linked to the patients. After approval, the study was carried out. At the conclusion of the study, it was found that as many as 27% of the specimens studied had been wrongly reported earlier. The error ran both ways, benign lesions of the thyroid had been reported as malignant and the patients treated accordingly and worse, malignant lesions of the thyroid had been reported as benign and patients left without further treatment. The question which arose was what to do with the new information? Could one recall the patients and tell them of the mistake or leave them with the past diagnosis. Since some of the specimens were as recent as 3 years, it was conceivable that the patients were still around and unaware of their disease status. This problem had not been anticipated by the Ethics Committee as it was part of Academic Research for Educational purposes and there was nothing in the then guidelines regarding this issue.

It must be remembered that when consent is given for providing a biological sample, the consent is not open ended. It is for a specific purpose, generally for diagnosis and treatment or for research which has been discussed with the subject and a proper informed consent is obtained. It is not an open consent for any future research on the specimens without further consent for the same unless this issue has been discussed with the subject, mentioned in the participant information sheet and their informed consent obtained. In this context, it is relevant to remember the case of Henrietta Lacks. Cells from her cervical cancers had the property of vigorously growing in cell culture and were named HeLa cells. The descendants of Henrietta had to go to court to receive the benefits of subsequent hugely successful commercialization. She had not been told during her life time of the possibility of commercial use of her cells and her consent was not obtained.

The subject should be informed at the time of providing the sample about the fate of residual sample, its duration of storage, whether the sample would be shared with other researchers or subject to future research for academic purposes or commercialization and proper consent obtained in writing. It must be remembered that the subject has the right to prevent use of biological samples (DNA, cell lines, etc.) and related data at any time during or even after completion of the research [8]. The subject should be made aware and proper consent obtained in writing after mentioning whether the subject would benefit by future profitable commercialization of the sample.

As a policy, academic research may be carried out after total anonymization of samples which have been in archives for a long period, and whose use for future research has not been expressly denied by the subjects, with the understanding and proviso that any significant finding which could affect the welfare or the health of the subject/patient who provided the sample must be conveyed to them, if their contact details are accessible from records.

#### 6.4.1.8 Process of Recording Interaction between Researcher and Subject

An important requirement to protect the interests of both the researcher and the subject is the method of recording the interaction between the two. It is necessary to video record the process of providing information to the subject and obtaining informed consent. This is particularly of significance in research on vulnerable populations. However, for stigmatizing diseases such as HIV or leprosy, the consent process should be only audio recorded.

#### 6.4.1.9 Training Medical Students in Obtaining Informed Consent in Research

Training in research skills should be viewed as a part of training medicos in patient care and research in a continuum of medical education. Communication ability is a trainable skill. The fact that communication for medical researchers is essential and there is a need for training has been realized worldwide and there are several such training programs [11–14]. Although the principles of bioethics and medical research ethics are essentially the same universally, for training programs to be effective, they should model themselves on the specific context of the situation in the country based on population awareness and the socio-economic milieu.

Factors to be considered include presentation style, body language, providing a comfortable environment, utilizing clear language, and establishing overall rapport with the subject [11]. The issues which need to be focused on in these training programs have been mentioned in a Global Health Centre publication [12] as follows:

1. The origin of the movement towards ethical behavior in human research with examples from the past showing adverse consequences of non-conformal behavior to focus attention on the importance of the issue.
2. Why, therefore, informed consent is desirable both in the interest of the subject and the researcher?
3. What information needs to be provided to the subject by the researcher with special emphasis on the language that should be used ensuring comprehension?
4. The fact that it is research and participation is fully voluntary with the subject able to refuse consent or withdraw at any time without adverse consequence to continued care.
5. Knowledge of "*who is*" and "*who is not*" eligible to give consent and special care to be taken in "*vulnerable*" groups of subjects.

The strategy for training medicos in communication skills in general has been discussed elsewhere, in this book. A schematic view of training emphasis has been shown in Fig. 6.1.

In India, the current process leaves much to be desired. It is quite common to see participation information sheets mention merely that the subject is being included because "*he/she fits the inclusion criteria*" or merely mention the reason for inclusion as "*you are suffering*" from ".... *disease*" on which we are working. It is also not uncommon to see risk levels mentioned as "*nil*."

Training for communication with patients and subjects has to start right from the beginning of medical education.

The Medical Council of India has realized this fact, and has included it right along with principles of bioethics from the first month after admission as part of the Foundation Course for the MBBS program [15, 16]. It would, thereafter, continue as a "*continuous vertical core curricular thread*" throughout the MBBS program. At the MBBS level one can introduce basic principles of bioethics, patients, and subjects rights in medical research and basic elements of required communication during researcher-patient/subject contact.

If undergraduate students are encouraged to participate in research such as the ICMR STS projects, and do small projects, they would learn by doing along with their supervisors. Alternatively, a small research program can be made mandatory for undergraduates in all health care disciplines.

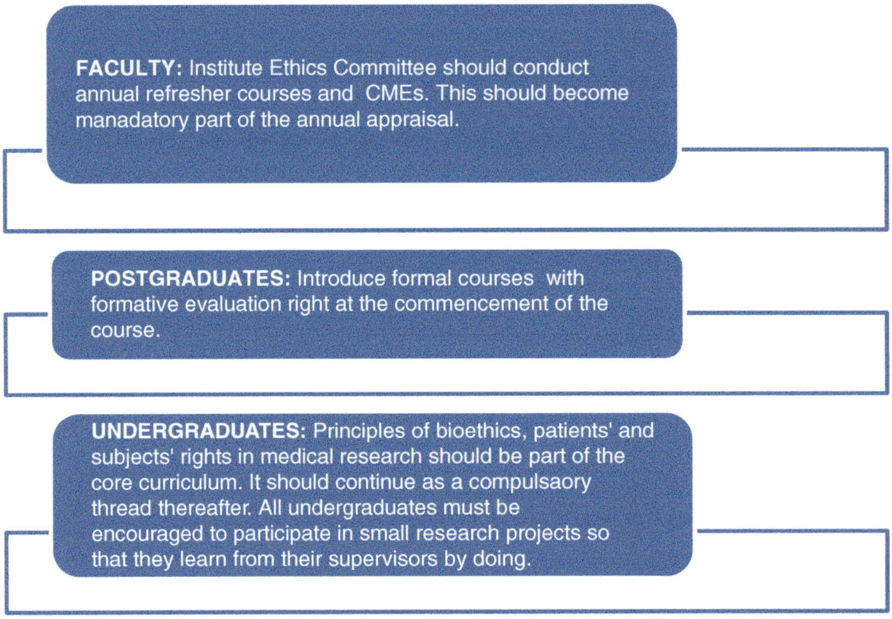


**Fig. 6.1** Approach to the training of medicos during different levels of medical education

At the postgraduate level there needs to be a formal course right at the entry level which ensures such competence.

### 6.4.2 Tips for Organizing Educational Strategies

The art of communication is a skill, which is learnt by doing and practice and therefore, small group activities would be far more suitable than lectures.

- Use case scenarios and real life examples for teaching purposes.
- Use audio recording of the process of obtaining informed consent by researchers, as videos may affect the confidentiality.
- Use standardized patients, supplemented with audio/video recording of the process of informed consent, taking care to show good and bad examples to drive the lesson home to the students.
- Role plays are very effective in internalizing the lesson learnt. They would have a more lasting effect in bringing attitudinal changes. Most of the messages can be brought out by organizing role play, which is enjoyable activity.
- All such training should be in small groups, and there is no role for large group teaching in this process since the aim is development of a skill and not transfer of knowledge.

- Evaluation process has to be part of the training. For the undergraduates, formative evaluation can be more feasible and effective to enhance learning of the relevant skills.
- For postgraduates, training in research methodology is mandatory. It can be re-emphasized in the session on training for dissertation writing. The formal course can be evaluated by a summative test at the end of the course. Day-to-day activities can be part of the formative evaluation.
- For faculty the concerned Institute Ethics Committee should conduct annual refresher courses to update them on the research guidelines. Real problematic cases encountered by them can be used as examples to provoke discussion and suggest problems to solve the concerned issue.
- The current ethical guidelines of the country should be part of the departmental library, and a certificate should be obtained from the researcher that he has gone through it and has conformed to the guidelines in submitting the proposal.

From the detailed discussion in this chapter of scope, it is possible to extract 12 tips which may be helpful for those interested in this field (Box 6.3).

**Box 6.3 Twelve Tips for the Researcher to Improve Communication**

1. Do not be overbearing, come down to patient's level.
2. Get patient to relax. In getting assent from children have the parents by the side.
3. Talk in their "*lingo*."
4. Do not use medical or research jargon.
5. Speak in small sentences.
6. Pause to hear their point of view or their opinion.
7. Patiently clarify their doubts.
8. Seek feedback to see whether they have understood.
9. Ask questions to see whether comprehension is complete and unambiguous.
10. Record above process by audio.
11. Back translate in to English.
12. Print both versions for their signature after allowing them time to read and clarify once again, if required.

### 6.4.3 Conclusions

- Conducting a research study should be a mandatory part of the training of medical researchers.
- This training should start from the undergraduate course itself as a mandatory core curricular thread and continue thereafter through the postgraduate course as a compulsory module and involve periodic refresher courses for faculty and other researchers.

- A predetermined standard of performance should be a mandatory requirement as a part of the annual appraisal of both faculty and postgraduates.
- The national guidelines should become part of the departmental learning resource material available for all researchers to consult.
- A case scenario based learning and a formative evaluation process as part of the service would motivate continued updating of knowledge.

## 6.5 Evaluate

Having gone through the chapter reflect the situation in your institute and make a roadmap for strengthening the skill of taking informed consent in research.

How that is going to differ from the skill of taking informed consent in patient care and educational research?

## References

1. Densen P. Challenges and opportunities facing medical education. Trans Am Clin Climatol Assoc. 2011;122:48–58.
2. Lehmann J. The importance of communication in clinical research. https://www.imarcresearch.com/blog/bid/262014/The-Importance-of-Communication-in-Clinical-Research. Accessed 12 Aug 2019.
3. Beran T. Advances in medical education. The importance of communication and collaboration. Can Med Educ J. 2012;3(1):e1–3.
4. Gota V, Nookala M, Yadav A, Menezes SR, Kannan S, Ali R. Quality of informed consent in cancer clinical trials in India: pattern and profile. Natl Med J India. 2018;31(6):334–8.
5. Deaths in the trial of the HPV vaccine. Indian J Med Ethics. 2010;7(3):144. https://ijme.in/articles/deaths-in-a-trial-of-the-hpv vaccine/?galley=pdf. Accessed 12 Aug 2019.
6. Fact finding of HPV vaccine "demonstration project" in Andhra Pradesh. http://www.samawomenshealth.in/fact-finding-of-hpv-vaccine-demonstration-project-in-andhra-pradesh/. Accessed 12 Aug 2019.
7. Krishna Kumar R. Ethics on trial. 2001;18(16). https://frontline.thehindu.com/static/html/fl1816/18161230.htm. Accessed 12 Aug 2019.
8. Indian Council of Medical Research. National ethical guidelines for biomedical and health research involving human participants. 2017. https://www.icmr.nic.in/sites/default/files/guidelines/ICMR_Ethical_Guidelines_2017.pdf. Accessed 12 Aug 2019.
9. Indian Council of Medical Research. National ethical guidelines for biomedical and health research on children. 2017. https://www.icmr.nic.in/sites/default/files/guidelines/National_Ethical_Guidelines_for_BioMedical_Research_Involving_Children_0.pdf. Accessed 12 Aug 2019.
10. Ministry of Health and Family Welfare. New drugs and clinical trial rules. 2019. https://cdsco.gov.in/opencms/opencms/system/modules/CDSCO.WEB/elements/download_file_division.jsp?num_id=NDI2MQ==. Accessed 12 Aug 2019.
11. Cadman ME, Murphy JH, Brintnall-Karebelas J, Cadman ME, Murphy JH, Brintnall-Karabelas J, et al. Training program for improving the informed consent discussion between clinical researchers and their subjects. J Empir Res Hum Res Ethics. 2014;9(4):71–5. https://doi.org/10.1177/1556264614546096.
12. Logan M, editor. Introduction to informed consent. Global Health Training Centre. https://globalhealthtrainingcentre.tghn.org/introduction-informed-consent/. Accessed 12 Aug 2019.

13. Shahnazarian D, Hagemann J, Aburto RS, Office for the Protection of Research Subjects (OPRS). Informed consent in human subjects research. University of Southern California. https://oprs.usc.edu/files/2017/04/Informed-Consent-Booklet-4.4.13.pdf. Accessed 12 Aug 2019.
14. University of Texas, Health Science Centre. Informed consent training. https://www.uth.edu/ctrc/training/informed-consent-training.htm. Accessed 12 Aug 2019.
15. Medical Council of India. Competency based undergraduate curriculum for the Indian medical graduate, vol. 1, 2 and 3. 2018. https://www.mciindia.org/CMS/information-desk/for-colleges/ug-curriculum. Accessed 12 Aug 2019.
16. Medical Council of India. Foundation course for the undergraduate medical education program. 2019. https://old.mciindia.org/UG-Curriculum/FOUNDATION-COURSE-MBBS-17.07.2019.pdf. Accessed 12 Aug 2019.

# Prescription Communication Using 5-R Framework

7

Nirmala N. Rege and Raakhi K. Tripathi

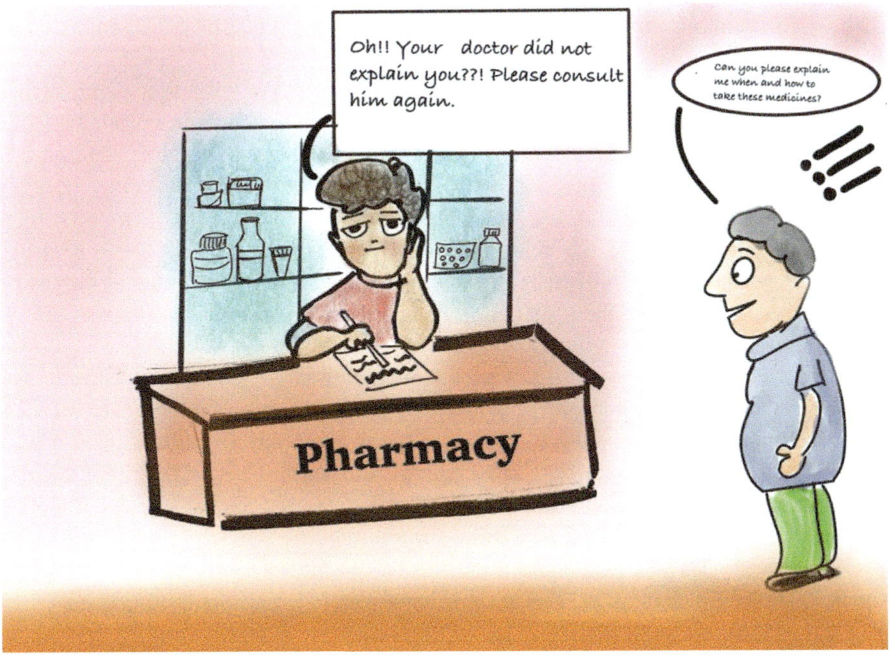


Prescription communication can be improved by using a structured framework—Rege and Tripathi

N. N. Rege (✉) · R. K. Tripathi
Department of Pharmacology and Therapeutics, Seth GS Medical College and KEM Hospital, Mumbai, India


S. C. Parija, B. V. Adkoli (eds.), *Effective Medical Communication*,
https://doi.org/10.1007/978-981-15-3409-6_7

## 7.1 Assess Need

Medical Council of India has identified communicator as one of the required roles for an Indian Medical Graduate (IMG) [1]. A graduate is expected to demonstrate competency in rational prescribing, which demands certain skills to be inculcated by a graduate. These prescribing skills include not only writing appropriate prescriptions but also communicating to the patient salient information about the prescribed drugs, instructions about their use, advice about special modes of drug delivery, important warnings, and when to visit for follow-up [2].

However, the existing curriculum lacks standardized training and assessment of communication skills [3].Current training of pharmacology is drug centred and focuses on providing information to the students about the drugs. The assessment in pharmacology also tests the cognitive domain. There is no emphasis on informing and instructing patients about drug therapy. The clinical training also neglects this aspect as it is focused on mainly the diagnosis, investigations, and selection of medicines. Thus there is no training in "*how*" and "*how much*" to communicate to a patient about the given prescription.

It has been reported that 30–80% of patients do not take the drugs as prescribed [4]. One of the important causes of non-compliance is inadequate communication with patients. A recent questionnaire-based study conducted in a North Indian city revealed that the patients were aware of the therapeutic effects of the drugs, but they lacked information regarding the side effects and the follow-up [4]. Similar studies are reported from the UK, the USA, and other countries [5, 6].

Our experience reveals that the only information given to patients is regarding the name of the drug, frequency of administration, and duration of therapy. This too is not delivered by all the physicians.

Poor communication regarding patient's medications increases inappropriate use of drugs which results in adverse effects, poor therapeutic outcome, and in turn, increased burden on the health care system [6]. An apt verbal communication with patients at the time of writing prescription can minimize these problems and strengthen the doctor–patient relationship. It may also reduce the observed friction between doctor and patients due to non-communication or miscommunication.

A systematic review indicates that very few studies have concentrated on the skill of communicating a prescription to a patient [7]. Various methods of teaching communication skills related to prescription writing and interviewing patients have been discussed [3] but prescription communication is the need of the hour.

WHO Guide to Good Prescribing is a promising model which has been shown to be effective in a wide variety of settings. Taking cue from the WHO guide, a 5-R framework (Reasons, Regimen, Risks, Revisit instructions, and Revision statements) has been developed through modification of criteria laid down by Ledford, et al. for communicating prescribing information to patients in shortest time available (4–7 min) using appropriate level of language that can be understood by him/her [8, 9].

## 7.2 Brief

In this chapter, we:

- Explain the 5-R framework to communicate any prescription.
- Describe the training and assessment strategy for prescription communication.
- Familiarize the readers with the checklist and rating scales for the content and quality of the communication.

## 7.3 Contextualize

### 7.3.1 Scenario

Mrs. R, a 26-year-old married lady attends the OPD of Dr. Comini. Mrs. R mentions that for the last 4 days, she has to run to the bathroom every 15–20 min to pass urine, and experiences a burning sensation whenever she passes urine. The quantity of urine is small, turbid, and foul-smelling. There is suprapubic burning. She denies a history of fever or flank pain. She is married 6 months back. Her menstrual periods are regular and LMP (Last Menstrual Period) is 7 days back. She does not give a history of similar episodes in the past. She does not give a history of diabetes, stone disease, or straining at micturition. Mrs. R reports that she is allergic to eggs, sulpha drugs, each of which have caused her to develop a rash around her mouth and face, as well as a low-grade fever. Mrs. R has no history of suffering from any cardiac, liver, kidney, or muscle disorders.

On physical examination, the patient's blood pressure was 130/90, heart rate was 88/min, respiration rate was 17/min, and the patient's temperature was 98.2 °F. Urine routine and microscopy examination reports revealed: Appearance—turbid; Colour—amber; Proteins—trace; Sugar—absent; Microscopy—plenty of pus cell/Hpf; RBC—5–10/Hpf and bacteria. Dr. Comini diagnoses Mrs. R to be suffering from uncomplicated lower urinary tract infection. As a treating physician, she has written the following prescription for Mrs. R (Box 7.1).

***Exercise***: Read the given scenario. Go through the written prescription. Demonstrate how you will explain the prescription to the simulated patient along with information and instructions related to drugs. Think about it!

Refer to Box 7.2 for the content to be communicated to the patient for the above case scenario.

## 7.4 Describe

While communicating a written prescription to a patient, both the elements, the content of prescribing information and quality of communication are important. The content has to be logical and sequential so that patient can remember the information given.

## Box 7.1: Prescription Form

Dr Comini
M.B.B.S; M.D
Reg. No.: 123456
Full address: KEM Hospital, Parel, Mumbai-400012; Contact: +91 1234567890

Prescription serial number: 01 Date: 13/03/2019
Patients full name: Mrs R
Patient's address and phone number: B3, Nagpada, Mumbai-400008; Contact: +91 3838383838
Sex: Female Age: 26 years Weight: 56 kg

Rx
- Tab. CIPROFLOXACIN 500 mg twice daily for 7 days
- To drink plenty of fluids
- Follow up after 7 days with urine, routine and microscopy report; if symptoms persist, visit earlier.

*Dr Comini* (13/03/2019)

## Box 7.2: Script for the Case Scenario

| Written script to be communicated verbally | 5 Rs |
|---|---|
| Mrs. R, from your complaints, most probably you are suffering from urinary tract infection. This infection is common in young women. There is no need to identify the organisms as various studies have shown that in 90% cases, the causative bacteria are *Escherichia coli*. Hence I am prescribing you an antibacterial drug - Ciprofloxacin, which will kill these bacteria. | Reason |
| Please take ciprofloxacin tablet 500 mg orally with a full glass of water - one in the morning and one in the evening - 12 hours apart for 5 days. Drink more than 10-15 glasses of water every day while you are taking this medicine, which should maintain your urine flow more than 3lit per day. Frequently void the urine. This may help to clear the infection faster. In addition, you need to clean the private parts properly each time after urination.<br>Ciprofloxacin should be taken preferably at the same time each day two hours after food. Do not take it with milk or milk products, or with calcium-fortified juice and antacid. They could make the medication less effective. Your symptoms may improve within 48-72 hours before the infection is completely cleared. But you should continue and complete the full course of ciprofloxacin as some organisms may remain alive to cause infection at a later date, which may be difficult to treat.<br>If you miss a tablet, take the missed dose as soon as you remember. Skip the missed dose if it is almost time for your next scheduled dose. Do not take extra medicine to make up the missed dose. Do not take this medicine for a longer period than recommended. Store the blister pack at room temperature away from moisture and heat. | Regimen |

| | |
|---|---|
| This drug is relatively safe. Occasionally, you may get some stomach discomfort, vomiting, mild diarrhea; vaginal itching or discharge; mild dizziness; or mild headache. If any of these effects are severe and persistent, contact me immediately. Ciprofloxacin may impair thinking or reactions. Be careful if you drive or do anything that requires you to be alert. Ciprofloxacin can rarely cause serious side effects, such as:<br>• Sudden pain, swelling, bruising, tenderness, stiffness, movement problems, or a snapping or popping sound in any of your joints suggestive of tendon rupture. You may have to give rest to the joint until you receive medical care.<br>• Neurological symptoms such as numbness, tingling, burning pain, or being more sensitive to temperature, light touch, or the sense of your body position and rarely, convulsions.<br>• Ciprofloxacin rarely can cause allergic reactions, e.g. hives or the first sign of a skin rash; fast heartbeat, difficulty breathing; swelling of your face, lips, tongue, or throat.<br>• Stop the drug immediately if you get any of these symptoms and contact me.<br>• Please avoid taking any medication, including vitamin or calcium/iron supplements within 6 hours before or 2 hours after you take ciprofloxacin. Inform me about all other medicines that you may use, during your treatment with ciprofloxacin. Avoid excess tea or coffee.<br>• Ciprofloxacin can make you more sensitive to sun rays. You are advised to use a stole or a cap or a sunscreen or calamine lotion to prevent exposure to sunlight. Inform me promptly if you have severe burning, redness, itching, rash, or swelling after being in the sun. | **Risks** |
| If your urinary complaints persist till day 2 of your treatment, please report to the clinic immediately, otherwise visit after 7days of therapy along with urine routine and microscopy report.<br>I hope you have understood what I told you. | **Revisit** |
| Do you have any questions?<br>Will you repeat the important information I told you.<br>Good! Remember----- (If the patient forgets to report, repeat the points she has forgotten).<br>Do not worry, you will be all right soon. See you next week. | **Revision statements** |

### 7.4.1 What Is the 5-R Framework?

The 5-R framework provides the structure so that the medical graduate will not forget the essential points to be communicated. These 5-Rs are as follows:

- **R**eason for prescribing a drug based on the disease condition: why the drug is prescribed and what it is supposed to do—cure/control the disease.
- **R**egimen prescribed: These include the name of the drug, dosage form, route of administration, frequency, duration, and dosing instructions. It also includes what should be done if a dose is missed and the information regarding storage.
- **R**isks associated with the drug use: These include (a) the commonly seen adverse reactions, which may be milder, disappear with time, and mostly require no spe-

cific measures, (b) serious adverse reactions, which require discontinuation of the drugs, and (c) possible interactions with concomitant drugs.
- **R**evisit instructions: These include when the patient should come for routine follow-up and if needed, what laboratory report he/she should carry at the time of the visit.
- **R**evision statements: It is necessary to revise the given information with the patient so that the doctor is ensured that the patient has understood the content. These statements remain almost the same for all prescriptions.
  - I hope you have understood what I told you.
  - Do you have any questions?
  - Will you repeat the important information I told you?
  - "*Good!*" (Appreciate patient's response and add to what he/she said, if necessary.
  - Reassure the patient. For conditions of short duration, it may be "*Do not worry, you will be all right by next week*", whereas for those, who need life-long therapy like diabetes or hypothyroidism, "*Follow the advice given and I assure you that you will enjoy a good healthy life despite the medication. Do not hesitate to contact me if you need any help*".

### 7.4.2 Suggested Training Strategy

Based on our experience of using the 5-R framework we recommend the following plan (Fig. 7.1):

1. *Organize a joint meeting of faculty of pharmacology with clinicians*: Organize an in-house workshop on rational prescribing for the junior faculty and residents involving clinicians.
2. *Select clinical conditions for developing scenarios*: The criteria for selection includes the followings:
   (a) Common conditions based on morbidity and mortality data.
   (b) Conditions detected in an OPD setting.

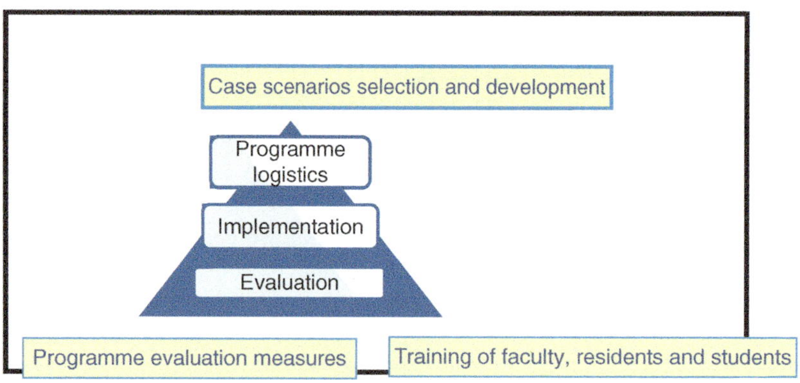


**Fig. 7.1** Plan for prescription communication programme

(c) Cases requiring single drug prescriptions.

For example, nutritional iron deficiency anemia, fever following vaccination, lower UTI, hypothyroidism, *Trichomonas* vaginitis, treatment naïve obese patient with type 2 diabetes mellitus, essential hypertension, temporal lobe epilepsy, a child with diarrhea can be tried.

3. *Develop case scenarios*: These should include case description, prescription, and script to be used by the students to communicate prescription to the patients.
   (a) Case description**:** Write brief history, examination findings, laboratory reports, and diagnosis.
   (b) Prescription**:** Write on a separate page using the standard prescription format.
   (c) Script-writing for communicating prescription: Use a 5-R framework. Write in a simple, non-medical language. Avoid jargon.

   The script for the case scenario given in Box 7.1 is presented in Box 7.2. The column on the right depicting 5-Rs is shown for the readers only (Box 7.2).
4. *Validation of the case scenario and the script*: This could be carried out by involving a group of pharmacologists and clinicians.
   (a) Edit and read aloud the script to check the time taken for delivery. Pilot test with residents to confirm whether they can reproduce the script in 4–7 min without looking at it.
   (b) Obtain final approval of the validation committee for editing.
   (c) Translate into the local language.
   (d) Develop an OSCE checklist and scoring system for content: This checklist varies with the prescribed drug. It is also essential to decide which risks are "*essential to communicate*". The weightages to different sections of 5 R framework are decided by consensus based on explanations for disease conditions and reasoning, number and severity of risks, administration intricacies, etc. The sum total, however, for the script for each drug should be kept constant.
5. *Train residents*: Organize a workshop for residents to train them to serve as standardized patients. They should be conversant with case scenarios and scripts (in English and local languages). Familiarize them with the standardized patient's satisfaction questionnaire (SPSQ), which they would be filling as a patient (Box 7.3).
6. *Train undergraduate students*: Organize a structured program for the undergraduates, depending on the number of students, time available, number of faculty available, and previous exposure of the students to any communication skill workshop (Fig. 7.2). The details of program logistics have been shown schematically in Fig. 7.3.

*Practice session 1*: Appoint three facilitators for this session (Table 7.1).
*Practice session 2*: In this session, the process mentioned above is repeated with different cases. This session covers more case scenarios as the students know how to proceed. It is ensured that each student enacts as student–doctor at least on two occasions. Students are briefed that same checklist is used for assessment. The content checklist based on the 5-R framework to be filled by the students has been shown in Table 7.2.

**Box 7.3: Standardized Patient Satisfaction Questionnaire (Standardized Patient Has to Tick the Most Appropriate Response Regarding the Behaviour of the Doctor)**

| |
|---|
| Rate the behaviour of the doctor on a five-point scale |
| **Excellent = 5, Good = 4, Satisfactory = 3, Fair = 2, Poor = 1** |
| 1. Making you feel at ease… (being friendly and warm towards you, treating you with respect; not cold or abrupt) |
| 2. Showing care and compassion… (seeming genuinely concerned, connecting with you on a human level; not being indifferent or detached) |
| 3. Being positive… (having a positive approach and a positive attitude; being honest but not negative about your problems) |
| 4. Speaking slowly------ (keeping pace with your understanding; without hurrying) |
| 5. Explaining things clearly… (explaining clearly, giving you adequate information; not being vague) |
| 6. Explaining things in language that is easy to understand ---- (Not using medical terms without explaining what they mean) |
| 7. Explaining the risks involved in the medicine prescribed without scaring or creating anxiety |
| 8. Informing a plan of action … (discussing the regime, what to do in case of adverse events or disease worsening or if you miss the doses) |
| 9. Helping you to revise relevant points regarding medicines… (exploring with you what you have understood; encouraging rather than only "*lecturing*" you) |
| 10. Listened carefully to what you repeated ---- (listening and reinforcing what is said correctly or adding if forgotten) |
| 11. Overall, how will you rate your satisfaction after your consultation with this doctor? |

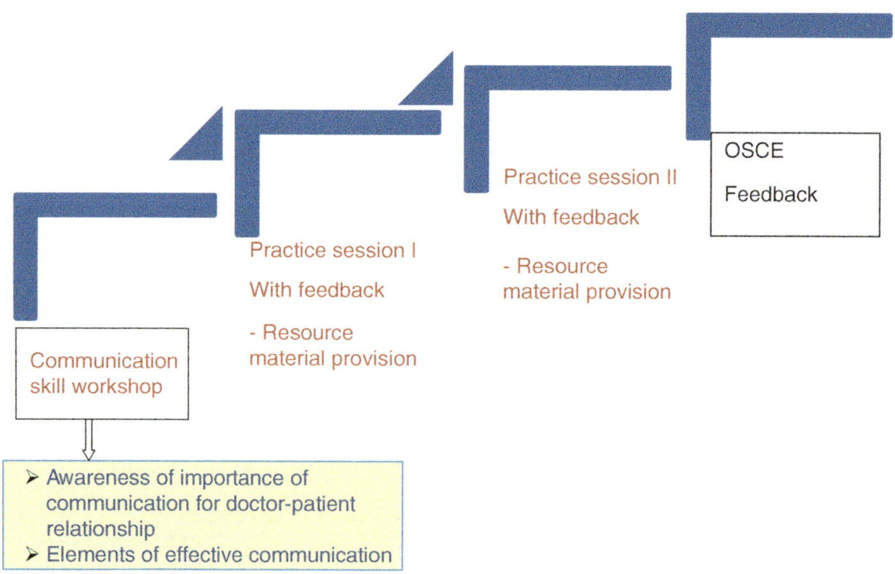


**Fig. 7.2** Structured programme of Department of Pharmacology and Therapeutics, Seth GSMC and KEM Hospital

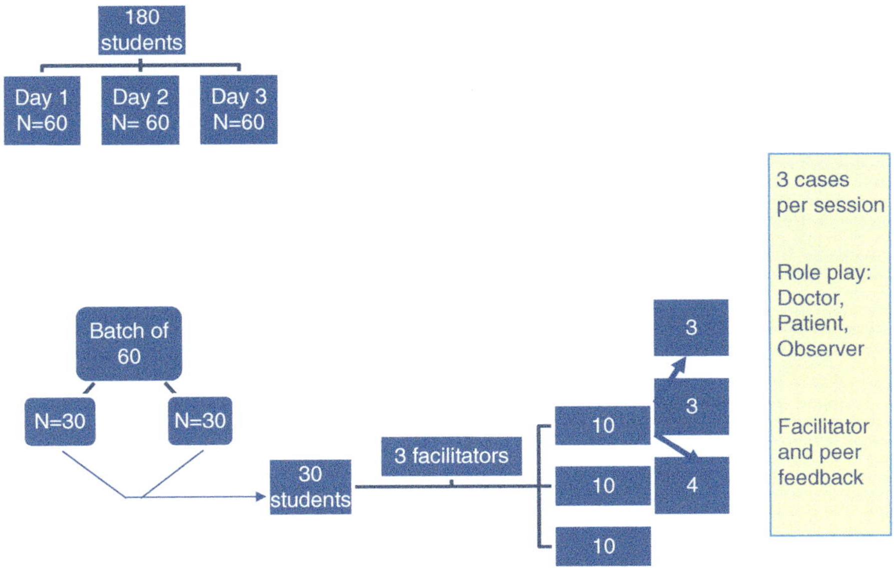


**Fig. 7.3** Programme logistics

**Table 7.1** Session plan in the practical class

| | Process elements | Time |
|---|---|---|
| 1 | *Introduction*<br>– Brief the students about the 5-R framework. Also, explain that they can use local language as per their choice<br>– Divide the students in the batch of ten with one facilitator | 10 min |
| 2 | *Group with facilitator*<br>– Further division can be done into three groups by the facilitator (Fig. 7.3)<br>– The student group is given a case scenario (3 different scenarios to 3 different groups), the script to be communicated, and the checklist (3 copies per group) | 5 min |
| 3 | *Each trio in the subgroup*<br>– Each group is told to decide the roles to be played, the doctor, the patient, and the observer<br>– Each group reads the case and the script<br>– Each student fills up the checklist (Table 7.2). This makes them understand that the material given fits into the 5-R framework<br>– After this, the student–doctor along with the student—simulated patient does a role play, in which the script is communicated to the student–patient. The student–observer checks whether the points in the script are communicated in a logical sequence as per the filled content checklist<br>– The facilitator rotates in three subgroup observing what is going on | 20 min |

(continued)

**Table 7.1** (continued)

| | Process elements | Time |
|---|---|---|
| 4 | *Group with a facilitator for the plenary session*<br>– All the three groups gather for plenary session, and each group repeats the role play<br>– The feedback for the content is given by the student–observer for the group and the facilitator and quality by the rest of the two groups. While giving feedback, a 2 × 2 model (what is good and what can make the interaction better) is used<br>– The facilitator adds if anything has been missed and reinforces the correct points | 30 min (10 min per group; 4 min presentation and 6 min discussion) |
| 5 | *Repeat session*<br>Each group now receives a different scenario and the process in the individual group is repeated with now the trio doing different roles in the individual group | 20 min |
| 6 | *Sum up for the entire batch of 30 students* | 5 min |

**Table 7.2** Content checklist based on 5-R framework to be filled by the students using the script

| Content | Item | Comment |
|---|---|---|
| 1. Reasons | 1. Explained disease | |
| | 2. Explained the reason for prescribing the medication | |
| | 3. Mentioned when the drug effect is expected to occur | |
| | 4. Mentioned the need to complete the course | |
| 2. Regimen | 1. Stated the drug regimen | |
| | a. Dose | |
| | b. Frequency | |
| | c. How long | |
| | 2. Advised when to take in relation to food | |
| | 3. Specified about missed doses | |
| | 4. Adjuvant therapy | |
| | 5. Stated the storage conditions for the prescribed drug | |
| 3. Risks | 1. Explained how to recognize the common adverse effects | |
| | 2. Stated actions to be taken for ADR | |
| | 3. Stated the serious ADRS that need prompt contact with the doctor/discontinuation of drugs | |
| | 4. Advised about concomitant disease and drugs | |
| 4. Revisit instructions | 1. Stated when to come for follow-up | |
| | 2. Stated when to come early due to disease worsening | |
| | 3. Specified which investigation reports the patient should bring when he/she comes for follow-up | |
| 5. Revision | 1. Asked the patient whether everything is clear | |
| | 2. Asked whether the patient has any questions | |
| | 3. Ask the patient to repeat the most relevant points | |
| | 4. Repeated what the patient has forgotten | |
| | 5. Reassurance | |

### 7.4.3 The Assessment Strategy for Prescription Skill

This is achieved by implementing the following components:

1. *Prepare the OSCE checklist* as mentioned earlier.
2. *Evolve consensus regarding scoring* as described earlier.
3. *Assess the content of prescription communication* using OSCE format.
4. *Give instructions for assessment* as follows:
   (a) Observe the student doctor—standardized patient encounter focusing on the content delivered by the student doctor.
   (b) A checklist for the same has been provided to you.
   (c) Please √ (tick) the points the student doctor communicates to the standardized patient. Points not communicated are marked by X.
   (d) Please do not interact with the student or the standardized patient.
5. *Assess quality of communication by the faculty assessor*: This can be done by using a rating scale (Table 7.3). It mainly captures the behaviour of the student doctor during the interaction, delivery of information, and the way the conversation is organized to serve its purpose.
6. *Assess the quality of communication by the standardized patient*: This is to be carried out by the residents in that role. For this purpose, develop a standardized patient satisfaction questionnaire (SPSQ) (Box 7.3).
7. *Encourage global assessment by the faculty*: The following indicators can be used by faculties incorporating incompetent, borderline, and competent with respect to prescription communication (Table 7.4).

   Though this scale gives overall categorization of the student, the earlier checklist and rating scales can point out the areas that the student needs to strengthen and make the feedback session more effective.
8. *Share post-assessment feedback with students*: The checklist, questionnaire, and rating scales can be shared with the students, and they can be briefed in a class about overall performance as a group. They can meet the faculty assessor if any clarification is needed.

### 7.4.4 Evaluation Strategy for Prescription Communication Programme

At the end of the prescription communication programme, the perception of students can be collected regarding the practice sessions and learning that took place on a 5 point Likert scale (Box 7.4). Improvement in OSCE scores also serves as an evaluation indicator, provided baseline OSCE is performed. Faculty feedback using a questionnaire or through interviews can also be collected in terms of the usefulness of the programme, feasibility, adequacy of student learning, improvement in communication skills in meeting the expectations from the programme.

**Table 7.3** Rating scale for assessing the quality of prescription communication

| Item | Score rating | Score given by faculty (0–5) |
|---|---|---|
| Rapport with the standardized patient | The student is<br>*0*—Condescending, offensive, judgmental<br>*1*—Shows minimal courtesies only<br>*2*—Borderline (unsatisfactory); somewhat deficient in communication<br>*3*—Borderline (satisfactory); communication just adequate<br>*4*—Polite and interested<br>*5*—Warm, polite, empathic | |
| Information giving | *0*—No attempt or inappropriate attempt to give information; e.g., not truthful<br>*1*—Awkward and/or incomplete attempts to give information<br>*2*—Borderline unsatisfactory, somewhat at ease, attempts to give information but somewhat deficient<br>*3*—Borderline satisfactory, somewhat at ease, attempts to give just adequate information<br>*4*—Gives information easily, somewhat attentive to the patient's understanding<br>*5*—Confident and skillful at giving information, attentive to patient's understanding, truthful | |
| Organization of the encounter | *0*—Scattered, shot-gun approach<br>*1*—Minimally organized conversation; logical flow deficient<br>*2*—Borderline unsatisfactory, logical flow is somewhat deficient<br>*3*—Borderline satisfactory, logical flow is just adequate<br>*4*—Logical flow with a sense of purpose<br>*5*—Purposeful, integrated handling of the encounter | |

**Table 7.4** Global assessment of the prescription communication competency

| Competency rating | Performance indicators | Grade |
|---|---|---|
| Incompetent | Performs the task inappropriately and ineffectively, indicating a lack of knowledge and/or undeveloped interpersonal and information delivery skills | A |
| Borderline | Performs some components of the task effectively, some development of interpersonal and information delivery skills | B |
| Competent | Performs the task precisely and perceptively, consistently integrating all components with a demonstration of interpersonal and information delivery skill | C |

**Box 7.4: Student Feedback Questionnaire**

| |
|---|
| Please rate the statements on the Likert scale: |
| **Strongly agree = 5, Agree = 4, Neutral = 3, Disagree = 2, Strongly Disagree = 1** |
| **Opinions of the students regarding participation in role plays** |
| 1. The role-playing exercise helped me to distinguish between less and more effective clinician-patient communication related to drug prescribing. |
| 2. Assessing the clinician's role during the role-playing exercise enhanced my understanding of how to use the communication checklists. |
| 3. The role-playing exercise helped me become comfortable with role-playing. |
| 4. The checklist provided structure to discussions with patients. |
| 5. I became aware of patients' concerns regarding drugs. |
| 6. I felt comfortable practising communication skills in front of classmates. |
| 7. The right amount of time was allotted for this exercise. |
| 8. Overall, these sessions were worthwhile. |
| **Perceptions of students about learning, satisfaction, and acceptability** |
| 1. The programme provided appropriate type and amount of information to patients regarding prescribed drugs. |
| 2. I learned something that I will use in future interactions with patients. |
| 3. I can relate to patients' concerns and desires. |
| 4. I shall be able to answer patients' concerns regarding the undesirable outcome. |
| 5. The programme made me aware of my strengths in communicating with patients. |
| 6. The programme made me aware of my weaknesses in communicating with patients |
| 7. I am satisfied with the way in which these sessions were conducted. |
| 8. This exercise improved my confidence in communicating with patients. |
| 9. I would like to participate in this type of exercise again. |
| 10. Overall, the experience was worthwhile. |

### 7.4.5 Conclusions

- The structured prescription communication programme can result in the improved ability of medical students to communicate relevant information regarding the prescription. They also demonstrate improved confidence.
- The standardized patients have shown a higher degree of satisfaction regarding the prescription communication style of the students.
- There is also an evidence of satisfaction among faculty members about the training programme.
- However, the process needs an investment of time. Involving clinicians is a challenging task, but such interactions are highly fruitful as the case scenario is based on real-life experiences.

## 7.5 Evaluate

Having read this chapter, now you can take some homework. Try to prepare a case scenario with a prescription for hypothyroidism. Now attempt to write the communication content of the prescription, fill in the 5-R checklist and allot marks to various points with a total score of 25.

## References

1. Medical council of India. Competency based undergraduate curriculum for the Indian Medical Graduate, vol. 1, sect. 1; 2018. pp. 19–20.
2. de Vries TPGM, Henning RH, Hogerzeil HV, Fresle DA. Guide to good prescribing. A practical manual. Geneva: WHO; 1994.
3. Nath Modi J, Anshu, Chhatwal J, Gupta P, Singh T. Teaching and assessing communication skills in medical undergraduate training. Indian Pediatr. 2016;53(6):497–504.
4. Singh J, Singh N, Kumar R, Bhandari V, Kaur N, Dureja S. Awareness about prescribed drugs among patients attending out-patient departments. Int J Appl Basic Med Res. 2013;3(1):48–51.
5. Ferner RE, Aronson JK. Medication errors, worse than a crime. Lancet. 2000;355(9208):947–8.
6. Tarn DM, Heritage J, Paterniti DA, Hays RD, Kravitz RL, Wenger NS. Physician communication when prescribing new medications. Arch Intern Med. 2006;166(17):1855–62.
7. Kamarudin G, Penm J, Chaar B, et al. Educational interventions to improve prescribing competency: a systematic review. BMJ Open. 2013;3(8):e003291. https://doi.org/10.1136/bmjopen-2013-003291.
8. Ledford CJW, Childress MA, Ledford CC, Mundy HD. The practice of prescribing: discovering differences in what we tell patients about prescription medications. Patient Edu Couns. 2014;94(2):255–60.
9. Nirmala R, Tripathi R, Salagre S, Furman G. Five-R framework for prescription communication skills learning. Med Educ. 2017;51(11):1170–1.

# 8 Effective Podium Presentation is More Than Showing Power Point Slides

Nalin Mehta

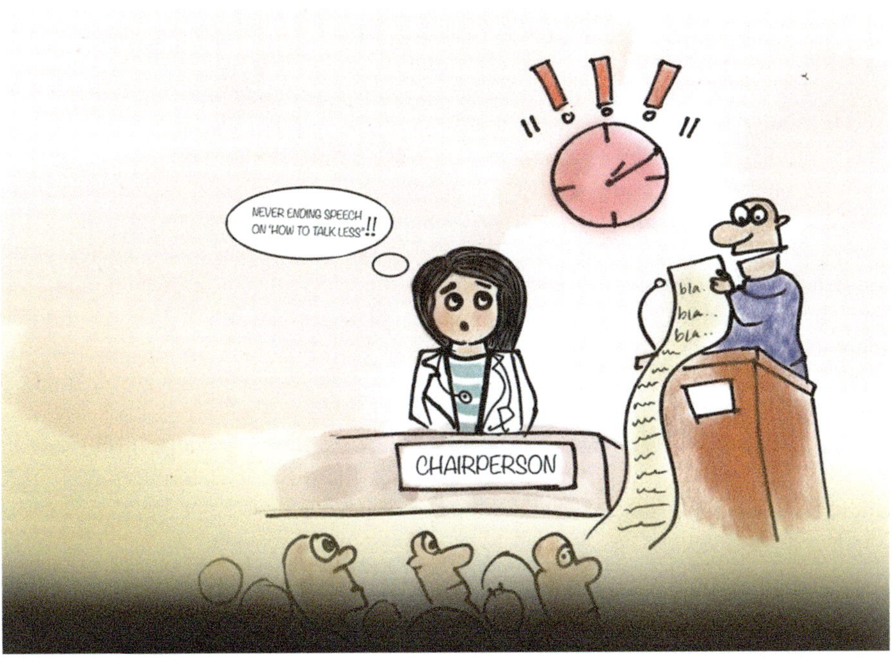


Three simple rules to make a fabulous presentation: 1. Practice 2. Practice 3. Practice!—Nalin Mehta

N. Mehta (✉)
Department of Physiology, All India Institute of Medical Sciences, New Delhi, India



S. C. Parija, B. V. Adkoli (eds.), *Effective Medical Communication*,
https://doi.org/10.1007/978-981-15-3409-6_8

## 8.1 Assess Need

Effective communication is seen as a potential instrument for strengthening teamwork, enhancing the quality of service, leading to higher patient satisfaction. However, the role of communication in enhancing the effectiveness of a medical professional, his/her message, and its impact has not been fully exploited in spite of the huge volume of literature piling up in this field. Effective communication in an educational setting is vulnerable because it influences the learning outcome of thousands of audience who would like to learn and apply new knowledge and best practices for enhancing their professional development. Unfortunately, medical professionals are never taught the basic techniques of teaching during their undergraduate or postgraduate courses [1]. Teaching is thrust upon them as a mandatory requirement since they are expected to teach, and they usually end up believing that they can teach. In this backdrop, the tips and tricks for effective podium presentation assume a great significance.

One of the foremost aspects of current teaching, especially in medical colleges, as well as in Continuing Medical Education (CME) platforms is the prolific use of power point (PPT) presentations. We are passing through an age where most people become handicapped without this ubiquitous audio-visual aid! 'Technology' has virtually become the middle name of every human being. Be it a student symposium or a guest lecture, the PPT has spread its wings everywhere. Albeit the extensive use of glamorous, flashy, animated power point slides or video clippings, one is not sure whether the key message of the speaker has gone across the audience. The matter gets further complicated because the audience who are present in a lecture hall are all different individuals with varying degree of previous knowledge, interest, motivation, and styles of learning. Making an effective presentation is, therefore, neither a matter of cookbook recipe nor a rigorous manual for the flight crew.

We have all seen great presentations and also suffered or slept through some highly forgettable ones. What was it that made the difference? An exploration of these issues is, therefore, the need of the hour to come out with practical tips, especially for the beginners who wish to emerge as great speakers who can make an impact on the audience.

## 8.2 Brief

In this chapter, an attempt has been made to offer a few practical tips for making an effective podium presentation. These tips can be applied judiciously:

- Before making a presentation (planning).
- During actual presentation (execution).
- After making a presentation (follow-up).

## 8.3 Contextualize

### 8.3.1 Scenario

Dr. Comini, Officer-in-charge of Medical Education Unit, invites an eminent guest speaker to make a presentation on 'Tips for effective presentation'. Unfortunately, the speaker flashes a regret message late in the evening just before the fixed day that he is ill and cannot participate. However, he sends a brief text along with PPT and suggests Dr. Comini to take his session without affecting the quality of the program fixed earlier.

This was a great challenge for Dr. Comini to explore something which she had never done before. Luckily she had exhaustive content information on 'How to organize a community camp' as a part of her curriculum. What she did was to fit into the content with the tips for effective presentation sent by the guest speaker.

This worked very well. Her presentation included preparation before organizing the camp, action to be taken while organizing, and activities needed after the camp. She aligned her talk into three segments: a good start, followed by an interactive session using both verbal and non-verbal communication ending in an effective closure, and take-home message. The presentation was liked by everyone, and no one complained that the eminent speaker disappointed them. Indeed they were happy to discover the strengths of Dr. Comini and the power of standard guidelines and tips given by the eminent speaker.

***Exercise***: Imagine and make a mental list of the tips which might have been given by the expert.

## 8.4 Describe

### 8.4.1 First Things First

There is no substitute for good content. However, an effective speaker is more than a content master. An effective presentation, therefore, is a combination of good content, delivered in an effective manner to create a lasting impression on the audience. Flashy slides, enthralling animation, breath-taking videos, and so on do not replace the subject matter! They can at best beautify and enhance the presentation, but it is the quality of the academic content or the lack of it is what draws attention.

It goes without saying that a presenter has to be cautious about making himself or herself presentable properly before the gathering. One need not have to splurge on a new wardrobe, but a comfortable, neatly pressed attire and polished footwear will help in gaining the audience initial attention (https://www.acponline.org/membership/residents/competitions-awards/acp-national-abstract-competitions/guide-to-preparing-for-the-abstract-competition/giving-the-podium-presentation).

A good framework for ensuring effective podium presentation should involve specific points to be considered before starting a session while running the session

**Table 8.1** The suggested tips which can be followed during three stages of presentation

| Before starting the session | During the session | After the session |
|---|---|---|
| Identify your target audience | Give a memorable start | Assess the outcome and seek student feedback |
| Plan your lesson, prepare well and practise | Engage in voice modulation | Share your presentation |
| Know your venue well | Use body language | |
| Prepare resources and handouts in advance | Make rational use of media | |
| Be prepared for the worst | Interaction holds the key | |
| | The lighter side of it all | |
| | Elicit feedback and reinforcement | |
| | Bring the session to an effective closure | |

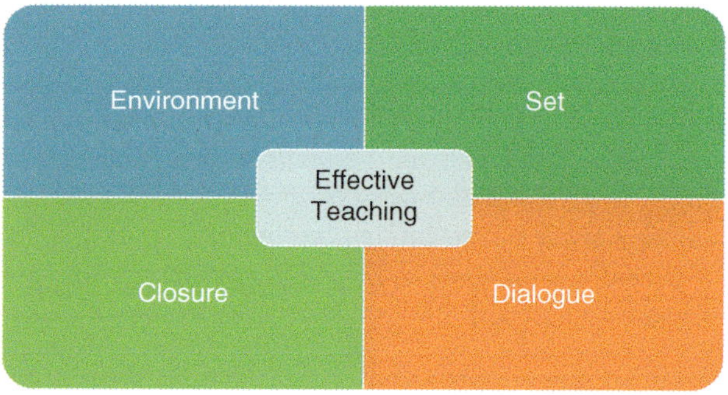


**Fig. 8.1** ESDC approach

and at the end of the session (Table 8.1). These are derived from good teaching practices based on experiential learning discussed in the literature [2], besides the author's personal experience over three decades. A good teaching session must address the four quadrants: environment, set, dialogue, and closure, known as the ESDC approach [3] (Fig. 8.1). This covers the ambience of the hall, the way you kick start, interact with the audience and end up with a clear message.

## 8.4.2 Before the Session

### 8.4.2.1 Identify Your Target Audience

It is most important to consider the level of the audience, whether they are undergraduates, postgraduates, or faculty. This will help in customizing the talk in tune with the audience previous knowledge and experience. In fact, preparing for undergraduate sessions takes a longer time. One needs to carefully filter the information and emphasize on the 'must know' areas. The 'desirable to know' and 'nice to know' issues can be touched by raising questions and asking the audience to ponder over those issues later.

#### 8.4.2.2 Plan Your Lesson, Prepare Well, and Practise

Preparation of a detailed lesson plan stating the objectives of your session, the lead questions, and the content, suggested audio-visual aid and the way in which you wish to begin, move ahead, and close are important aspects of a good lesson planning. Templates of lesson plans are available and discussed elsewhere in this book. Borrowing old presentations, especially PPTs prepared by others will not be helpful, and at times may lead to disaster if someone questions its accuracy or relevance in the present context.

A beginner is faced with a dilemma as to how many slides to carry. For an hour-long lecture, not more than 25–30 slides are recommended unless you plan to show images, in which case you may include more.

#### 8.4.2.3 Know Your Venue Well

It is always a good idea to inspect the venue and familiarize yourself with the position of the podium, lighting of the arena, location of electricity points, quality of A-V aids, microphones, a projection device, functioning of slide presenter and most importantly the compatibility of the laptop with the projection. Often hyperlinks fail to open. It is better to make sure that the presentation works and the back-up plan is in place.

#### 8.4.2.4 Prepare Resources and Handouts in Advance

Nowadays, with the availability of Learning Management Systems (LMS), it is easy to share the resources in advance, or as and when needed. However, well-prepared handouts have their own advantage if the technology meets with glitches. The distribution should be planned well to avoid wastage of time. One has to make sure that the handouts are well made ideally, 2–4 slides printed on each side of an A4 size sheet, with space for the students to take notes.

#### 8.4.2.5 Be Prepared for the Worst

Have a back-up plan ready in place just in case the projection fails you at the last moment! A sheet of paper with main points that you wish to discuss should be a good guide as you go back to 'chalk board era' to complete the task.

### 8.4.3 During the Session

1. *Memorable Start*: Well beginning is half done. Always make an impressive and confident start to get the attention of the class. The use of questioning, case scenarios, short video clip or anecdotes works very well. An introductory slide with topics and sub-topics is a must.
2. *Voice Modulation*: A monotonous tone, especially in the post-prandial session, is most likely to induce sleep. This can be overcome by a good voice modulation or effective use of pace and pause which many great speakers use.
3. *Use of Body Language*: Effective use of eye contact, movement, and facial expression are potential tools to energize the session. One should avoid hiding

behind the podium ('sticky feet syndrome') or purposeless movement ('lion in a cage syndrome'). One should use controlled movement and reasonable proximity in engaging the audience.
4. *Rational Use of Media*: Images, videos, and schematic diagrams are helpful for effective teaching provided they are accompanied by good explanations. They should not be a substitute for the session. Also, animations should not be overdone and kept under full control with a slide changer in the hand of the speaker. Saying 'next slide please' may irritate the audience!
5. *Interaction Holds the Key*: The most crucial aspect of a presentation lies in one's ability to 'engage' the students in a meaningful dialogue. Asking questions, soliciting questions, and handling the question-answer are the real challenges for a presenter. One needs to strike a balance between time for interaction and time for completing the session in time.
6. *The Lighter Side of it All*: A little bit of humour is always appreciated during the class. However, the jokes should not be cracked at the cost of the audience. The sensitivities of the audience coming from diverse cultural background should be considered before cracking a joke or narrating anecdotes. The Jargons should be avoided.
7. *Elicit Feedback and Reinforcement*: It is important to keep track of where the students are! By resorting to questioning, one can give ample opportunity to the audience to clarify their doubts. Repetition helps reinforcement.
8. *Closure*: The role of summarizing and closing the session is perhaps most important. The audience eagerly look forward to the last slide! It is a good idea to suggest a few resources for those who want to probe further.

### 8.4.4 After the Session

1. *Assess the Outcome and Seek Student Feedback*: Feedback is the most powerful tool to check audience reaction so as to bring about future improvement. The feedback form can be administered anonymously to obtain an unbiased opinion. Survey monkey and Google forms are the most commonly used mechanisms to elicit feedback or to assess the learning outcome of presentations.
2. *Share Your Presentation*: A number of electronic sharing mechanisms are now available in the form of portals and websites, LMS, slide share, blogs, and other means of social media including WhatsApp groups and Google groups which are free of cost. While sharing materials which have been borrowed from some other sources, one has to be careful about the copyright issues.

Putting the bits and pieces together it emerges that making an effective presentation involves attention to a number of factors including hard technical skills and soft skills of the presenter.

A frequent matter of debate in the educational circle is whether an effective presentation is an in-borne skill or acquired. Though effective presentation skill for a long time has been associated with a few talented individuals, educationists are now convinced that it can be acquired with effort and practise [4]. Everyone can be an effective presenter provided he/she masters the rules of the game.

In the words of Marcela Cintra, 'Teachers can be born with a passion for learning, for teaching, for education. Nevertheless, if no action is taken towards the development of more effective and innovative techniques … we risk becoming obsolete. How many advances in other domains have we heard of in the past decades and how much have we done for education at the same time? These are questions that may help us to distinguish between teachers who feel entitled to recognition because they chose to follow a vocation and those who work hard to improve their effectiveness in the classroom' [5].

A practical and potent strategy to develop teaching skills is the use of microteaching. Microteaching is a potential instrument for beginners to develop their presentation skills one by one in a safely designed environment. The trainees are called upon to practise a skill for five minutes, followed by self-evaluation, feedback given by peers and supervisors using a structured checklist. A detailed discussion on microteaching is perhaps beyond the scope of this chapter. Some of the progressive institutes have even introduced microteaching as a requirement for the postgraduate training, which has reaped immense benefit for a junior faculty member to gain competence and confidence in teaching [6].

### 8.4.5 Conclusion

- An effective presentation involves attention to technical aspects besides the skill of a presenter to motivate and interact with the audience.
- Before making a presentation, one must know the audience well, fine-tune the content and check the venue for the facilities available. A back-up plan is a must.
- During the presentation: Make a good beginning. Follow an interactive style. Practice pacing and pausing. Operate audio-visuals skilfully and judiciously. Use light humour to elevate the audience mood.
- After the presentation, summarize your talk, obtain feedback, leave an assignment, or a take-home message to stimulate further reading

## 8.5 Evaluate

Now that you have an idea of what an effective presentation entails, here is a quick reality check exercise—just click open one of your PPT of a class you took more than a year ago and critically appraise it keeping in mind the following points whether:

a. The objective of the presentation clearly mentioned.
b. The contents tailored to the audience level; organized sequentially.
c. The slides are well designed, following the rules; original or borrowed from open access/copy left sources.

## References

1. Sathe MJ. Evaluation of medical education unit trained teachers by students. Int J Healthc Biomed Res. 2016;4(4):58–63.
2. Kolb DA. Experiential learning: experience as a source of learning and development. 2nd ed. Englewood Cliff, NJ: Prentice Hall; 1984.
3. Bullock I, Davis M, Lockey A, Mackway-Jones K, editors. A structured approach to teaching. 2015. https://doi.org/10.1002/9781119088769.ch2. Available at Wiley online library https://onlinelibrary.wiley.com. Accessed 23 Sept 2019.
4. Education Reform, Teaching the teachers. The Economist. 2016. Boston, Newark and New York.
5. Marcela Cintra in Reflections about Education. https://www.richmondshare.com.br/are-good-teachers-born-or-made/.
6. Muthukrishnan SP, Mehta N. Microteaching enhances teaching skills of resident doctors of India: a pilot study. Medical education. Natl Med J India. 2019;32(1):29–31.

# Part III

# For Junior and Mid Faculty: Hold Them Strong!

# 9 Teaching, Learning, and Assessing Communication Skills

Tejinder Singh and Rajiv Mahajan

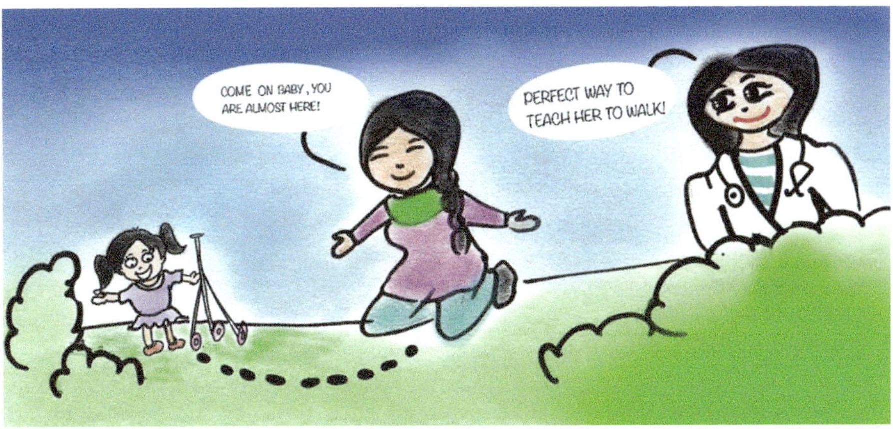


The patient will never care how much you know until they know how much you care.—Terry Canale [1]

T. Singh (✉)
Departments of Pediatrics and Medical Education, Sri Guru Ram Das Institute of Medical Sciences and Research, Amritsar, Punjab, India

R. Mahajan
Department of Pharmacology, Adesh Institute of Medical Sciences and Research, Bathinda, Punjab, India


S. C. Parija, B. V. Adkoli (eds.), *Effective Medical Communication*,
https://doi.org/10.1007/978-981-15-3409-6_9

## 9.1 Assess Need

Effective communication with patients is always considered as one of the most important components of health care. Communication skill is regarded as a soft skill, and for ages, it has been proposed that such skills are "*caught*" by observing the role models, mentors, and teachers. However, with the changing paradigm of medical education, with the changing outlook of the society towards the medical profession, with easy access of the medical information to the patient, and with the incremental rates of litigations against medical professionals, the focus has certainly shifted to equip our undergraduate students with these skills during graduate training itself.

Studies have shown that effective doctor–patient communication results in better health outcomes ranging from emotional health, symptom resolution, to pain control [2]. Patients experiencing good communication with their doctors are more satisfied and compliant [3]. A relationship between effective doctor–patient communication and enhanced psychological adjustments and better mental health of the patients, a decrease in length of hospital stay, and therefore the cost of individual medical visits and fewer referrals have also been reported [4, 5]. An effective and patient-centric communication facilitates the exchange of information and includes patients in decision-making [6]. As reported in literature, a patient-centered communication leads to better satisfaction of patient as well as doctor and satisfied patients are less likely to complain against doctors or file a litigation [7]. Satisfied patients are valuable for doctors in terms of better job contentment, less work-related stress, and reduced burnout. On the other hand, ineffective communication skills are associated with medication errors, malpractice claims, and litigations against doctors [8].

Till now, it has been advocated that students "*caught*" soft skills like communication skills from role models, teachers, and seniors; but changing paradigm in medical education is putting more stress on the "*taught*" phrase of soft skills too, thereby meaning that soft skills like communication skills have to be taught to the students. Considering the importance and benefits of communication skills in medical practice, most competency frameworks have included communication as one of the essential and important competency. These include the concepts of the Medical Council of Canada (1993), Educational Commission for Foreign Medical Graduates (1998), the United States Medical Licensing Examination (2004) [9], "*five-star doctor*" mooted by the World Health Organization [10], and Indian Medical Graduate as defined by the Medical Council of India (2018).

## 9.2 Brief

In this chapter, we will discuss:

- The methods to teach and train medical students in effective doctor–patient communication during graduate medical training.
- The brief outline of an effective doctor–patient communication curriculum and the ways to incorporate it in graduate medical training.
- Important models of effective doctor–patient communication.
- The methods of assessment of communication skills during graduate medical training.

## 9.3 Contextualize

### 9.3.1 Case Scenario

Dr. Comini being Professor of Department of Medicine has noticed that one of her residents Dr. ML, who is clinically very competent and has good diagnostic and decision-making skills, is constantly getting poor patients' ratings. His conduct and performance in the department are very good. While his colleagues describe him as a soft-spoken and compassionate guy, patients often have expressed dissatisfaction with him. On the other hand, her other resident Dr. PC, whom she knows is lacking in clinical and diagnostic skills, always manages to satisfy the patients. She is confused but went ahead to investigate the matter further.

On probing, she comes to know that though Dr. ML cares for patients and is very good in the way he provides medical care to each and every patient, the way he patiently listens to patients' concerns and queries and answers them instantaneously; but he tends to use technical terms and jargons while communicating with patients and relatives. He is not in the habit of asking for patients' understanding and assumes that the patients understood his interactions in a perfect manner. On the other hand, Dr. PC, is a local guy and uses vernacular language and talks to the patients in their own words. He builds a personal rapport with the patients. This skill of communicating with patients in their own language and ability to build an interpersonal relationship allow Dr. PC to get excellent patients' satisfaction.

***Exercise***: Now think and decide—what will you do in such a situation? What you will plan to do with your graduate students in future, in order to ensure that they do not face a similar problem while working in the field after graduation.

## 9.4 Describe

Medical educationists for a long time assumed that medical students acquire the art of communication merely by watching their seniors as role models and mentors. However, over the years, it has been realized that the communication skills thus acquired are not adequate. All senior teachers and physicians are neither good role models, nor do they show ideal communication skills at all the times in their working conditions. Though students pick up some tricks-of-the-trade while observing their teachers and make their ideal picture, formal training will definitely help them to fine-tune the learned behavior [11].

The obvious questions then arise—how to train medical undergraduates in communication skills? Can we have a structured program for the same? How to find opportunities to apply them in practice and how to assess our undergraduates for communication skills? We will try to answer these queries in the next sections precisely.

The curriculum for training undergraduate students in communication skills should be part of the medical training. As such, teachers must have teaching-learning and assessment methods for communication skills in their armamentarium. They must be conversant with the methods to assimilate the curriculum with the existing one seamlessly.

### 9.4.1 Teaching Methods

For communication skills training, conventional teaching methods like didactic lectures, seminars, and symposium will not be effective. Students need hands-on training, and as such methods imparting experiential learning should be used [11]. These methods must have a scope for giving feedback to the students. Some important methods and their unique features have been listed in Table 9.1.

#### 9.4.1.1 Role Plays

In role plays, students enact a particular role as per the script designed. Not much training is required in enacting role plays, and there is ample scope for rehearsals, creativity, and improvisation. The same script can be used with different sets of students in other sessions. Teachers and peers can always give feedback, thus making it an ideal assessment and learning platform for communication skills. Any potential doctor–patient encounter can be converted into a role play, such as interaction in an outpatient or indoor setting, counseling session, breaking bad news, taking informed consent, or organizing a community service camp. Though no extraordinary acting skills are required for enacting a role play, however, it can prove a hindrance for some students, which is a major drawback of role play.

#### 9.4.1.2 Video Recordings

Pre-designed video recordings of "*good*" and "*not-so-good*" doctor–patient communications showed to the students can be a good teaching-learning method. They

**Table 9.1** Some important teaching methods used to impart communication skills training to undergraduates along with their features

| Teaching method | Characteristic features | Advantages |
|---|---|---|
| Role plays | - Students enact a particular role as per the script<br>- Teachers and peers give feedback after the session | - Easy to conduct, not requiring much training<br>- Can be repeated in other sessions with different students<br>- Training for non-verbal communication too |
| Simulated patients (SP) | - SP is trained for a particular scenario<br>- SP is given enough time to learn first | - Same SP can be used multiple times for the same or different scenario<br>- Trained SP can give feedback too |
| Cinemeducation | - Use of videos/cinema for showing good and bad doctor–patient interactions<br>- Feedback by the teacher afterwards | - Can be watched by students themselves for self-directed learning<br>- The same video can be used multiple times with multiple learners |
| Video recordings of real interactions | - Recorded videos of learners' interaction with patients<br>- Take informed consent of patients being filmed | - Feedback by the teachers on the observed behaviors of the learners<br>- Self-assessment possible |

can make comparative notes and can reflect further on both types of interactions. Such videos are easily available on the internet. At the same time, students' interaction with the patients can be recorded, after taking due consent and these videos can then be used for self-assessment by the learners as well as for feedback by the teachers. These video recordings of the learners' interaction with the patients act as "*assessment for learning*."

#### 9.4.1.3 Simulated Patients

Trained simulated patients (SPs) can be used for communication skills training of undergraduate students. Training of SPs requires administrative support for hiring and making payments. SPs are, in a sense, higher form of role plays, where the role of the patient is being played by a person exclusively trained to be a patient. Also, the script is not under the control of the students (Table 9.1).

#### 9.4.1.4 Communication Skill Lab

Many medical colleges have established communication skill lab (CSL), similar to the ones established for the training of clinical skills. Salvatori et al. have described the creation of two simulated scenarios, one reflecting inpatient and other reflecting outpatients' encounters, for communication skill training using standardized patients in inter-professional educational environment [12]. Dealing with cultural issues, a difficult patient, and family conflict were the communication challenges involved in this team-based approach of communication skills training. Several medical colleges have introduced CSL in which undergraduate medical students are posted for two days during their first year and five days during their second year and third professional years. The module is delivered through debates, role plays, and powerpoint presentations [13]. Training of students in small groups, frequent change of scenarios giving wider scope, an opportunity of feedback from teachers, and repeated practice leading to deliberate practice are some of the advantages of the CSL.

For conceptualization of basic facts about communication skills initially, methods such as interactive lectures, small group discussion, buzz groups, and reflective writing can be used. Medical Council of India (MCI) released a longitudinal training module named "*Attitude, Ethics, and Communication*" (AETCOM) module for training of undergraduate medical students in ethics and communication skills in 2018 [14]. Thus formal training in communication skills is now a reality.

### 9.4.2 Assessment Methods

Assessment of communication skills should be based on observable skills. It is more of "*assessment for learning*" with ample opportunities for feedback. Salient features of assessment of communication skills in undergraduate students have been highlighted in Fig. 9.1.

While planning for assessment of communication skills, integrating it with an assessment of other domains like clinical competencies must be considered. Isolated assessment of communication skills will often lead to faking of skills by the

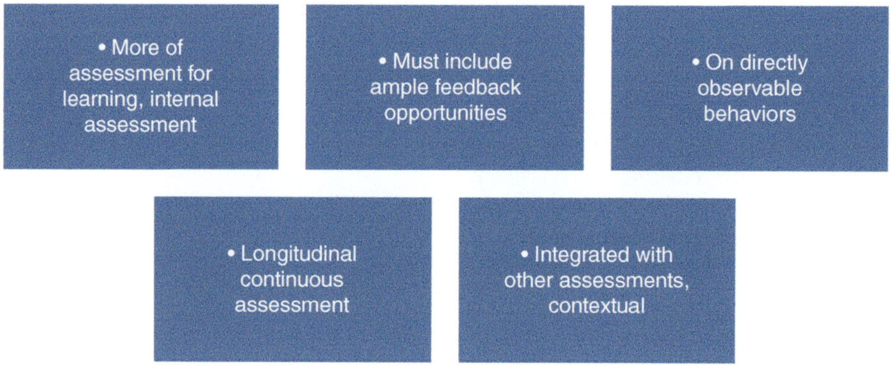


**Fig. 9.1** Salient features of communication skills assessment

**Fig. 9.2** Tools to assess communication skills (Based on Miller's Pyramid). *MCQs* Multiple choice questions, *EMQs* Extended matching questions, *OSCE* Objective structured clinical examination, *SPs* Simulated patients, *MSF* Multiple source feedback

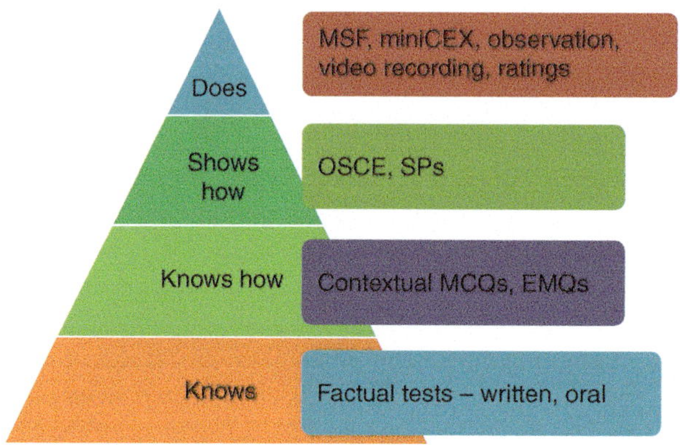


students. Communication skill assessment methods must be aligned with Miller's pyramid (Fig. 9.2).

Very specific rating scale—Kalamazoo consensus statement assessment tools can be used for patient ratings as a part of multi-source feedback (MSF) for assessment of communication skills. This scale has also been adapted for developing a rating scale for assessment purposes for AETCOM module by MCI. Kalamazoo Essential Elements Communication Checklist includes seven core communication competencies and 24 sub-competencies. Student's performance is rated on the competencies and sub-competencies using categorical ratings: done well, needs improvement, not done, not applicable. In Kalamazoo Essential Elements Communication Checklist, which has been adapted, the rating scale has been modified from categorical ratings to global ratings on a Likert scale (1 = poor to 5 = excellent) [12]. The third tool is Gap–Kalamazoo Communication Skills Assessment Form. This form has been designed by integrating the Kalamazoo Consensus Statement framework and

360-degree assessment models to develop a multi-rater form. This form has four versions—clinician/ faculty, patient/family, peer facilitator, and self-assessment. This assessment tool includes the original seven competencies of the Kalamazoo Consensus Statement framework and two additional dimensions: demonstrates empathy and communicates accurate information [13].

### 9.4.3 Models of Doctor–Patient Communication

Teachers use a variety of models for teaching and assessment of communication skills, and a model that allows the seamless accomplishment of both tasks is regarded as the best. All models for communication skills, particularly for doctor–patient communication, have three major components—giving information to the patients, paying attention to the emotions of the patients, and shared decision-making. Emotional support, empathy, and making patients a partner in the decision-making are some additional components of some more complex models. The key elements and steps involved in any doctor–patient interaction in a clinical setting have been outlined (Box 9.1).

**Box 9.1: Key Elements of Doctor–Patient Communication in a Clinical Setting**

- Listening to patients' problem.
- Searching for patients' concerns and expectations.
- Paying attention to patients' emotions and provide psychological support.
- Giving clear, specific information in a language and wording understandable to the patients.
- Asking for patients' understanding.
- Trying to build consensus for further testing (if required).
- Trying to build an environment for shared responsibilities and making patient an informed partner in treatment goal achievement.

Though many models—Bayer Institute for Health Care Communication E4 Model, the Three Function Model, the Calgary-Cambridge Observation Guide, Kalamazoo Consensus Statement to name a few—are in use, the key elements remain the same. The learner may start training by learning and following the steps of any model; a trained and expert doctor will ultimately coin his/her own approach and will communicate in a more automated way rather than in a mechanical, stepwise fashion; as it happens with any other clinical skill [11].

### 9.4.4 Curriculum for Communication Skills

Any proposed curriculum for communication skills must be a longitudinal program, running across all the phases of undergraduate medical training. As literature has pointed out, communication skills decline during the latter part of the medical program, so a longitudinal program packed with frequent reinforcements must be designed. This curriculum must be integrated with other academic curriculum and must be contextualized. Though a curriculum can be designed to target specific topics, like—breaking bad news, counseling to patients having psycho-social problems, genetic counseling, counseling for family planning; a curriculum having a wider range of generic competencies for students' training must be implemented at the undergraduate level. Some of the generic communication competencies have been described in Box 9.2.

**Box 9.2: Important Generic Competencies for Communication Skills**
- Ability to build interpersonal relationships.
- Respect for patients, peers, teachers, and other health care professionals.
- Care for patients' confidentiality and privacy.
- The basic interviewing technique, history taking, and clinical examination.
- Basic documentation techniques and data gathering.
- Proper prescription writing skills.
- Ability to take informed consent.
- Ability to work in a team.
- Basic counseling skills.

The AETCOM module prescribed by MCI is a longitudinal training and assessment program that has communication component. This document has four generic communication competencies, viz.*"Demonstrate ability to communicate adequately, sensitively, effectively, and respectfully with patients in a language that the patient understands; demonstrate ability to establish professional relationships with patients and families that are positive, understanding, humane, ethical, empathetic, and trustworthy; demonstrate ability to communicate with patients in a manner respectful of patient's preferences, values, prior experience, beliefs, confidentiality and privacy; and demonstrate ability to communicate with patients, colleagues, and families in a manner that encourages participation and shared decision-making"* [14]. For professional year 1, five modules for 34 h have been designed. Professional year 2 has eight modules for 37 h, professional year 3 has five modules for 25 h, and professional year 4 has nine modules for 44 h. The whole curriculum has five modules—The Foundations of Communication 1–5 spread over all professional years, specifically designed for communication skill training. These communication modules require a total of 27 h. Specific teaching-learning methods, case scenarios, assessment plan along with checklist, and format of log-book have been well documented in this curriculum. This curriculum is complete in itself for undergraduate training, though we strongly believe that efforts should be reinforced and fortified during internship period too, through direct observation and multi-source feedback of the internees, supplemented with formative assessment and feedback.

### 9.4.5 Conclusion

- Communication skills must be taught to the medical students right from the first year itself.
- The program designed must provide opportunities for experiential learning to the students.
- Communication skills must be assessed both formatively and summatively.
- The program should be designed for longitudinal, continuous training throughout the undergraduate teaching program.

## 9.5 Evaluate

Having read this chapter, now you are in a position to take up a small assignment for self-directed learning and assessment. Identify the specific learning objectives for the four generic communication skill competencies as given in AETCOM module for different doctor–patient communication situations and scenarios. Align teaching-learning and assessment methods with these competencies to develop a comprehensive curriculum plan.

## References


1. Tongue JR, Epps HR, Forese LL. Communication skills for patient-centred care: research-based, easily learned techniques for medical interviews that benefit orthopaedic surgeons and their patients. J Bone Joint Surg Am. 2005;87A(3):652–8.
2. Stewart MA. Effective physician-patient communication and health outcomes: a review. Can Med Assoc J. 1995;152(9):1423–33.
3. Ha JF, Longnecker N. Doctor-patient communication: a review. Ochsner J. 2010;10(1):38–43.
4. Maguire P, Pitceathly C. Key communication skills and how to acquire them. BMJ. 2002;325(7366):697–700.
5. Little P, Everitt H, Williamson I, Warner G, Moore M, Gould C, Ferrier K, Payne S. Observational study of the effect of patient-centeredness and positive approach on outcomes of general practice consultations. BMJ. 2001;323(7318):908–11.
6. Chandra S, Mohammadnezhad M, Ward P. Trust and communication in a doctor-patient relationship: a literature review. J Healthcare Comm. 2018;3(3):36. https://doi.org/10.4172/2472-1654.100146.
7. Brinkman WB, Geraghty SR, Lanphear BP, Khoury JC, Gonzalez del Rey JA, Dewitt TG, et al. Effect of multi-source feedback on resident communication skills and professionalism: a randomized controlled trial. Arch Pediatr Adolesc Med. 2007;161(1):44–9.
8. Levinson W, Roter DL, Mulloly JP, Dull VT, Frankel RM. Physician-patient communication: the relationship with malpractice claims among primary care physicians and surgeons. JAMA. 1997;277(7):553–9.
9. Tamblyn R, Abrahamowicz M, Dauphinee D, Wenghofer E, Jacques A, Klass D, et al. Physician scores on a national clinical skills examination as predictors of complaints to medical regulatory authorities. JAMA. 2007;298(9):993–1001.
10. Boelen C. The five-star doctor: an asset to health care reform? World Health Organization. https://www.who.int/hrh/en/HRDJ_1_1_02.pdf. Accessed 17 May 2019.

11. Modi JN, Anshu, Chhatwal J, Gupta P, Singh T. Teaching and assessing communication skills in medical undergraduate training. Indian Pediatrics. 2016;53(6):497–504.
12. Salvatori P, Mahoney P, Delottinville C. An interprofessional communication skills lab: A pilot project. Educ Health. 2006;19(3):380–4.
13. Jagzape TB, Jagzape AT, Vagha JD, Chalak A, Meshram RJ. Perception of medical students about communication skills laboratory (CSL) in a rural medical college of central India. J Clin Diagn Res. 2015;9(12):JC01–4.
14. Medical Council of India. AETCOM – Attitude, Ethics and Communication competencies for the Indian Medical Graduate, 2018. https://old.mciindia.org/UG-Curriculum/AETCOM_book.pdf. Accessed 7 June 2019.

# Communication in Large Classrooms: Issues, Challenges, and Solutions

# 10

Jyoti Nagmoti

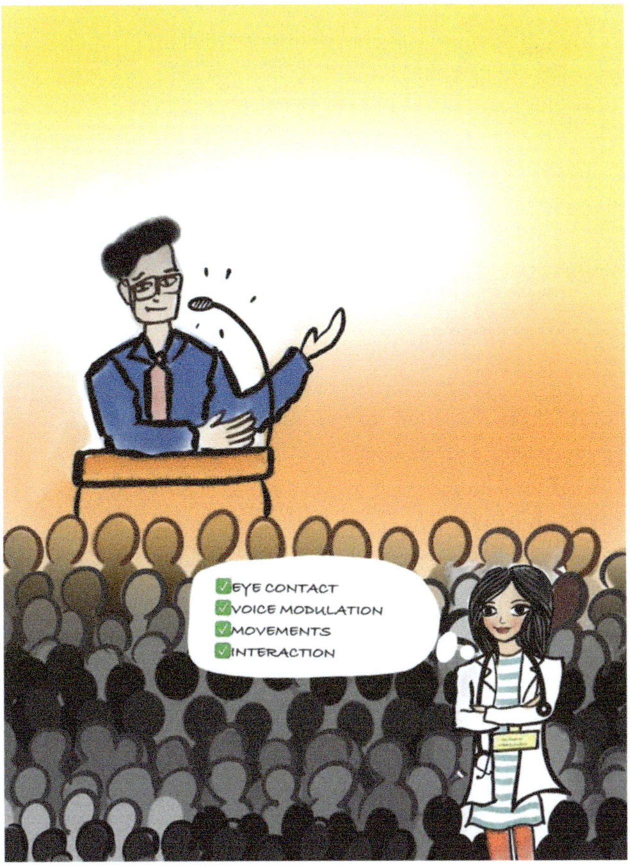


Persuasive communication skill is an essential competency of a teacher that can be acquired through training and reflective practice.—Jyoti Nagmoti

J. Nagmoti (✉)
Department of Microbiology, J.N Medical College, KLE Academy of Higher Education and Research (KAHER), Belagavi, Karnataka, India



S. C. Parija, B. V. Adkoli (eds.), *Effective Medical Communication*,
https://doi.org/10.1007/978-981-15-3409-6_10

## 10.1 Assess Needs

Communication is not just about transmission of information, but it is all about connecting with the class, creating a deeper understanding of message, and leaving the audience enthused! Lectures are the common modes of communication in academia; however, they are generally criticized for being passive, inefficient to promote higher order thinking skills (HOTS), lacking outcome-based approach, and having limited scope for feedback on learning [1]. Nonetheless, one cannot underestimate the power of lectures since they are the most feasible means to address a large audience.

Evidence shows that many faculty members lack the requisite knowledge and skills in educational science and technology. To be effective, the educators need to switch from less interactive traditional practice to a more interactive lecture (IL) format [2]. IL is a complex interplay between teacher, student, and the content [1]. It is principle driven, student centered, and outcome oriented. It requires meticulous lesson planning, effective monitoring, active participation of teacher and the trainee, and assessment of learning [3]. Conducting effective IL in large classrooms is a challenging issue.

## 10.2 Brief

This chapter will address:

- What is interactive lecture?
- Why does it work better?
- How to engage effective IL?
- Issues and challenges involved in IL.
- Solutions.

## 10.3 Contextualize

### 10.3.1 Case Scenario

Dr. Comini, a mid-level faculty, is neither trained in pedagogic science nor prepared for handling large class. However, having joined as a faculty member, the Head of the Department who is facing the problem of shortage of faculty assigns lectures to Dr. Comini.

Initially, she feels terribly helpless while engaging the class. She is deeply concerned about what to teach? How much to teach? How to make students learn the best? Dr. Comini had no clue. Fortunately, a workshop organized by the Medical Education Unit came as a game changer for her. This workshop came handy to sensitize young teachers to learn the principles of adult learning. It also gave ample opportunity for the participants to practice different methods of interactive teaching

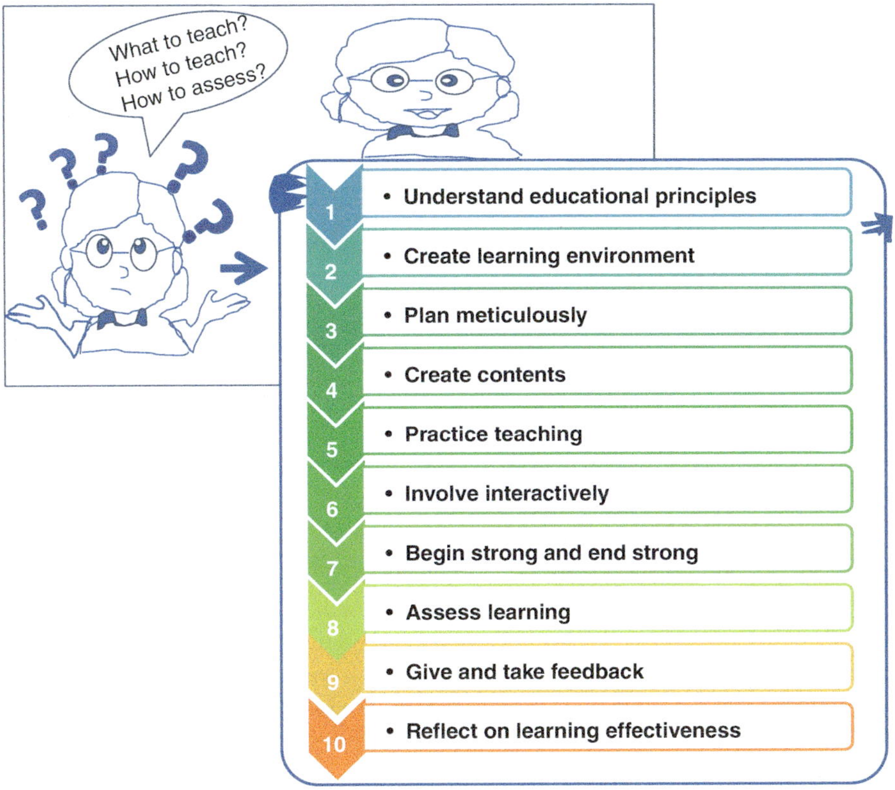


**Fig. 10.1** Tips for teaching in large class

in the form of demonstrations, individual and group exercises besides video sessions and role plays.

When Dr. Comini returned after the workshop to take her normal class, the students were dazzled to see a drastic transformation in her style of teaching!

***Exercise***: Discuss whether effective teaching in a large class is in-born ability or acquired by practice (Fig. 10.1).

## 10.4 Describe

### 10.4.1 What Is Interactive Lecture?

Interactive lecture is a planned interplay between teacher, active learner, and the contents in a supportive environment aimed to achieve lesson objectives. Success of IL depends on the ability of a teacher to effectively connect with students and the content. Interactive lectures are outcome oriented. They encourage knowledge retention, application of new knowledge, promotion of higher order thinking skills

**Table 10.1** Differences between traditional and interactive lectures

| Traditional lecture | Interactive lectures |
|---|---|
| Teacher centered | Learner centered |
| Often one way and passive | Interactive learner engagement is the key |
| Usually content driven | Principle driven |
| Learning is mainly through auditory | Learning is multisensory |
| Assessment of student learning is not a priority | Assessment of student learning is a priority |
| Taking feedback is not a usual practice | Timely feedback is an integral part of IL |
| Reflection on learning is usually not adopted | Reflection on learning by student and teacher to achieve metacognition is encouraged |
| May not spark interest and student motivation | Leaves the students motivated and enthused |
| May not promote self-directed lifelong learning | Promotes self-directed lifelong learning |

(HOTS), problem-solving, and creative thinking. Here, the knowledge application is known to be facilitated through multisensory approach among different types of learners [3, 4]. IL differs from traditional lecture in number of ways as enumerated in Table 10.1.

General steps involved in IL include lesson planning, interactive learner engagement, assessment of learning, feedback, and reflection (Fig. 10.2). Here, the teacher engages the audience in different ways. The teacher also assesses students' learning through various verbal and nonverbal responses of the learners. Further, the teacher provides timely and constructive feedback to the students on their learning progress and at the same time receives feedback on his/her teaching effectiveness. In other words, IL provides scope for adopting reflective practice for both teacher and students to advance their abilities [5–7].

Some of the interactive techniques like one-minute reflection paper, short character memoir, or learning logs are known to encourage metacognition which means thinking about one's own cognitive process. Metacognition is a reflective skill that promotes learners creativity, critical thinking, and problem solving, thus leading to enhanced learning outcomes [8].

### 10.4.2 Why Do These Work Better?

Interactive lectures are based on strong learning theories like Kolb and Gagne [9, 10]. IL promotes deep learning because of the involvement of a teacher in meticulous lesson planning, careful content creation, and active engagement of the learner through verbal and nonverbal communication.

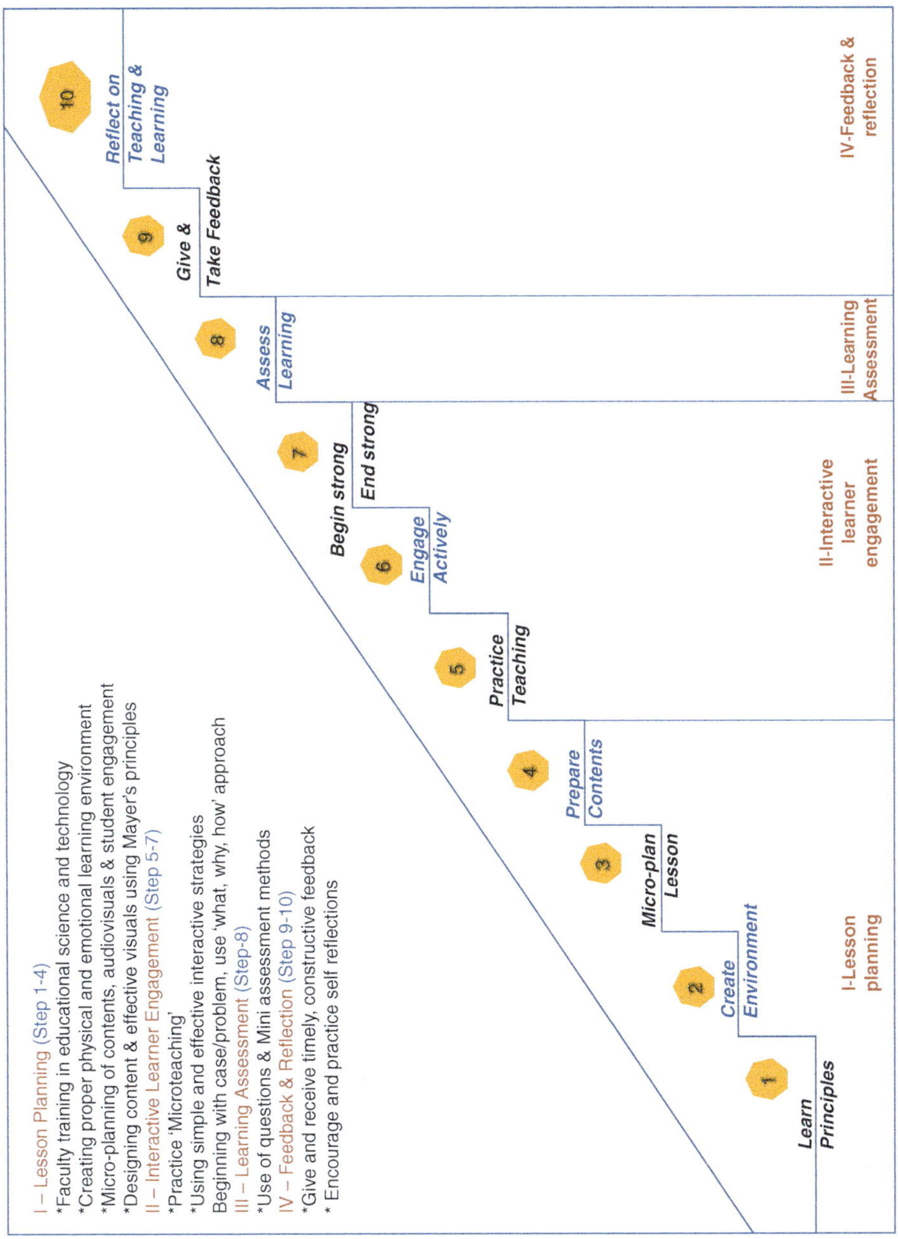


**Fig. 10.2** Steps on effective engagement of interactive lectures

### 10.4.3 Issues and Challenges

Issues and challenges in a large classroom can be multifactorial [5]:

- Teacher's perceptions, experiences, and beliefs may not be favorable to IL.
- Lack of willingness to change the role from "*knowledge provider to knowledge facilitator.*"
- Lack of awareness of diverse learning styles of students.
- Inadequate training in educational science and technology.
- Varying ability of the teacher to plan, create learning resources, and involve the learners.
- Teacher's attitude, fear of losing control over the class.
- Learners' expectations, deficiencies, stress levels, and fear of poor performance.
- Wrong belief that interactive techniques are time-consuming and are meant for postgraduate training rather than undergraduate training.
- Non-availability of supportive learning infrastructure, like hall, seating arrangements, projection facilities, and ambience needed for IL.

### 10.4.4 Solutions to Overcome Challenges: Engaging Effective IL

#### 10.4.4.1 Understand the Educational Principles

Understanding "*How people learn*" is the basic requirement. Adult learners have prior knowledge and experience. They are motivated to learn by the relevance and immediate application of a topic.

Other guiding principles include (a) sharing of reading material in the form of handouts and resources is essential while dealing with a new topic, (b) gaining attention, eliciting prior knowledge, and connecting learning to its practical application, and (c) self-reflection and feedback from peers often motivate the adult learners.

#### 10.4.4.2 Create Supportive Learning Environment

Creating supportive physical and emotional learning environment can enhance learning [9, 10]. Physical environment includes hall size, seating arrangements, projection facilities, stage, flip charts, whiteboard, smart board, and other devices. Ensuring the availability of high speed internet connectivity is a must to bring novelty to the classroom interaction. It is worthwhile to be familiar with the facilities available at the venue prior to class. Planning for back up is equally important.

#### 10.4.4.3 Plan Lesson Meticulously

Adequate planning is an important prerequisite of IL. Preparation of a lesson plan is a must. Each lesson should be built upon few main concepts. Students actually retain only a small portion of the information presented to them [11]. Therefore, specific learning objectives (SLO) should be derived based on the general lesson

**Table 10.2** Lesson plan template

| | | | | |
|---|---|---|---|---|
| Topic<br>Level of the students | | | | Date<br>Time |
| Lesson Objective | | | | |
| **Segment** | | **Duration** | **Student engagement strategy** | **Teaching aids, infrastructure, student preparation, distribution of learning resources, handouts** |
| I. Introduction<br>("What and Why" of the topic) | | 1/4th class time | 1.<br>2. | |
| | | | Segment summary | |
| II. Body<br>("How" of the topic) | | 2/4th class time | 1.<br>2.<br>3.<br>4. | |
| | | | Segment summary | |
| III. Closure<br>(Reinforcement and scope) | | 1/4th class time | Grand summary<br>1.<br>2. | |
| Assessment | Learning | | | |
| | Teaching | | | |
| Feedback | Learners | | | |
| | Teacher | | | |
| Reflection | Learners | | | |
| | Teacher | | | |

objectives and each SLO should be addressed effectively. A template of lesson plan has been shown in Table 10.2. Adequate planning helps to avoid running out of time and missing important ideas from content! It is always good to keep plan-B ready in case of unanticipated events like power failure or technical hiccups!

#### 10.4.4.4 Carefully Craft the Contents

Since the advent of technology, powerpoint presentation (PPT) is popular among educators. However, their judicial use is an art; they can either make or mar ones' presentations! Mayer's multimedia presentation principles come handy to design and present the PPT slides effectively (Table 10.3) [12, 13].

First few slides may contain the lesson objectives and contents followed by, logically built material on what, why, and how components of the topic under consideration. Carefully embedded pictures, animations, video clips, and cases can work as "*lid opener*" to arouse interest in the lesson. Well-designed PPT can help not only in better understanding of complex topics but also in facilitating long term retention since they are based on multisensory learning. Videos can work the best to achieve attitudinal objectives. One can selectively pause the videos and engage in discussion to ensure understanding of basic concepts, and reinforce key messages [3].

**Table 10.3** Application of Mayer's multimedia principles for designing and delivery of powerpoint presentations

| Mayer's multimedia principles | *PPT slide designing/delivery |
|---|---|
| *Multimedia principle:* People learn better from words and pictures than words alone | Include relevant and interesting pictures, flow charts, and tables stuffing with text alone |
| *Coherence principle:* People learn better when extraneous words, pictures, and sounds are excluded than included | Exclude any extraneous words and pictures |
| *Spatial contiguity:* People learn better when text and pictures are placed close by than far from each other | Place text and pictures close to each other |
| *Temporal contiguity:* People learn better when text and pictures are presented simultaneously than successively | Present text and pictures simultaneously |
| *Signaling principle:* People learn better when essential material is highlighted | Highlight the important and essential key points and stress on them during presentation |
| *Modality principle:* People learn better from images with narration than images with text read out | Present images with narration |
| *Personalization principle:* People learn better when words are delivered in conversational manner than formal style | Deliver the contents by engaging learners in a conversation |

**PPT* Powerpoint presentation

#### 10.4.4.5 Practice Teaching

Learning IL skills in a large classroom is akin to learning any other skill like swimming or driving. Practice makes perfect. Effective teaching skills can be honed through the practice of microteaching which is a unique method of training in a safe environment. Microteaching is a scaled down form of teaching practice in which only one skill is practiced at a time, under observation by a supervisor and small group of peers who will give feedback after each presentation. A typical microteaching cycle includes "*teach, review, reflect, and reteach*." It is an unique method to practice and obtain constructive feedback from others to refine one's own teaching skills (Fig. 10.3) [14].

#### 10.4.4.6 Connect Interactively

In teaching, "*how we teach*" is as important as "*what we teach*" gaining students' attention and getting them involved in learning through activities is the key feature of IL. Connecting with learners through verbal and nonverbal cues and effective use of media and materials determine the success of IL. Verbal tools are the language and words that one chooses to convey message. Quality of voice through which message is conveyed [3] is an important attribute of effective communication. Engaging the audience in a loud conversational tone conveys confidence. Varying the tone or pitch helps to break the monotony. Sometimes, a pause can be very effective to gain attention, to allow reflection on learning and to have smooth transition between the lesson segments. One should avoid rhetorical fillers like um, aah, okay, well, you know, etc.

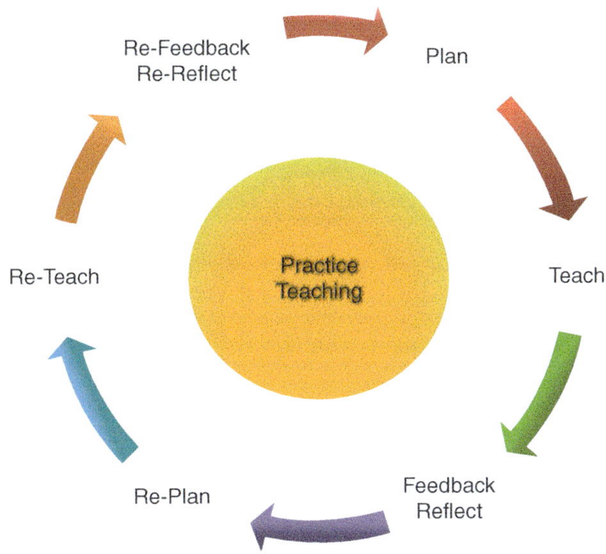


**Fig. 10.3** Microteaching cycle

Nonverbal cues are more of teacher's personal attributes like appearance, presence, movement, and gesture. Evidence shows that, people perceive two-thirds of whole communication through nonverbal cues or body language [3]. When the verbal communication contradicts nonverbal, the audience value the nonverbal rather than verbal! Overall body language, attire, eye contact, movements enhance the effectiveness of IL. Nevertheless, a smile adds value and exhibits teacher's confidence. Role played by chalkboard, whiteboard, and smart boards besides flip chart and the audience response systems cannot be underemphasized.

#### 10.4.4.7 Begin Well and End Up with a Clear Message

Every effective presentation has three parts, the beginning referred to as "*set*," the main body of presentation, referred to as "*dialogue*," and the final summary or conclusion, referred to as "*closure*."

In the first segment, preview the lesson objectives and provide road map of what will happen in each segment. Beginning with a quote, question, anecdote, or a case scenario can act as a lid opener. This segment should generally address "*what*" and "*why*" about the topic. First few minutes of a lesson are crucial because the audience attention span and interest rates are high. Therefore, this opportunity can be used to "*jump start*" the lesson by exhibiting our passion, sparking curiosity, and to stay emotionally connected with the audience.

Transition to second segment should begin by a brief wrap up of the first segment. Here, engaging the learners in discussion on "*how*" to find solutions helps in fostering self-directed learning. The learners can be engaged in buzz sessions, or group activities to solve, analyze, compare, and contrast the learning issues. It is important to vary the stimulus and introduce a variety of activities to sustain audience interest which is likely to dip down during this segment (Table 10.4).

**Table 10.4** Interactive strategies for the large classrooms

| Interactive technique | Description |
|---|---|
| *Brain storming* | Students randomly contribute ideas to an open ended question |
| *Jigsaw technique* | Small groups discuss on different topics, groups are shuffled so that at least one expert is present in new group and teaches that group |
| *Think-pair-share* | Students share their viewpoints with neighbor and share with the class |
| *Concept map* | Students write the keywords, organize them, and connect them to understand concepts |
| *Notes taking* | Students write down the skeletal points and take home points of a lesson |
| *One-minute paper* | In one minute, students write down on a specific question |
| *Muddiest point* | Students write down the points which they were unable to understand |
| *Role plays* | Some students are assigned roles of a concept and they enact, others critique and ask questions |
| *Picture prompt* | Images/pictures are shown without explanation and students are asked to identify and explain |
| *Pro and con grid* | Students make a list of the pros and cons of a topic |
| *Harvesting* | At the end of the class students reflect on what they learned, so what (implications), now what (applications) |
| *Crosswords puzzles* | Student or teacher builds crossword puzzles using key terms of a topic |
| *Pictionary* | Students/teachers draw images of the key terms or concepts and the rest will guess |

Last segment is equally important because the audience show high interest at this point of time. This segment can begin by a quick summary of second segment followed by the wrap up of all three segments. After the grand summary, refer back to the lesson objectives and check whether they were achieved. This helps to close the loop from objectives to outcomes [15]. Finally, provide the key take homes and suggestions for further reading.

#### 10.4.4.8 Assess Learning

A long teaching session can include mini-assessment activities which can provide feedback to both learners and the teachers. Multiple tools can be used for assessment such as questioning (preferably rapid fire MCQs), mini-quizzes, or asking audience to summarize. Questions can work like a magic wand; they can be used at any time during the class, irrespective of the number of students to encourage active learning. Brainstorming and whipping questions work the best. Students' responses can be captured through clickers or similar smartphone apps, analyzed, and displayed.

Asking questions help in multiple ways; to find out previous knowledge, to check the learning progress and to enhance interactivity. On the other hand, allowing questions during the class can make the learners feel comfortable and creates the impression that the teacher is supportive and approachable. Handling questions is an art. Reward each response and appreciate the students' efforts. One should always address the question, not the questioner [16]. In case the teacher does not get a response, it is better to paraphrase the question and try again. Even if the answer is not forthcoming the teacher can answer. In case the teacher has no correct answer to a question posed by the audience, it is humble to redirect the question to the audience. If none replies, the teacher can either ask the students to go online and find out a satisfactory answer or declare politely that he/she would get back with correct answer.

#### 10.4.4.9 Give and Take Feedback

Feedback is an important component that guides teaching and learning [17]. IL provides the scope for receiving and giving feedback on teaching and learning. Feedback helps both students and teachers. Students should be given timely, specific, and constructive feedback in order to motivate and enhance learning. On the other hand, teachers should receive feedback from learners on the effectiveness of teaching-learning. Feedback can be obtained informally by observing students reactions, body language, and response to the question or on a written feedback questionnaire. The practice of giving and receiving feedback can be enhanced by microteaching combined with analysis of video recorded lectures.

#### 10.4.4.10 Reflect on Process and Outcome

Adopting reflective practices by students and teachers on teaching-learning process can benefit both. Reflection can be aided by asking students to write narratives in a diary or e-portfolio which is current trend in a competency based medical education. Thus, reflection by students and teachers can go a long way in fostering metacognition, better retention, and transfer of knowledge.

### 10.4.5 Conclusions

- Interactive lectures can greatly help to overcome the challenges of handling large classrooms.
- It is possible to convert the traditional lectures into IL to enhance learning.
- Engaging in effective IL is a skill, which can be acquired by conscious efforts.
- One has to pay attention to a good start, an interactive dialogue, and ending up with a clear summary.

## 10.5 Evaluate

After reading the chapter, make a plan for converting your conventional lecture in to an interactive lecture. Try out with your students. Assess its impact and share your experience with your colleagues.

## References

1. Steinert Y, Snell LS. Interactive lecturing: strategies for increasing participation in large group presentations. Med Teach. 1999;21(1):1021–3.
2. Hafler JP. Effective presentation: tips for success. Nat Immunol. 2011;12(11):1021–3.

3. Teaching and persuasive communication class presentation skills. A hand book for faculty, teaching assistants & teaching fellows. Brown University; 2005. http://www.brown.edu/sheridan_center.
4. Svinicki MD, Wilkerson L. In: Hafler JP, editor. Extraordinary learning in the workplace. Faculty development for workplace instructors. Netherlands: Springer; 2011. p. 131–64.
5. Wilkerson L, Irby DM. Strategies for improving teaching practices: a comprehensive approach to faculty development. Acad Med. 1998;73(4):387–96.
6. Winstone NM. Reframing perceptions of the lecture from challenges to opportunities: embedding active learning and formative assessment into the teaching of large classes. Psychol Teach Rev. 2012;18(2):31–41.
7. Huxham M. Learning in lectures: do 'interactive windows' help? Active Learn High Educ. 2005;6(1):17–31.
8. Lovett MC. Teaching metacognition 2008; [PowerPoint slides]. Retrieved from http://web.uri.edu/teach/files/Metacognition-ELI.pdf.
9. Kolb DA. Experience as the source of learning and development. 2nd ed. Englewood Cliffs: Prentice Hall; 1984. p. 1–256.
10. Gagne R, Briggs L, Wager W, editors. Principles of instructional design. 3rd ed. New York: Holt, Rinehart and Winston; 1998.
11. Bourne PE. Ten simple rules for making good oral presentations. PLoS Comput Biol. 2007;3(4):e77. https://doi.org/10.1371/journal.pcbi.0030077.
12. Mayer RE, Moreno R. Nine ways to reduce cognitive load in multimedia learning. Educ Psychol. 2003;38(1):43–52.
13. Nagmoti JM. Departing from powerpoint default mode: applying Mayer's multimedia principles for enhanced learning of parasitology. Indian J Med Microbiol. 2017;35(2):199–203.
14. Ananthakrishnan N. Microteaching as a vehicle of teacher training its advantages and disadvantages. J Postgrad Med. 1993;39(3):142–3.
15. Cooper PJ. Speech communication for the classroom teacher. 4th ed. Scottsdale, AZ: Gorsuch Scarisbrick Publishers; 1991.
16. Rafe SC. How to be prepared to think on your feet. New York: Harper Business; 1990.
17. Jason H, Westberg J. Providing constructive feedback: a CIS guidebook for health professionals. Boulder, CO: Center for Instructional Support; 1991.

# Publishing Effectively and Ethically 11

Tony George Jacob and Peush Sahni

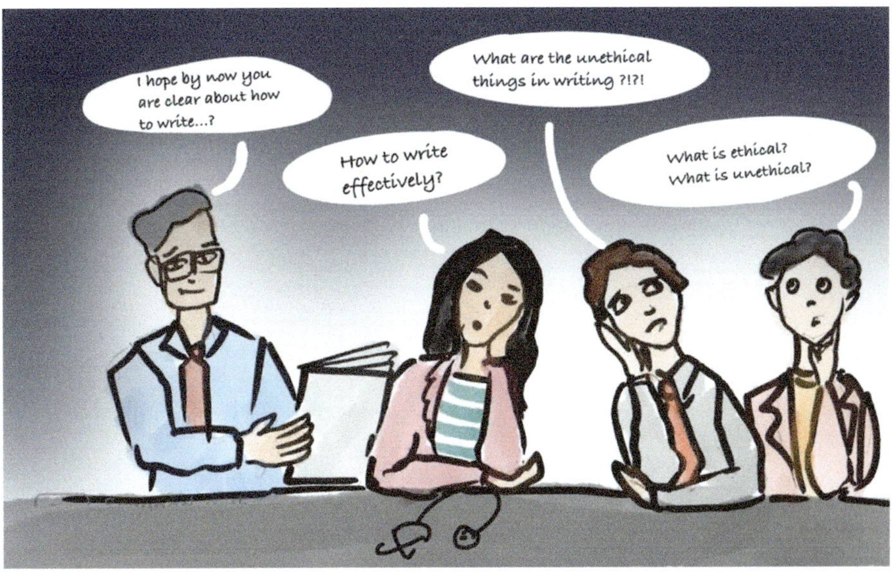


If it ain't published, it never happened! [Anonymous]

T. G. Jacob
Department of Anatomy, All India Institute of Medical Sciences, New Delhi, India

P. Sahni (✉)
Department of Gastrointestinal Surgery and Liver Transplantation, All India Institute of Medical Sciences, New Delhi, India



S. C. Parija, B. V. Adkoli (eds.), *Effective Medical Communication*,
https://doi.org/10.1007/978-981-15-3409-6_11

## 11.1 Assess Need

Writing is a science and an art. In the same vein, writing and publishing a scientific manuscript also has a method to it and is an art. However, scientific writing straddles the twin-worlds of literature and science. Like all literature, there is and should be a story to tell; a story that has a background, characters, plot, discoveries, and finally a conclusion to make. Like any piece of good literature, the scientific paper can also be riveting, be read again and again, and quoted in other writings, oral presentations, and dinner table conversations.

There are varied reasons and motivations to publish: contributing to global literature to inform policies or to improve practice; competing for promotion, grants, or recognition; or satisfying a mandatory requirement. However, what is disturbing is the concerns expressed regarding the quality of scientific publication. The *Economist* in October 2013 reported that much of scientific literature is alarmingly non-replicable and hence, unreliable [1]. Further, it raised concern that though science and its proceedings should be self-correcting over time, but in effect, it is not. There is a need, therefore, to inform the scientific community regarding the attributes of a good scientific paper and how to achieve it in a systematic manner.

## 11.2 Brief

In this chapter, we discuss:

- How do we determine the research question?
- Introduction, Method, Results and Discussion (IMRaD) format.
- The content/components of each section.
- Guidelines and tips for organising these components in a coherent manner.

## 11.3 Contextualize

### 11.3.1 Scenario 1

Dr. Comini gets admitted to a postgraduate course in a premier medical institute. She has to select a topic under the supervision of a guide, who would be normally allotted by the department. Fascinated by the digital revolution, she is genuinely interested in exploring the mobile application to be used by rural women in accessing health facilities. The only available guide in the department is Dr. A, who is passionate about research in the field of genomics. The Dean (Research) has announced areas, which are of priority for the institute are either public health, nutrition, or application of IT leading to patents and technology-transfer. He thinks that patents would contribute to high scores in the institute's accreditation and ranking.

***Exercise***: How can you help Dr. Comini in resolving her dilemma to take a wise decision?

### 11.3.2 Scenario 2

This story is related to a problem faced by Dr. Comini during her postgraduate course. Every PG student has to work in a particular area of interest to meet the mandatory requirement of a dissertation to be submitted during the final year. Dr. Comini, inspired by her mentor, got interested in the area of dyspepsia. During the course of clinical postings, she makes a consistent observation that patients taking a large amount of fried food have a sensation of bloating and acid reflux. In spite of this observation, she has no clue as to how to articulate a research question.

***Exercise***: List the requirements needed for Dr. Comini to move ahead in this field of research.

The primary requirement here would be confirming the observation in a large number of people across a geographically and ethnically varied population.

The secondary requirement may be giving a group of people, in experimental conditions, a fixed diet of food containing different percentages of fat content and observing and recording the effects over a period of time, while comparing it to individuals that were administered a diet completely devoid of fat. The third level of investigation maybe finding the cause for this observation through animal models, histopathological and physiological studies. Lastly, once the cause is found, one can intervene with some lifestyle modifications, pharmacological agents, or surgical procedures to relieve this symptom in affected individuals.

***Exercise***: Imagine how this story outlines the eventual discovery and utilisation of antacids, histamine-receptor blockers, vagotomies, and proton-pump inhibitors to treat dyspepsia.

## 11.4 Describe

It all begins with a question, which arises from the lacunae found in the existing literature or practice from general observation that requires validation by reliable repetition. Hence, most scientific literature should be based on a background of data and justification for the work done and reported. In the case of a postgraduate student performing research as a mandatory requirement, the subject of research is most commonly determined by the area of interest of the guide.

### 11.4.1 The IMRaD Format

With the global increase in the number of scientific publications, the editors of journals decided to make such publications more precise and concise to reduce the cost of publication, and increase access to authors and readers. Hence, from long essays of earlier centuries evolved the current IMRaD format, that has transformed manuscript writing [2] (Fig. 11.1).

This format is followed, almost uniformly, by all biomedical journals. There may be some variations in the journal style and specific requirements, but

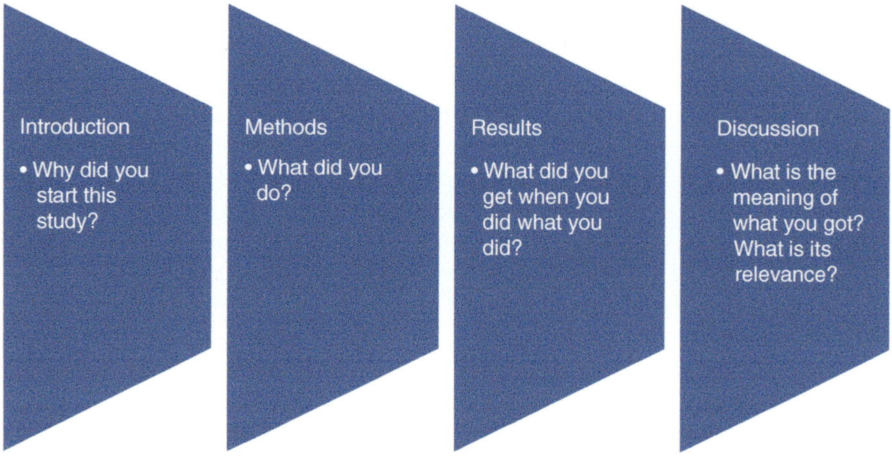


**Fig. 11.1** The IMRaD (Introduction, Methods, Results and Discussion) format

**Table 11.1** The contents of the introduction and the suggested guidelines

| Contents | Guidelines for writing |
|---|---|
| • Importance and magnitude of a particular problem, prevalence and incidence, burden of disease, current knowledge on the subject.<br>• The lacunae in the existing literature.<br>• Statement of the hypothesis.<br>• Aim of the study. | Avoid the passive voice.<br>Avoid complex sentences (with clauses and sub-clauses).<br>Devote each paragraph to only one topic or idea.<br>Link last sentence of a paragraph with the first sentence of the next paragraph. |

overall if the manuscript is prepared using this format, one can easily reformat it according to the style of the targeted journal with little effort.

#### 11.4.1.1 Introduction

This section should be written in the form of an inverted pyramid. It starts with a broad base that describes the importance of the problem in focus, what is known and what is not known, and usually ends with a statement of the aim of the study. The introduction, not more than 500–600 words, should provide context and motivation to the reader to read the paper entirely. The introduction should be written in the present tense and active voice. It is worthwhile to revisit the introduction after the remaining sections are written to check for its relevance and appropriateness. The contents of the introduction along with the guidelines to be followed [3] are listed in Table 11.1.

#### 11.4.1.2 Methods

This section describes how the research was done in order to answer the questions raised at the end of the introduction. Many consider this section as the most important part of the manuscript. The details in this section should allow a reader

**Table 11.2** The contents of methods section and the guidelines for writing

| Contents | Guidelines for writing |
|---|---|
| • The population—the characteristics of the subjects of the study; inclusion and exclusion criteria, definitions, the method of recruitment, the duration of the study, the gender and age, source of the subjects—hospital/community based.<br>• Intervention or exposures—drugs and their dosages if used; methods of randomisation, controls.<br>• Measurement of outcomes/results: either clearly defined clinical outcomes or laboratory values. The variable (continuous or categorical), the unit of measurement, the definition of qualitative findings, details of kits and instruments used, and timeline of study.<br>• Data analysis/statistical treatment of data: summary of data depending upon the outcome variable (continuous or categorical); the tests of significance and the level of significance. Any method to calculate sample size, assumptions, and corrections made to the data.<br>• Guidelines and ethics: This precedes the conduct of the study; certificate of clearance from a registered Institutional Ethics Committee. | Write in the past tense. |
| | Avoid complex sentences. |
| | Avoid minor details that were included in the protocol of the study. |
| | Summarise complex study design with the help of flowcharts and diagrams. |
| | Include tables for a list of reagents and chemicals, or conditions of analysis, bacterial species, cell types, list of antibodies and their concentrations, primers for PCR, etc. |
| | Use figures to define specific features (clinical, histopathological, or microscopic) to be recognised or melting curves in qRT-PCR, etc. |
| | Randomised control trials require registration and reporting according to CONSORT guidelines. |

anywhere in the world to replicate the study. However, the details should be adequate and not the replica of a laboratory user's manual. This section allows the reader to understand the validity of the study and the results reported in the paper. It is better to write this section in a logical and chronological order.

The first paragraph in this section summarises the overall study design. Sometimes, the study design may have already been described in the introduction if it were unique or different from previous studies. The main body deals with the population characteristics, intervention, measurement of outcome, data analysis, and ethical guidelines followed in the research [4].

The contents of the methods section, along with the guidelines for writing this section are summarised in Table 11.2.

#### 11.4.1.3 Results

This section answers the question—what did you get when you did what you did?

In this section, details are welcome, but some of it may later be moved to supplementary files to fit the word count limit. Three components that need to be used in the results are text, tables, and figures.

One can avoid repetition of data in the text if it is already there in the tables. The synergy between these components makes reading and understanding of the manuscript much easier. The key message of the table and any significant results presented in the tables may be repeated in the text with exact $p$-values mentioned in the brackets (instead of using the generic statement $p < 0.05$). Summary of detailed numerical data is actually better represented in a table than histograms and pie charts.

**Table 11.3** The contents of the results section and guidelines for writing

| Contents | Guidelines for writing |
|---|---|
| • Description of the study subjects and groups with the number of cases recruited followed up to the conclusion of the study, the exclusions etc. This can be represented as a flowchart.<br>• The results of the various measurements made in the methods.<br>• The probability or *p*-values mentioned in brackets as actual *p*-values.<br>• Tables along with footnotes, explanatory notes, and legends.<br>• Figures in various forms: charts, photographs, line diagrams, graphs, or data charts (bar diagrams, scatter plots, pie charts). | Write in the past tense. |
| | Avoid mismatch of numbers in the text tables, and figures. |
| | Keep the methods section handy, so that everything that is listed in the methods is covered in the results. |
| | Avoid interpreting results in this section. |
| | Avoid including results that were not generated by the methods listed in the methods section. |
| | Pay special attention to the tables and graphs; Follow the requirement of journals. |
| | Review the data again and get it peer-reviewed. |

The results section includes the description of study subjects, results of various measurements, the probability or *p*-values, and tables [5]. We have outlined the contents of the result section, along with the guidelines for writing in Table 11.3.

#### 11.4.1.4 Discussion

This section emphasises and puts into perspective the important aspects of the study. Here too, it makes sense to follow the sequence of the results. However, there may be points in the methods that may need to be discussed in terms of pros and cons, or advantages and disadvantages. This section also allows the authors to look and admit retrospectively to the limitations of their own study, acknowledge them, and mention whether any corrective measures were taken by them or can be taken up in a future study. The authors may have a tendency to go overboard with the discussion. This can be limited by the thumb rule that the discussion should not be longer than any other section of the manuscript.

The content of the discussion section should revolve around answering the following questions, in a coherent manner rather than like answering a checklist [6].

- What is the summary of the main results?
- How do your results compare with the results of earlier studies? Be frank and bold enough to show negative results.
- How convincingly have you answered your research question? This should be based on the data available in the literature vis-a-vis, your data.
- What are the strengths of your study? Be modest and avoid exaggeration such as 'for the first time in the world…'
- What are the limitations of your study? All studies have limitations, and there is no harm in admitting honestly.
- What is the generalisability of your study? To what extent?

- What are the implications of your study with respect to adding new knowledge, practice or policy?
- What conclusions can you draw from your study? This usually encapsulates the core findings of the study in just 1–3 sentences.

#### 11.4.1.5 References

Before starting any research work, we recommend that researchers begin creating a list of references in the digital format with the help of software available to manage references. There are many free and paid software available that can make the task of citing references easier. The examples of free ones are *Zotero* and *Mendeley*. They allow the authors to build a reference base from which they may keep adding citations as they type into their manuscript. They all come with user guides and are easy to navigate.

#### 11.4.1.6 Abstract and Title

These two segments are usually written after the entire manuscript is prepared. The abstract is limited by the journal requirements regarding word-limit and structure. The usual length of an abstract is 250 words and is written in a free-flowing manner. However, there are ways of writing a good and complete abstract:

- Highlight the important points in each segment of the manuscript.
- Copy and paste them into a new document; the parts derived from the introduction will go into the background, and so on…
- Read the pasted highlights (words, phrases, and sentences) and string them into complete sentences.
- Read again and cut down to the word-limit.
- Check whether there are any missing results or new results that appear in the abstract but are not there in the manuscript.
- Format according to the instructions to the authors from the journal.
- Always reconfirm after every modification in the prepared manuscript is made whether the abstract still matches it.

### 11.4.2 Conclusions

- It is possible to write and publish effectively provided one follows the rules of the game embedded in the IMRaD format.
- First, write the methods in the past tense.
- Next, compose the figures and tables in the order of the methods.
- Find out the relevance of the results from published literature and discuss them.
- Write the introduction from the review of literature in the inverted pyramid form—starting with the general background and need for study and ending in the statement of aim.

- Compose the abstract by selecting highlights from each section and paring it down to the word-limit.
- Compose the title and title page.
- Format according to the style of the targeted journal.

## 11.5 Evaluate

After reading this chapter, have a look at a scientific manuscript written by you or your colleague. Critically go through if they are according to the IMRaD format? Point out the flaws considering the content of each section and the prescribed guidelines.

## References

1. Trouble at the lab—Unreliable research. The Economist, October 18, 2013.
2. Batmanabane G. The IMRAD structure. In: Sahni P, Aggarwal R, editors. Reporting and publishing research in the biomedical sciences. New Delhi: The National Medical Journal of India; 2015. p. 2–4.
3. Ghoshal UC. The introduction section. In: Sahni P, Aggarwal R, editors. Reporting and publishing research in the biomedical sciences. New Delhi: The National Medical Journal of India; 2015. p. 5–8.
4. Aggarwal A. The methods section. In: Sahni P, Aggarwal R, editors. Reporting and publishing research in the biomedical sciences. New Delhi: The National Medical Journal of India; 2015. p. 10–23.
5. Aggarwal R, Sahni P. The results section. In: Sahni P, Aggarwal R, editors. Reporting and publishing research in the biomedical sciences. New Delhi: The National Medical Journal of India; 2015. p. 24–44.
6. Fletcher RH, Fletcher SW. The discussion section. In: Sahni P, Aggarwal R, editors. Reporting and publishing research in the biomedical sciences. New Delhi: The National Medical Journal of India; 2015. p. 45–57.

# 12 How to Handle General Public, Media, Press, and Very Important Persons

Tashi Tenzin

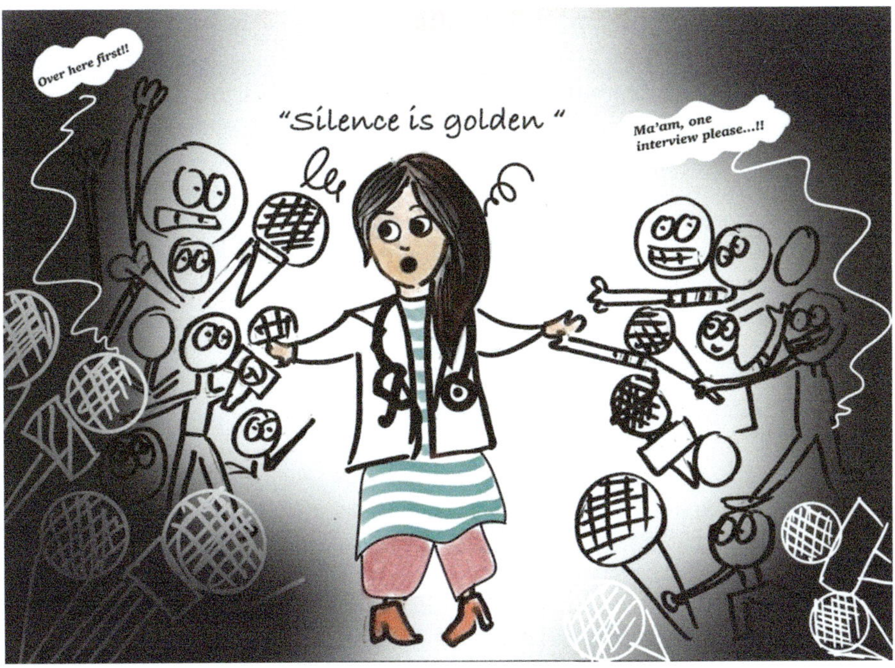


Your customer does not care how much you know until they know how much you care.
—Damon Richards

T. Tenzin (✉)
Faculty of Postgraduate Medicine, Khesar Gyalpo University of Medical Sciences of Bhutan, Thimphu, Bhutan
e-mail: tashitenzin@kgumsb.edu.bt



S. C. Parija, B. V. Adkoli (eds.), *Effective Medical Communication*,
https://doi.org/10.1007/978-981-15-3409-6_12

## 12.1 Assess Need

Globally, healthcare is considered a service industry. Whether it's a public run or private-owned, healthcare centers must have patient centric care at their core. Patients are not alone. Their families and close ones are equally important while providing care to them. Taking care of a patient and their close ones need an empathetic approach in a timely manner. Survival and progress of healthcare companies are based on the quality of care they provide and the daily interactions between staff and patients, other people, and agencies. Therefore, effective communication is the key for successful relationship with others.

Medical centers all over the world face a shortage of trained human resources. Additionally, healthcare organizations in the developing world are criticized for poor communication skills. Most healthcare professionals have inadequate knowledge and skills to handle the general public, the press, the media, and Very Important Persons (VIPs). There is a need for comprehensive policies, guidelines, and standard operating procedures to handle them effectively. Since all employees in a healthcare company are potentially customer service representatives, they need training on attitudes, ethics, and communication. Similarly, the views reported by press and media plays a critical role in determining whether potential patients seek our services in the future.

The standard medical textbooks do not deal with topics on handling the general public, press, media, and VIPs. Lack of dedicated communication and information services lead to erroneous reporting in the press and media. Healthcare providers and institutions are also expected to disseminate information on medical and health-related issues to the community in a professional manner. Effective communication is important routinely and more so at the time of emergencies and crises. Health institutions must move from reactive to proactive communication with the public [1]. Therefore, training on the handling of our customers and visitors needs special focus.

While management and leadership are much more than communication, there is little doubt that communication skills are at the heart of effective leadership [2]. The importance of communication for the success of leadership has been shown throughout history. Winston Churchill had once said, "*the difference between mere management and leadership is communication*." Leadership is said to be action-orientated, not just by virtue of a title or a certain rank [3].

## 12.2 Brief

Objectives of this chapter are:

- To sensitize all healthcare providers, the importance of public relation or customer care principles through good communication skills.
- To set a guideline for clinicians, faculties, managers, and leaders how to deal with the public, media, and VIPs through effective communication.

## 12.3 Contextualize

### 12.3.1 Scenario 1

Dr. Comini is now, a Chief of premier medical institute, meets with a tricky situation of handling media. There was breaking news reporting the death of many babies in its neonatal intensive care unit. The national newspaper blamed the "*lack of infection control*." The hospital management attributed the deaths to premature births of babies who are potentially immune-compromised. The media and public demanded an inquiry. The government assigned an independent investigation team to carry out the outbreak study. The investigation revealed several issues such as managerial lapses, inadequate infection control measures, premature babies, and miscommunication. The media, however, projected the fault of hospital management. This was a challenge for Dr. Comini to convert the problem into an opportunity.

She was tactful to deal with the situation. First, she spent time with the affected families and counseled them on the loss of their babies. Then she conducted a proper press conference, where she brought out the real issue, viz. the lack of staff in critical care which is the root cause of the mishap. In fact, she had repeatedly proposed to the government earlier to recruit more staff in the critical areas like NICU, but her requests had been ignored. Immediately after this episode, the government sanctioned additional staff and resources to prevent the recurrence of such incidences in the future.

***Exercise***: Deliberate how communication skill, like handling press media assumes a great significance in health care institutes, especially in handling disaster preparedness.

## 12.4 Describe

Establishing a healthy relationship with the general public and media is perhaps the most important necessity for an organization in a competitive world. Customer satisfaction is the foremost goal of any service organization. It is all the more important in medical care, where the customer becomes the reason for our existence (Box 12.1).

> **Box 12.1: The Importance of Customer Satisfaction as Portrayed by Mahatma Gandhi**
> A customer is the most important visitor on our premises; he is not dependent on us. We are dependent on him. He is not an interruption in our work. He is the purpose of it. He is not an outsider in our business. He is part of it. We are not doing him a favour by serving him. He is doing us a favour by giving us an opportunity to do so.—Mahatma Gandhi

In the case of health care establishments where the resources are limited, communication errors are more likely to happen because of the interdependence of all units and staff. It is necessary to define certain terms that are relevant to this chapter (Table 12.1).

**Table 12.1** Definition of terms related to media and communication

| Terms | Definition |
|---|---|
| Communication | Communication is a very complex process of sharing information, ideas, and feelings, through the intricate use of a myriad of elements. This includes verbal utterances (words), written or pictured text, graphics, gesticulations, tone, expression, and specific actions to name a few |
| General public | Patients, their families, and other people who are likely to use the services |
| Very important persons | Key stakeholders including member of parliament, elected representative, overseas dignitary, member of the royal family, hospital trustees, board members, prominent physicians, and community leaders, and others as designated by the organization |
| Media and press | Media include print (press), TV channels, and electronic media which takes various forms. With the revolution in information technology media has enlarged its scope even to include social media like portals, websites, blogs, podcasts, WhatsApp, Facebook, Twitter, Instagram, and other mechanisms of sharing information |
| Celebrity | Famous, high profile figure who might be well known to the public and therefore to patients and their families |

### 12.4.1 Guiding Principles

Many well-established organizations have policies and standard operating procedures in place, for handling public and visitors [4]. The guiding principles for communication with the general public, media, press, and VIPs should be:

- clear, open, honest, transparent, and consistent with the vision, mission, and values.
- appropriate for all audiences and written in simple language.
- equally accessible to all.
- facilitating engagement of all audience providing support to overcome barriers to people's involvement.
- well planned, timely, and targeted.
- cost-effective, of high quality, and making the best use of resources.
- innovative and be responsive to change.
- people-friendly, based on trust and treating them as equal partners.
- choosing the right format and use channels and mechanisms that work.
- encouraging feedback from all stakeholders.

### 12.4.2 Handling the General Public

The policies on dealing with public relations today are in place in almost all areas of business. Without a doubt, healthcare being one of the most important areas of social activity, public relation is a must. As it deals with lives at critical times, services are exposed to numerous critics. Therefore, building and maintaining good relationships with every individual will pay huge dividends (Fig. 12.1).

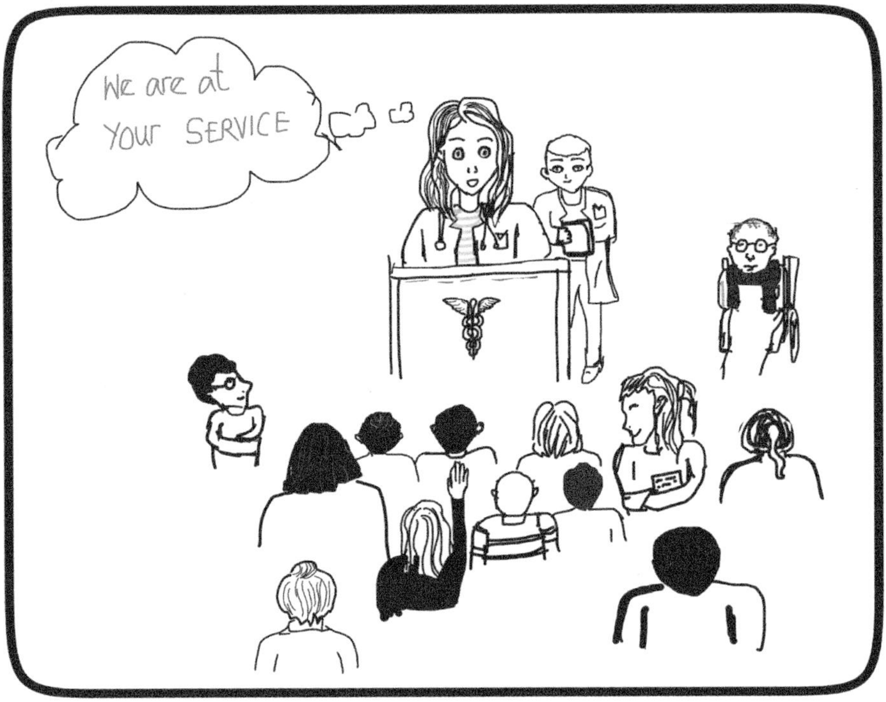


**Fig. 12.1** Chief executive officer briefing the public in a hospital lobby

### 12.4.3 Handling Press and Media

Many organizations allow only designated people to interact with the media. Chief Executive Officer may respond depending on the importance of issues. Other staff may require to seek approval to grant interviews to the media and press. Healthcare centers attract press and media mostly for the wrong reasons. They hardly publish and report good things happening most of the time. One mishap is good enough for casting a negative image of the service. Therefore, it is essential to follow a strict procedure to ensure that calls are handled appropriately. Make sure that you designate only one person on the staff to respond to calls.

#### 12.4.3.1 Tips for Handling the Media

Tips for handling media include the followings [5]:

- Be prepared for the media, both as individuals and as an organization.
- Be familiar with your organization's media policy.
- Understand how the media works and therefore how to handle them.
- Be better prepared for facing media interviews, collect and keep data handy.
- Feel more confident in handling the media; handle it professionally.

- During the interview, allow the press media to seek further clarifications as needed.
- Always thank the interviewer and the media office for the opportunity.

#### 12.4.3.2 Handling a Crisis

Everybody dreads the occurrence of crisis in an organization [5]. It happens in big or small measure. There is no need to get panic. Media may sometimes misquote a statement. During the crisis, it is better to seek sympathy from the media. A healthy relationship with the media helps.

For minor misquote, just call the journalist and explain the problem and get it corrected. If serious damage is likely to be caused to the reputation of the organization, it warrants to take up the issue with the authorities to correct their error. Sometimes, journalists do not admit their mistake for fear of losing their reputation. However, as a leader, you need to intervene, work tactfully in a collaborative approach rather than blaming the media.

During the crisis, it is important to communicate necessary information early to the constituent members, board members, staff, and funders rather than hearing it from the media. It is necessary to work out the best ways to communicate with each group either through letters or phone calls, or an emergency meeting.

### 12.4.4 Handling Celebrity and VIPs

Celebrity and VIP visits play significant role in enhancing the image of any organization. Healthcare centers must have a policy to handle VIPs. To have the celebrities and other VIPs as a patient is a complicated matter. In a situation often referred to as the "*VIP syndrome*," his/her special social or political status and our perceptions of it induces changes in behavior and clinical practice that can lead to poor outcomes [6–10]. To deal with this syndrome effectively it is advisable to follow the following rules:

- Vow to value your medical skills and judgment,
- Have an excellent command over the medical aspects of the situation, and
- Practice medicine in the same way for all your patients.

The visits of celebrities, VIPs, and media representatives must be organized and managed in accordance with the procedures outlined in the policy. We must ensure that there is no risk to the safety and security of patients and staff arising from such visits. All visits by media, VIPs, or celebrities should be handled and managed by the public relation or relevant unit with prior approval of the chief executive. Such visits should always be accompanied throughout their visit to the healthcare center, where there is a possibility of contact with vulnerable patients/visitors.

The policy must outline protocols that should cover preparation before visits, action to be taken during visits and after visits. It must also outline the code of conduct for the employees concerning maintaining the confidentiality and the safety of patients and visitors alike. Before visits, the designated unit may appraise the visitors on the visiting protocols in advance. It is better to identify and arrange a suitable reception area for a briefing to avoid or minimize disruption to the normal functioning of the services. During the visit, ensure that no visitor is left unaccompanied. Staff need to be reminded to behave professionally. They should continue to work in their usual role while supporting the management of the visit. Any concerns raised during the visit must be noted and appreciated. On completion of the visit, visitors must be thanked for the honor and opportunity to serve them (Box 12.2).

**Box 12.2: Active Listening Techniques**

- Use verbal responses like 'really?', 'I see', 'what happened next?'
- Comment directly on what is being said.
- Restate the speaker's ideas in your own words ('do you mean….?').
- Encourage the person to express feelings ('I guess you must have felt…').
- Encourage more information ('tell me about….').
- Don't pass judgment.

### 12.4.5 Communication Modalities

#### 12.4.5.1 Website

Use of well-designed websites is very useful communication tools to reach out to the institute's mission, services, programs, and their messages on health education. The contents should be updated and refreshed regularly.

#### 12.4.5.2 Social Media

Use of social media like Twitter and Facebook for public health messages, campaigns have found a strong place in any business nowadays. It will continue to play a more significant role in reaching out locally and nationally. Feedback provided by patients, the public, and stakeholders through social media channels helps in the course of our future actions. We must take constructive criticism positively and do not react to such posts.

#### 12.4.5.3 Video

The hospitals may use videos on YouTube to tell people about their experiences as patients and to support our public engagements. We may also use videos to explain more about some of our initiatives, health campaigns, and public health educations.

#### 12.4.5.4 Face-to-Face

We may also conduct regular face-to-face communications with stakeholders, patients, and the public through meetings, presentations to key groups, and attending relevant local public events. Public opinions and feedback can be collected even from internal staff meetings [11].

#### 12.4.5.5 Newsletters

Some major health institutes produce bulletins for staff and members. These can be shared with partners and subscribers.

#### 12.4.5.6 Surveys and Questionnaires

Surveys and questionnaires are some of the most effective methods that we can use to gather feedback through both online and in printed format [11]. They help in soliciting continued support from community organizations and the public.

#### 12.4.5.7 Printed Materials

These consist of a range of information leaflets, publicity posters, health messages, newsletters, annual reports, and other documents. They can be widely distributed to promote services, invite people to give their feedback, or explain ways in which they can get involved to promote the institute's achievements and future plans. The printed materials can be made available in other formats, translated into other languages to ensure they reach all audiences.

### 12.4.6 Core Communication Skills for Leaders: The Need for Training

There are various ways of categorizing core communication skills. The literature includes active and passive listening skills, which are beyond the scope of this chapter. However, what is important to highlight here is the need for training the young doctors in preparing themselves for their future roles. Such training can be informally imparted through CME activities, mock drill activities, etc., or included as a part of the undergraduate curriculum in communication training.

### 12.4.7 Conclusion

The healthcare is a service industry and effective communication with patients, their families, the general public, press, media, and VIPs is a key factor for a good relation. Therefore policies, guidelines, protocols, and standard operating procedures must be in place for handling our patients, their families, media, and VIPs. Our future healthcare systems must excel not only in clinical care but also in leadership with good communication skills. The universities and healthcare institutes need to go beyond routine medical curricula to focus on promoting the importance of not only competent clinicians but also great managers and leaders.

## 12.5 Evaluate

After reading this chapter, reflect on a recent incidence of a tussle between the public and the service facility. What factors triggered this problem? What was the role of media played in this episode either to flare up the problem or to resolve it? What lessons did you learn from this episode?

## References

1. Tomic Z, Lasic D, Tomic T. Public relations in health care. Mater Sociomed. 2010;22(1):25–7.
2. Miller, P. Leadership Communication—the three levels. Singapore Institute of Management Today's Manager; 2012. p. 19–21. https://www.researchgate.net/publication/254664129.
3. Bennis W, Goldsmith J. Learning to lead: workbook on becoming leader. Reading: Perseus Books/Adison Wesley; 1997. Not in Vancouver
4. Leeds West Clinical Commissioning Group. Communications, engagement and equality and diversity strategy. 2015–2017. https://www.leedsccg.nhs.uk/content/uploads/2014/.../IFI12.-CommsStrategy2015.
5. Judith B. How to talk to the media—make the most of every media opportunity in press, radio and television. London: How to Books Ltd; 2000.
6. Smith MS, Sesser RF. The emergency care of the VIP patient. N Engl J Med. 1988;319(21):1421–3.
7. Block AJ. Beware of the VIP syndrome. Chest. 1993;104(4):989.
8. Mariano EC, McLeod JA. Emergency care for the VIP patient. Intensive care medicine Berlin: Springer; 2007. https://doi.org/10.1007/978-0-387-49518-7_88. Accessed 27 Dec 2010.
9. Schenkenberg T, Kochenour NK, Botkin JR. Ethical considerations in clinical care of the "VIP". J Clin Ethics. 2007;18:56–63.
10. Weintraub W. "The VIP syndrome": a clinical study in hospital psychiatry.1964. J Nerv Ment Dis. 2012;200(6):457–69.
11. Black, J. Five steps to delivering effective employee feedback. 2009. http://articlet.com/article2549.html. (Retrieved June 15, 2009)

# 13 Social Media and Medical Education: Issues, Influences, and Impact

Anshu

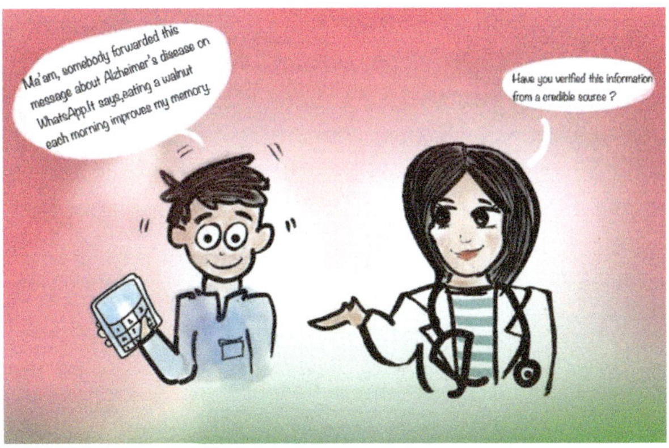


We need to pro-actively embrace social media to engage with patients and other stakeholders, build collaborative networks, and disseminate correct information.—Anshu

---

Anshu (✉)
Department of Pathology, Mahatma Gandhi Institute of Medical Sciences, Wardha, Maharashtra, India


S. C. Parija, B. V. Adkoli (eds.), *Effective Medical Communication*, https://doi.org/10.1007/978-981-15-3409-6_13

## 13.1 Assess Need

Social media seems to have infiltrated every walk of our lives. It is impossible to stay immune from its powerful impact. Like every other sphere of life, the world of medicine too has been influenced in several ways. There are two main areas where social media affects us:

First, the way our patients gather information about their health has completely changed. Information on almost every disease is easily accessible on the internet. Every person has the opportunity to gather information and ask questions. Some of these information are correct. Unfortunately, not everything that comes our way via social media is accurate. In view of this scenario, are health professionals prepared to communicate with patients differently and combat the misinformation? Are there issues of professionalism which arise on social networks?

Secondly, the way we learn and communicate within the health professions community has drastically altered. Books are no longer the only means of learning. Online resources and social media platforms are available on the go, and can be accessed at the bedside. How is the learning from these resources different from textbook learning? Also, are teachers adequately prepared to deal with this new generation of digital learners?

The infiltration of the social media can be both a boon and a bane in the health professions context.

## 13.2 Brief

This chapter will address the following key issues:

- What is the impact of social media on the manner in which patients gather health-related information and make decisions about their health? How do clinicians need to adapt to this changing scenario?
- How does the millennial generation of medical students learn differently? How do teachers need to adapt to this digital generation of learners and use social media to their advantage?
- What are the issues related to professionalism that can arise on social networks?

## 13.3 Contextualize

### 13.3.1 Scenario 1

A nervous 25-year-old woman visits her gynecologist. She says: "*I have spotting between my periods. I looked at Google last night and it says, it could be cancer…*" Her busy doctor is irritated and interrupts her, "*Listen, I am the doctor, not Dr. Google. Can you simply list your symptoms, and let me decide what you have?*"

***Exercise***: Reflect for a minute on the response given by the doctor. Do you subscribe to his views? How would you have dealt with this situation?

### 13.3.2 Scenario 2

At the dining table in the mess of a medical college hostel, there is talk of a rare case of progeria being admitted in the Pediatrics ward. A group of medical students visits the ward in the evening to see the patient. One of the students clicks a picture of the child on his phone, and posts it on a closed group of medical students, in order to discuss the case. The next morning someone forwards it to a friend outside the group, this time with a new tagline, calling the child, the real *Paa*, referring to a popular movie theme. Soon, the case is forwarded on several social groups, and goes viral. Layer by layer, more information is added, not all correct. The parents of the child find out and are dismayed at this invasion into their privacy and at this breach of confidentiality. They bring this up with Dr. Comini in the Pediatrics ward. The case is investigated and the medical student who clicked the picture is summoned for an explanation.

***Exercise***: What is the root cause of this whole "*mess*"? What action needs to be taken to prevent such problems?

## 13.4 Describe

### 13.4.1 Impact of Social Media on Health Seeking Behavior and its Influence in the Clinical Context

Every individual has the right to seek information about their personal health. With changing times and easy access, patients have begun to explore health-related information on the internet. In earlier times the practice of medicine was quite paternalistic, and patients depended upon doctors to diagnose, and make decisions related to their health. However, patients have the right to know about their health condition so that a process of shared decision-making can be initiated.

The problem arises because some online resources are verified and peer-reviewed by subject experts, while others are simply opinions with no evidence base. The inability to distinguish wheat from chaff creates problems for both doctors and patients. Patients come from all kinds of cultural and educational backgrounds, and have different concerns. Doctors need to be able to gauge their concerns, listen carefully, and give them adequate time. Clinicians need to be able to clarify questions that patients raise, and also convince them about the choices available at their disposal. Counseling and communication skills need to be given adequate weightage during the training of medical students. Acquiring this competency is integral to every clinician's training [1].

The second opportunity that the health profession has, is to share correct health information with patients and communities in an efficient manner. It is essential that this is done pro-actively, and all forms of misinformation are strongly combated. Medical organizations, peer-reviewed journals, and subject experts all need to have prominent presence in the social media, and present a credible face for the medical profession.

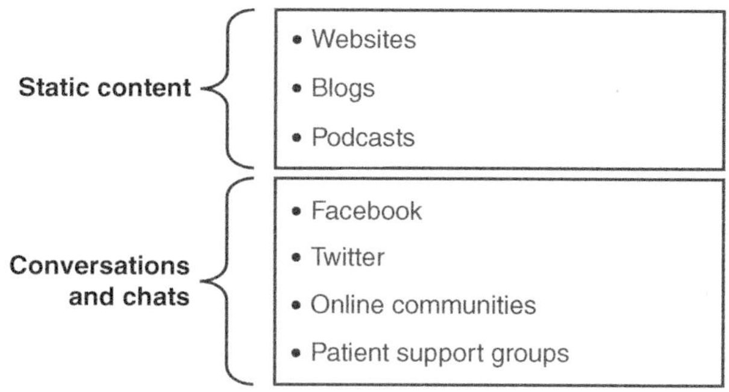


**Fig. 13.1** List of the methods for dissemination of information through social media

This information can be disseminated through the social media in two ways:

a. The first is through static content like websites, blogs, and podcasts. The information distilled in these sites needs to be in patient friendly language, and devoid of jargon.
b. The second is through conversations and chats happening on social media sites such as Facebook and Twitter. Building communities of patients or support groups for parents or caregivers is another way to build engagement. These days user-friendly apps have also made an appearance where health experts are available to converse with people, and guide them about their health (Fig. 13.1).

Both these ways are important to engage with patients, communities, and other key stakeholders such as the media. These open approaches also go a long way in reducing some degree of hostility and mistrust that the doctor community presently faces from society.

### 13.4.2 Impact of Social Media on the Learning of the Millennial Generation

The students of the millennial generation have been described by Marc Prensky as the *digital natives*, while teachers have been called *digital immigrants* [2]. He feels that these learners are used to receiving and processing information really fast and multitasking. However, students need to be taught how to identify credible sources of information which are peer-reviewed and distinguish them from opinions, which might not necessarily be scientific.

Social media has changed the way health professionals themselves access information. While often one is confronted with trivial content, if used judiciously these networks can be very promising platforms to facilitate knowledge transfer. Experts have the opportunity to share their knowledge with wider audiences. There are more opportunities to collaborate and expand our understanding of medicine. Most journals have a presence on social media these days where they disseminate key reports. This makes things easier, as not everyone is able to keep up with the exponential rise in medical

**Table 13.1** Advantages and disadvantages of social media

| Advantages of social media | Disadvantages of social media |
|---|---|
| 1. When used judiciously, can facilitate knowledge transfer | 1. Difficult to sift wheat from chaff. Not all information is credible |
| 2. Experts can share their knowledge with wider audiences | 2. Information which is not peer-reviewed is of lesser validity |
| 3. Key findings of important journals can be disseminated | 3. Curtailed reports with condensed word limits are prone to misinterpretation |
| 4. Useful for continuing professional development: Easier to keep up with scientific updates | 4. Useful only when one has basic foundation and knowledge of the subject |
| 5. Second opinions and consultations from experts possible | |

literature. By following RSS (Rich Site Summary) feeds, podcasts, blogs, and other networks it is possible to keep updated. This is particularly useful once one steps out of medical school for continuing professional development. When one needs a consultation from another expert, online methods of communication within the profession make life easier. Almost every specialty has closed groups on social media where complicated cases and diagnostic dilemmas are thrashed out daily. Such forums shrink the world and make latest advances accessible to health professionals working in remote areas. The advantages of social media have been listed in Table 13.1.

However, it must be remembered that this territory comes with its own problems. Receiving short, curtailed reports with fixed word limits can be prone to misinterpretation. Blogs which are not peer-reviewed have lesser validity than those which have undergone some form of peer review. There are others who argue that these methods work when students have a strong foundation of knowledge. Therefore, in the early stages of training, learning basic concepts from textbooks is mandatory for better understanding of any subject.

Prensky argues that the present generation of learners are no longer the people that our educational system was designed to teach [3]. They have access to various forms of digital learning, and the traditional classroom approaches need to change. Dreary lectures are clearly not the best way to engage learners. Teachers need to think of newer student-centric methods to capture the attention of this digital generation. The flipped classroom approach is being advocated by many educators [4]. The flipped classroom is an educational model where students are assigned didactic study content before they come to class. The time in the classroom is used for more active learning strategies. Such asynchronous and distributed learning formats are possible with the use of technology.

Not all faculty will find it easy to adapt to these changes immediately and there will be quite a learning curve. As Roger's law of diffusion of innovations predicts, some faculty will be quicker to adopt innovations than others. Faculty development and hand-holding will be essential for teachers to change their teaching strategies. However, sooner rather than later, educators will need to pull up their socks and reach out to learners.

Prensky points out that this generation of learners is differently wired and come with a very different set of cognitive skills compared to their predecessors. He says that in their quest for speed, they find less and less time for reflection. Where teachers can help, is by giving them more and more opportunities for reflection and critical thinking.

### 13.4.3 Social Media and Professionalism

This generation of learners needs to be taught about the problems that can arise with the social networks. Students need to be oriented and explicitly taught internet etiquette. Social networks are public platforms. All ethical principles need to be followed and professionalism needs to be maintained irrespective of what is shared online. The rules of online behavior remain the same as offline behavior.

The Mayo Clinic has shared a 12-word social policy which went viral [5] (Box 13.1). It clearly tells social media users the risks of being careless and callous online, since errors are magnified and quickly disseminated to a global audience. It underlines the need to maintain patient and institutional confidentiality, and remember the rules of privacy, consent, and professional behavior.

**Box 13.1 Mayo Clinic 12-Word Social Media Policy**

Don't Lie, Don't Pry
Don't Cheat, Can't Delete
Don't Steal, Don't Reveal

### 13.4.4 Conclusion

- Social media is here to stay. There is no way we can ignore it. We have entered an era where the traditional confines of the clinic or the classroom have been demolished. Ideas and information are derived from our interconnectedness with the rest of the world.
- It is important that the health professions community adapts technology at the earliest to its advantage. It can be used to engage with patients and the community, to disseminate correct information, and to keep abreast with the latest.
- For this to happen, both clinicians and faculty need to be quick to adopt technology and engage with patients and learners, respectively.

## 13.5 Evaluate

Having read this chapter think of any episode of misuse of social media by a medical personnel in your campus. Suggest in what manner one can take preventive measures to avoid such a problem from recurring.

## References

1. Anshu, Singh T. The art of talking to patients. In: Patwari AK, Sachdev HPS, editors. Frontiers in Social Pediatrics. 2nd ed. New Delhi: Jaypee Brothers Medical Publishers Ltd.; 2016. p. 199–210.
2. Prensky M. Digital natives, digital immigrants: Part 1. On the Horizon. 2001;9(5):1–6. https://doi.org/10.1108/10748120110424816.
3. Prensky M. Digital natives, digital immigrants: Part 2: do they really think differently? On the Horizon. 2001;9(6):1–6. https://doi.org/10.1108/10748120110424843.
4. Anshu. Is it time to shift to flipped classrooms? AHPE Bull. 2018;3(1):3–4. http://ahpe.in/is-it-time-to-shift-to-flipped-classrooms-dr-anshu/.
5. Leibtag A. A 12-word social media policy. Mayo Clinic Social Media Network; 2012. https://socialmedia.mayoclinic.org/2012/04/05/a-twelve-word-social-media-policy/.

# 14 Language Skills in Research Paper Writing

Balachandra V. Adkoli and Subhash Chandra Parija

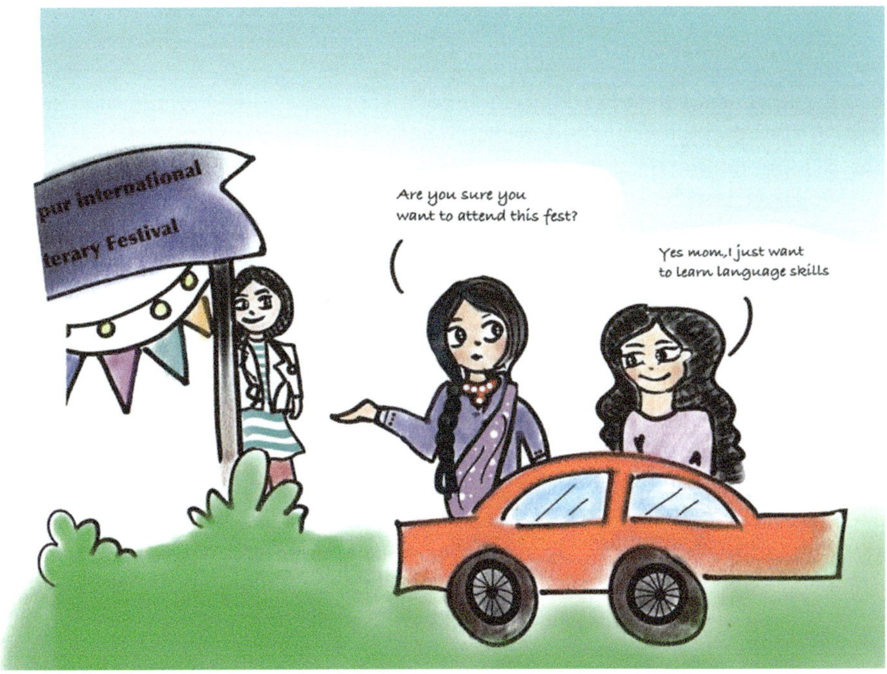


Language does matter in scientific communication—Adkoli and Parija

B. V. Adkoli (✉)
Centre for Health Professions Education, Sri Balaji Vidyapeeth (Deemed-to-be University), Pondicherry, India
e-mail: balachandraa@mgmcri.ac.in

S. C. Parija
Sri Balaji Vidyapeeth (Deemed-to-be University), Pondicherry, India



S. C. Parija, B. V. Adkoli (eds.), *Effective Medical Communication*,
https://doi.org/10.1007/978-981-15-3409-6_14

## 14.1 Assess Need

Scientific communication is a blend of scientific facts presented in a language that everyone can understand and appreciate. Experts claim that an effectively written research paper is more about a story, and not a study [1]. In fact, one of the virtues discussed in conducting research points to telling the story in a cohesive manner, which depends upon a powerful and skillful use of language [2].

Language is one of the major barriers to the growth of science and its dissemination to the public. A study reported from Bangladesh indicates that language is a barrier that affects the health service of the country [3].

Researchers in medical sciences are facing a stiff competition of publishing or perish [4]. The higher the impact factor of a journal, higher the rejection rate. Under such situation, poor language can affect the chances of acceptance. In fact, the research publication in natural sciences has been dominated by metropolises as reported by the journal *Nature* [5]. We hear about the stories of many dedicated researchers whose papers are referred back for resubmission after polishing the language of the paper.

Language is a valuable addition to enrich your paper. Just because of poor language, your paper will not be knocked down. However, poor language can irritate the editor to return your paper for resubmission. Mastering language skill is an asset for the rapid growth of a researcher or scientist.

Many journals and publishing houses have also started language services to enhance the readability of papers, often with additional charges. Courses are also available for enhancing editing skills [6]. However, they are expensive and may not ensure your full involvement to express what you really want to express.

Recognizing the need for promoting skills in scientific writing, a large number of individuals and organizations have started training their faculty in this area. However, the focus of such workshops is on improving the scientific quality of a paper. Not much of published information is available on improving the language component. Most of the writers from non-English speaking countries face problems in getting their articles accepted for publication in international journals, mainly due to poor use of language. We, therefore, wish to address this issue and offer some practical tips by way of citing examples. We hope the research workers, especially from non-English speaking countries, will benefit from this chapter.

## 14.2 Brief

In this chapter, we argue that:

- Language by itself is not a major criterion for acceptance of your paper. However, a paper with rich scientific content but poor language can eliminate the chances of publication.
- One needs to master the rules of the game.
- Self-review and peer feedback are vital instruments for enhancing the language as well as the quality of the article.

## 14.3 Contextualize

### 14.3.1 Scenario

This is a story of Dr. EF (English fan), who recently returned from Oxford University. Dr. EF was invited as a Guest Speaker in a rural medical college in India to address the students on high blood pressure. Being strongly influenced by the richness of English and its accent, he started by telling *"Hi, guys the most enchanting physiological phenomenon which is surmounted by complicated human dynamics affecting innumerable systems, impinging upon the human generation in all spheres of life, including biological, social, economic, and even anthropological dimensions of life is hypertension. Many call it as blood pressure, without understanding either the hemodynamic of blood or an in-depth insight into the ramification of thermostatic pressure…blab…blab…blab."*

Slides after slides rolled out. Dr. EF went on with his flow of choicest words. Most of the students looked blank but did not dare to stop him. However, Ms. Comini, sitting in the last row, who came from a non-English medium school, stood up and asked Sir, can you speak in English Sir? Dr. EF was spell bound. He got a real taste of what high blood pressure is!

***Exercise***: Study the scenario and analyze the root cause of this problem.

## 14.4 Describe

### 14.4.1 Language Is a Value Addition

To be accepted for publication, one needs to follow a structured format decided by the journal policy. In addition, there are several factors, such as handling an ethical issue, the originality of the contribution, its applicability, utility, and reproducibility of results. Besides, there are technical aspects like IMRaD structure, graphic representation of data, statistical analysis, and bibliographic style, which are important. All these collectively decide the fate of a manuscript. Nevertheless, it is the language of the manuscript which plays important role in making the submission acceptable to the editor or the reviewers.

It is indeed difficult to separate language component from the content of a scientific paper, as they are interwoven. What editors want is clarity of message, accuracy in presenting the information, and to some excitement or "*wow factor*" to make the paper interesting to the readers. The language should aid in making an impact on the readers. It should be coherent and efficient in terms of economy of words.

### 14.4.2 Master the Rules of the Game

Most scientific papers have a fixed sequence starting with Title to Abstract, Introduction, Methods (sometimes Materials and Methods), Results, Discussion, Conclusions (often recommendations for further research), and References.

However, a beginner will be more comfortable in writing methods section, followed by other sections—Results, Discussion, and Conclusion, Introduction, Abstract, and Title in that order (Fig. 14.1). The reader will find a more detailed account of the sequencing and organization in another chapter on 'How to publish ethically and effectively'. We will not repeat those details but offer a summary in the form of tips (Table 14.1).

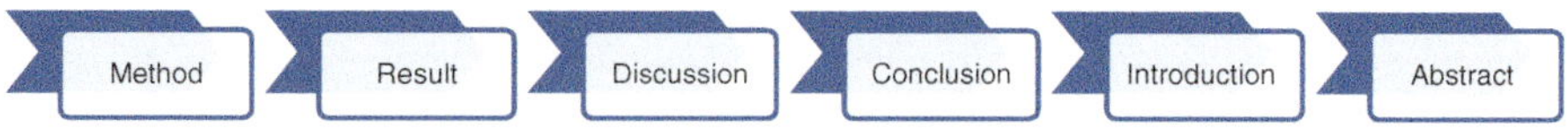


**Fig. 14.1** The order in which a manuscript is to be written

**Table 14.1** Components of various sections of a paper and tips for writing

| Section | Broad components involved | Tips for writing |
|---|---|---|
| Methodology | Involves ethical issues, tools designed or borrowed, how are they administered, how the data were collected and analyzed | Narrate as per the sequence in which they were done (moving through times)<br>Use past tense and preferably active voice |
| Results | This involves the presentation of data mostly in tabular or graphic form | Your text should only supplement the data avoiding repetition. Here, you will use mostly present tense<br>Go on writing research question-wise |
| Discussion | Summary of your findings,<br>How they are similar or different from others' findings, comment on your methods used, their strengths and limitations; make recommendations for further research | Begin with a summary of what all you did, using which method and what did you find.<br>Compare and contrast your results with others<br>Do not extrapolate or over-generalize your findings. Be neutral and modest in reporting results irrespective of whether they are positive or negative. Be reflective and self-critical. Support your statements with facts and figures drawn from your review of the literature<br>Discussion section involves both past tense and present tense, at times even future tense |
| Introduction | Birds'eye of the context in which research problem is embedded;<br>What is already known and what is unknown<br>How you will tackle the problem<br>Defining the objectives and scope of the study | Use "*helicopter approach*." Start with some broad, general statements to place your study in the present context of research or practice. Narrow down gradually to your actual study by defining the study aims, and objectives and research questions. Define your study population, sampling framework, and how that is decided |
| Abstract | Mostly based on IMRAD structure<br>Structured or sometimes unstructured according to the journal's policies | Tailor your abstract strictly according to the requirement of the journal. Use words economically and effectively. Do not crossword count limit.<br>Generate and list keywords keeping in mind the utility of your study |

#### 14.4.2.1 Appropriate Use of Past Tense, Present Tense, and Future Tense

Appropriate use of past tense, present tense, and future tense appears to be a problematic issue for many postgraduate residents when they write their dissertations. This is usually due to the fact that the residents submit their research protocols stating "*what will be done*", and later they copy-paste the same text while submitting their research dissertations. Care should be taken to avoid this mistake.

The methods section is invariably written in the past tense.

For example:

"*We obtained ethical clearance from the Institute Ethics Committee. In order to answer our research question, we chose to apply a quasi-experimental design.*"

"*Renuka et al. (2008) reported that the practice of Yoga benefitted nursing students in reducing stress.*"

The results section may require a mix of past tense and present tense.

For example:

"*The results of the analysis of variance clearly show the effectiveness of the treatment A over the treatment B.*" (Present tense) OR "*The analysis of variance showed a higher degree of effectiveness of the treatment A over the treatment B. However the values were not statistically significant.*" (Past tense)

The discussion section is generally written using the present tense.

For example:

"*There are many studies to support our findings.*"

"*Based on the study findings, we conclude that the practice of Yoga benefits nursing students in reducing stress.*"

However, the last part of the discussion section may involve the use of future tense.

"*Further research using multi-centric studies will prove whether the practice of Yoga can benefit nursing students in reducing stress.*"

#### 14.4.2.2 Use of Active Voice Vs Passive Voice

Most of the scientific literature in the South Asian context is found in the passive voice. However, the current trend is to use the active voice (Table 14.2).

### 14.4.3 Four Common Problems Faced in the Language

#### 14.4.3.1 Repetition

Some authors tend to repeat the same information in graphic form and text form, which is not a good practice in scientific writing. Reinforcement is needed only in

**Table 14.2** The use of passive voice and active voice

| Passive voice | Active voice |
|---|---|
| In the beginning, a detailed medical history of each subject was taken. All the subjects were then subjected to detailed intervention. A sudden increase was noticed after the intervention in many of the physiological parameters. | We took a detailed history of each subject. We then subjected them to detailed intervention. We noticed a sudden increase in many of the physiological parameters, after the intervention. |

**Table 14.3** An example of a repetitive statement

| Poor | Better |
|---|---|
| We calculated the body mass index of each person using the formula. For this purpose, we used a simple mathematical calculation involving two variables, viz. person's height and weight. The scientifically proven, standard formula which we used was BMI = kg/ $m^2$ where BMI is body mass index, kg is a person's weight in kilograms and $m^2$ is their height of the person in meters, squared. | We calculated body mass index by dividing a person's weight in kg by height in meters, squared. |

**Table 14.4** Examples of too long sentences; see how they can look better

| Poor | Better |
|---|---|
| In order to find out the difference in the effect of treatment between the outcome variable and the dependent variable, we also conducted a statistical analysis so that the difference becomes crystal clear. | We compared the treatment effect on the outcome variable and the dependent variable. |
| There is a broad consensus among scientists with respect to the statement that air pollution is a significant source of lung disease. | Air pollution is a significant source of lung disease. |
| Our study was aimed at making a careful assessment of the extent of anemia among the school going children who were admitted and studying in the schools situated in the Union Territory of Puducherry. | We assessed the prevalence of anemia among the school going children of Puducherry. |
| When the investigator probed the history of this patient who was 50 year about his spouse, he suddenly burst into tears stating that she had died in a road traffic accident last year, which appears to be the main cause of his depression, as has also been reported by previous studies. | We took the history of a 50-year-old male. When we enquired about his spouse, he suddenly burst into tears. She had indeed died in a road traffic accident last year. Since then, he appears to have gone into depression. A similar case has also been reported. |

teaching. A common pitfall noticed in scientific papers is the tendency to repeat the contents of the result section in the discussion section to re-emphasize the points. This can dilute the quality of your writing rather than improving the same. However, in order to reinforce the key message of an article, it may be necessary to write a brief summary. Some examples of repetition have been cited in Table 14.3.

### 14.4.3.2 Redundancy (Verbiage)

Redundancy refers to the use of language, which is unnecessary. It is called verbiage (in sync with garbage!). Long sentences are difficult to grasp. Often we notice long sentences, assuming that the readers would be impressed by the flowery language. It is not true. On the contrary, long sentences cause difficulty in comprehending. Besides, you are also wasting paper. A sentence consisting of a maximum of 8–10 words should be all right. A sentence consisting of more than 20 words should be avoided. We have shown some examples of long sentences and how they can be trimmed in Table 14.4. The last example in this table shows how you can break a long sentence into 3–4 short sentences to make it simple to understand.

**Table 14.5** Examples of ambiguous statements; you can make them unambiguous

| Poor | Better |
|---|---|
| Drinking lassi reduces heart disease. | Drinking one glass of lassi per day reduces the incidence of heart attacks in Indian males over 50—A cross-sectional study |
| The patients were asked to go to the lab for further necessary investigation. | The patients were directed to go to central lab (room no. 5) for lipid profile. |
| We conducted all the required tests, including physical examination, mental health assessment, etc., etc., for a detailed data collection. | We conducted mental health assessment using a Likert scale developed by Adkoli [1]. |

#### 14.4.3.3 Ambiguity

Ambiguity means lack of precision or accuracy of communication. There is no place for ambiguity in scientific communication. The title of the study should be comprehensive. Check out the following examples given in Table 14.5.

**Use of Punctuation**

Punctuation marks are the hallmarks of a good language. Wrong placement of a punctuation mark can distort the meaning which we want to convey.

See this example: "*A woman without her man is nothing*."

You wanted to convey that "*A woman: without her, man is nothing*"!

**Caution while using spell-check!**

Nowadays, everyone types text and relies on the spell-check application to correct the mistakes. However, at times, this habit can be dangerous as the software may not be able to decipher the correct alternative. See the following sentences which were twisted by the spell-check software.

A sentence "*Experiment was done in two fases*," got corrected as "*Experiment was done in two faces*"(instead of phases)! "*Breast feading*" was corrected as "*breast fading*" instead of breastfeeding!

The moral of the story is that human intervention is needed to check after the spell-check.

#### 14.4.3.4 Exaggeration

The authors of many scientific papers tend to exaggerate their findings, thinking that they are the pioneers in the field. On the contrary, such claims are not only egoistic but often far from the truth. See this statement.

"*We are reporting for the first time in the world that music therapy certainly reduces depression.*"

A modest way of telling the same is "*To the best of our knowledge, the evidence of the positive effect of music therapy on depression has not been reported in the literature (2000–2017)*."

### 14.4.4 Role of Self-Review and Peer Feedback

The role of feedback from peer scientists as well as lay public holds the key for enriching the quality of a paper. It has been cited as an important tip for the researchers [7].

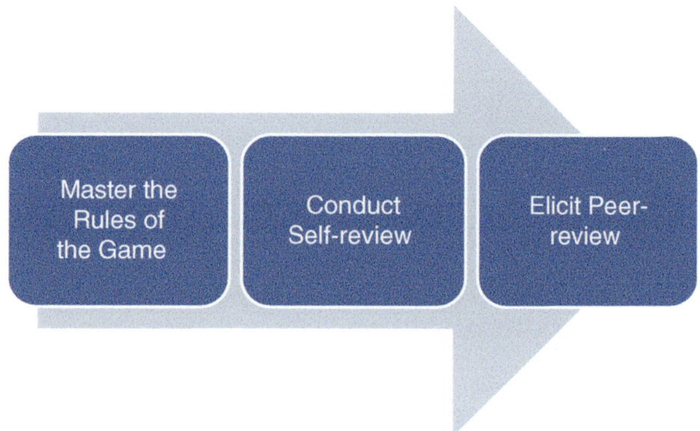


**Fig. 14.2** Three-point formula to enhance your language skills

Self-review of a write up after a gap of few days results in a magical improvement. This technique not only helps in improving sentence construction but also in reorganizing contents in a logical manner. Many writers prefer to do this exercise a week after a paper is written. While doing a self- review, it is better to check one aspect at a time. For example, check only sub-headings throughout the document for their uniformity in font size and style.

There is nothing like peer review in enhancing language quality. Those who are the potential target population are best suited for picking up your lapses. In fact, you will be benefitted by an ardent critique rather than a beloved friend. Consulting a language specialist can also help in polishing your manuscript. Self-review and peer review combined with the mastery of rules of the game constitutes a three-point formula for acquiring language skills (Fig. 14.2).

The problem in our setting is that most writers are hesitant to show it to their colleagues fearing criticism or chances of plagiarism. Often the colleagues are not sincere to give a balanced picture. This is owing to the lack of "*feedback culture*." There is an urgent need for the leaders to promote and support a feedback culture in which critiquing plays a major role. The habit of giving constructive feedback rather than making it a 'fault-finding exercise' is vital for achieving effective language skill. Language services on payment basis have started mushrooming everywhere. Many journals have started providing language services at a cost. This may relieve a researcher's burden to some extent. However, we strongly recommend that the researcher should try to do on his own so that he is able to express clearly what he wants to express.

### 14.4.5 Conclusion

- Language is a major barrier in research publication.
- While language cannot replace the importance of content, it is an important value addition.

- Language skill is not a genetic attribute; it can be learnt by everyone.
- Master the rules of the game.
- Encourage self-review, feedback, and constructive criticism from colleagues or potential readers.

## 14.5 Evaluate

Let us have an exercise or rather fun. Just browse again the rules of the game which you studied in this article. Write down for each rule, a wrong example, and its correct version. Share with your colleague over a cup of coffee. If he/she agrees you will enjoy more!

## References

1. Lingard L, Watling C. It's a story, not a study: writing an effective research paper. Acad Med. 2016;91(12):e12. https://doi.org/10.1097/ACM.0000000000001389.
2. O'Brien BC, Balmer DF, Maggio LA. Finding our way through shades of gray: 6 virtues to guide researchers in planning, conducting, and writing up research. J Grad Med Educ. 2017;9(5):555–9. https://doi.org/10.4300/JGME-D-17-00546.1.
3. Bhuiyan BA, Urmi IJ, Chowdhury ME, Rahman T, Hasan AS, Simkhada P. Assessing whether medical language is a barrier to receiving healthcare services in Bangladesh: an exploratory study. BJGP Open. 2019;3(2):1–9. https://doi.org/10.3399/bjgpopen18X101641. pii: bjgpopen18X101641.
4. Publish or perish. Nature. 2010;467(7313):252. https://doi.org/10.1038/467252a.
5. Mallapaty S. Metropolis of minds. Nature. 2017;550(7676):S157. https://doi.org/10.1038/550S157a.
6. Barreto SG. Editing for language and avoiding ambiguity in data presentation. In: Parija SC, Kate V, editors. Thesis writing for Master's and Ph.D. program, vol. 201. Singapore: Springer Nature Singapore Pte Ltd; 2018. p. 199–206. https://doi.org/10.1007/978-981-13-0890-1_18.
7. Dubé CE, Lapane KL. Lay abstracts and summaries: writing advice for scientists. J Cancer Educ. 2014;29(3):577–9. https://doi.org/10.1007/s13187-013-0570-1.

# Part IV

# For Leaders: Can't Go Wrong!

# Communication Skills for Organizing Workshops

# 15

Subhash Chandra Parija and Balachandra V. Adkoli

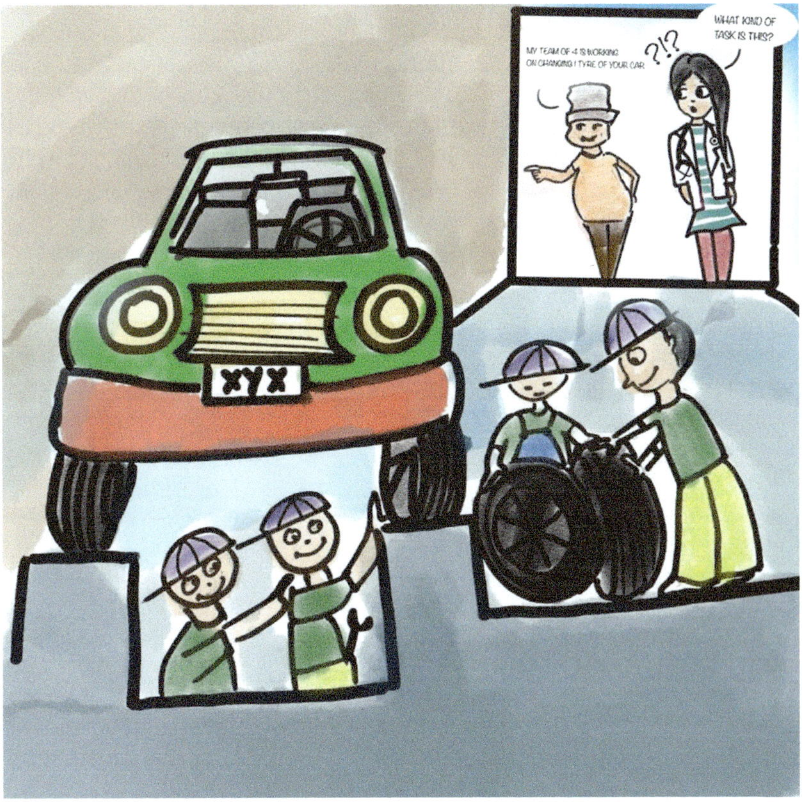


Communication skill assumes a great significance while organizing a workshop —Parija and Adkoli

S. C. Parija (✉)
Sri Balaji Vidyapeeth (Deemed-to-be University), Pondicherry, India

B. V. Adkoli
Centre for Health Professions Education, Sri Balaji Vidyapeeth (Deemed-to-be University), Pondicherry, India





S. C. Parija, B. V. Adkoli (eds.), *Effective Medical Communication*,
https://doi.org/10.1007/978-981-15-3409-6_15

## 15.1 Assess Need

With the growing emphasis on Faculty Development Programs (FDP), workshops have become a necessity rather than a luxury. Though FDPs can be offered in a number of ways, there is nothing like conducting a workshop. Workshop is one of the most useful innovations by educationists. Because, it engages the participants in active learning through hands-on experience, which is the fundamental principle of adult learning. In a workshop format, one cannot simply sit back, relax, and walk away with a certificate as it often happens in case of most Continuing Medical Education (CME) activities. One has to toil, engage in a group activity, or a hands-on experience for a successful completion of a workshop.

The quality of a workshop depends upon a large number of factors such as quality of resource persons, ambience, infrastructure, facilities, equipment, scientific content, or even the hospitality extended. However, effective communication between the organizers and the participants, or in between the organizers themselves can be a deciding factor. Instead of inquiring what went right or what went wrong after the completion of workshop, it is wiser to plan in advance, anticipate problems, and take precaution to avoid such faults. Unfortunately, specific guidelines are not available and most organizers learn by trial and error method. We therefore explored this area of felt need of the day.

## 15.2 Brief

In this chapter we attempt to:

- Identify the communication challenges involved at various stages of organizing a workshop which hamper its quality.
- Offer suggestions for overcoming these hurdles.
- Recommend measures for conducting a high-quality workshop.

## 15.3 Contextualize

### 15.3.1 Scenario

Dr. GP, a top-notch researcher with three decades of experience was happy when he was nominated by Dr. Comini, as the organizing secretary for conducting a workshop on Objective Structured Clinical Examination (OSCE) for the faculty of eight medical colleges in his State. Dr. GP believed in himself and did all planning single handed. The venue chosen was a clinical skill lab of the college, situated on the fifth floor of the main building. Being a senior faculty member he issued circular to various clinical departments to come prepared for running the various OSCE stations.

The student volunteers were also strictly instructed to come in time. He ordered the clinical faculty to send in all 25 cases (patients) to be recruited for demonstrating various skill stations. Dr. GP also invited the health minister to inaugurate the workshop in style in presence of public and press media.

The trouble began on the day of the workshop:

1. There was a big power failure in the concerned building, affecting the lift operation. The only mechanic who was supposed to be highly competent person was out of station on leave.
2. Dr. GP immediately shifted the venue depending upon the immediate availability. However, the new venue happened to be a store room which had no furniture or facilities to organize OSCE stations.
3. The patients who attended OPD on that day were mostly pregnant mothers or sick children. Those who were actually needed were the patients with diverse medical problems.
4. The patients faced a lot of hardship in reaching the new venue.
5. Many of the participants and even the faculty members were not aware of the venue change. They reached the originally planned venue and found that it was locked and hence wasted a lot of time in searching for the new venue.
6. The chief guest arrived two hours late due to traffic jam. He was not informed about the theme of the workshop. He delivered a speech on "*female infanticide*," which he had delivered recently, instead of speaking on OSCE.

***Exercise***: What flaws did you notice in organizing this workshop? What could have been done to avoid them?

## 15.4 Describe

FDPs have been recognized as foremost instruments of capacity building all over the world. They have been evolving over the years [1]. FDPs can assume a wide range of activities from traditional lectures to seminars, symposia, workshops, and conferences besides other activities leading to professional development [2]. However, workshops are commonest among group educational activities [3].

### 15.4.1 Communication Challenges in Conducting a Workshop

Educational workshop is an intensive and experiential activity targeting not more than 20–30 participants working under the facilitation of one or few resource persons. Workshop is as an outcome-based activity. An effective communication with the participants and amongst the organizing team is vital for the success of the workshop.

#### 15.4.1.1 Salient Features of a Workshop

- The workshop format underlines the "*hands-on*" experience including individual exercises, group work, and plenary presentations.
- It includes a variety of activities such as interactive lectures, demonstration, group discussion, role play, buzz groups, brainstorming, video session, and a lot more.
- These activities are derived from the sound educational principles including group dynamics.
- The workshop requires infrastructure and physical facilities congenial for active learning.
- The duration of a workshop may vary between half a day and nearly, one week.
- However, workshop planning may take several days, weeks, or even months.

#### 15.4.1.2 Communication Challenges Before the Workshop Organizers

A workshop generally involves three phases: planning phase, implementation phase, and evaluation phase. There are communication challenges encountered in each of these phases (Table 15.1).

Besides communication strategies, other things that matter are availability of resources at the disposal of the facilitators. A comprehensive workshop kit is an essential requirement (Box 15.1).

**Box 15.1 Workshop Kit**

Audio-visual equipment (Projection device, slide presenter, inbuilt pointer, battery cells).

Stationery items, scissor, tapes, stapler.

Soft board, marker pens, duster, flip charts.

Handouts, exercises, arranged ready for distribution.

Alarming bell (to stop the vocal participants)!

Toffees or any small prize material to cheer-up the participants.

Program evaluation forms, pre-test, and post-test questionnaires.

Bags or folders to be distributed to each participant.

Note: The participants may be given a decent jute bag (eco-friendly), which contains program schedule, badges, scribbling pad, pens/pencils, lunch coupons, list of all participants, and faculty with their contact numbers. If the participants bring their own laptops or smart phones, many of the handouts, exercises, and evaluation forms can be downloaded by the participants.

Access to high speed internet is much needed facility for organizing video-conferencing with a remotely placed resource person. It also helps in accessing any information from the internet or playing a video as and when required.

**Table 15.1** Communication problems usually encountered in conducting workshops

| The problem areas | Strategies to overcome |
|---|---|
| ***Planning phase*** | |
| The participants are not aware of what to expect from the Workshop | Plan well in advance; design a comprehensive flier or brochure stating the outcomes and benefits to the participants. One week before the event, send reading materials along-with a checklist stating the preparations required |
| Communication with resource persons | Use all channels of communication, emails, WhatsApp, telephone, and direct meeting wherever possible; negotiate with them regarding the details of the program as well as logistics |
| Organizing a workshop team | Ensure willingness and time commitment from team members before fixing teams. Ensure voluntary participation. State clearly the expectations and compensation (honorarium, certificates, credits, etc.) |
| Eliciting logistic support from administration | Establish good rapport with administrative staff<br>Give them checklist of requirements |
| Coordinating various tasks, such as registration, informing schedule, updating the information from time to time | Ride on technology, create portals and websites to drive all activities (from registration till evaluation)<br>Form WhatsApp groups, use e-facility, Google form, etc., for program evaluation |
| ***Implementation phase*** | |
| Ensuring interaction among participants | Start first session with "*breaking the ice*" session to encourage group dynamics; ensure appointment of facilitator, reporter, and a time keeper for each group |
| Adhering to the principles of adult learning | Use participatory methods, maintain a non-threatening environment, provide appropriate reinforcement, and get feedback about the process |
| Time management | Beware of time wasters, avoid long talks, moderate the interaction, and regulate break time |
| ***Evaluation and follow-up phase*** | |
| Evaluating the program effectiveness | Use simple forms, but create evidence of learning |
| | Use a variety of tools including social media |
| | Promote further networking and dissemination |

#### 15.4.1.3 Plan in Advance, it Pays!

The workshop organizer should organize preparatory meetings to design the schedule and various exercises for individual and group activities to be assigned during the workshop. This should be done at least a fortnight in advance.

At least one week before the workshop, all the reading materials should be sent to the participants along-with the instruction. With the easy availability of Google groups and WhatsApp groups, it becomes very handy for the organizers to communicate simultaneously with all the participants in the group. Opening a dedicated website or providing links to the existing pages helps in sharing resource materials before, during, and after the workshop. Even most of the activities such as registration of participants, sharing resource materials, evaluation, and certification can be aided by the web-based tools.

**Table 15.2** Important principles of adult Learning and their implications for workshop

| Principles of adult learning | Implications for workshop |
|---|---|
| Adult learners are self-directed learners. | Help them in setting their own goals, pursue at their own pace, in their own style. |
| Adults bring a wealth of information and previous experience.<br>They are motivated by new challenges. | Facilitate construction rather than instruction. |
| Adults are motivated by 'value attached' to the task and their self-efficacy. | Demonstrate the relevance of the task;<br>Help them to build self-confidence. |
| Adult learning is facilitated by feedback from the peers and self-reflection combined with practice. | Provide feedback and receive feedback. Promote reflection and practice all the time. |
| Adults can do better in a collaborative learning setting. | Engage them in group tasks; tap the power of media including social media to get them connected and work. |
| Adults are sensitive about their ego and self-pride. | Provide a non-threatening and respectful environment in which learning becomes a fun rather than a job. |

#### 15.4.1.4 Focus on Adult Learning Principles

Participants bring with them their rich experience, knowledge, skills, and attitudes, which should be tapped by the organizers. The foremost *mantra* to be followed by a workshop coordinator is to follow the adult learning principles. The adult learners need to be treated with full respect, no matter how "*novice*" they are. We have listed the essence of adult learning principles as applicable to a workshop format (Table 15.2).

#### 15.4.1.5 Follow Group Dynamics

The knowledge of group dynamics is essential for running a workshop [4]. Every group undergoes the stages of forming, storming, norming, and performing (followed by adjournment). Each group should appoint a facilitator, time keeper, and a reporter for an efficient group outcome. While grouping the participants, care should be taken to see that maximum interaction takes place among the group members. In general, groups are formed by assigning numbers to each individual. However, if the group is asked to discuss the content, it may be better to group the participants according their specialities. In most cases, it is better to regroup after every long session so that participants meet with new partners to enhance their learning.

#### 15.4.1.6 Emphasize Active Participation and Hands-on Experience

A good workshop program must have a wide range of activities to accomplish the expected outcomes. Some of the common activities have been cited in Table 15.3.

#### 15.4.1.7 Choose a Right Resource Person or Facilitator

The resource person or often called facilitator plays a key role in the success of a workshop. He or she need not be a subject expert, but a good communicator.

**Table 15.3** List of common activities used in the workshop

| Activities | Brief description |
|---|---|
| Individual assignments or exercises | Individual participant becomes highly active but there is no scope for sharing with others. |
| Think—pair—share | A participant starts thinking aloud, works with his/her neighbor, and shares idea. Both together learn and share with the whole group. |
| Brainstorm | The facilitator asks a thought-provoking question; elicits rapid response individually. No point is opposed, every point is well taken and listed for further evaluation. |
| Affinity mapping | Brainstorming is usually followed by prioritization of each point by sticking colored stickers (dots)<br>Participants may be asked to go round and round until a clear priority emerges. |
| Jigsaw | Here, the participants engage in a group activity. One participant from each group is invited to form a new group. The issues discussed in each group are focused in this mixed group. Solutions are found. The participants again go back to their original groups and try applying their solutions. |
| Buzz groups | Each group is assigned a task or few tasks. The group thrashes out the problem. One representative from each group is called to present their findings or views to the whole group. |
| Role play | Participants are assigned a particular theme and roles for each, then they are asked to write script and enact before the whole group. This is followed by de-briefing. |

Facilitator's main job is to motivate the participants to collaborate with each other and share learning. This requires role modelling, coaching, mentoring, handholding, and delegating the tasks to the learners in a gradual manner. At the end of the day, the participants should get a feeling that "*they*" have done the job and the time spent was worthwhile. Constant monitoring of the progress is a must to achieve the expected outcomes of the workshop.

#### 15.4.1.8 Evaluation of the Workshop and Follow-Up Activities

Proof of the pudding lies in eating. Evaluation is the most important component of the workshop. The success of a workshop needs to be evaluated by collecting evidence from diverse sources. One of the practical model is given by Kirkpatrick who deals with four levels of learning occurring in a workshop [5].

The workshops in the future are likely to be driven by technology. Simulation pedagogy and e-learning are bound to create new tools for the participants in developing skills including soft-skills. New developments such as Artificial Intelligence (AI), big data analytics, and machine learning may help us in conducting workshops in virtual class rooms. This will greatly enable the organizers to customize their workshops to suit individual needs, motivations, and interests. However, the core elements that make or mar the success of these activities lie in the purview of effective communication.

### 15.4.2 Conclusion

- Workshops are the robust methods for creating new knowledge or solving a problem by providing intense hands-on experience. Start planning well in advance.
- Use multiple modes of communication to work with the organizing team as well as the participants.
- Overcome the challenges during planning, implementing, and evaluating the workshop.
- Provide logistic support, create a good ambience, encourage interactivity using a variety of activities.

## 15.5 Evaluate

After reading the chapter now you are fully charged to take a test! Indeed, this is not a test, only a small rest! To arrest your interest.

Imagine about the next workshop which you are likely to organize in the near future. Imagine the type of participants you are likely to meet. Think about the communication challenges which you are likely to encounter. Come out with some out of the box solutions to face those challenges. Share your list with your trusted colleagues and find out how they feel about it.

## References

1. McLean M, Cilliers F, van Wyk JM. Faculty development: yesterday, today and tomorrow. Med Teach. 2008;30:555–84. AMEE Guide No. 36.
2. Steinert Y, Mann K, Centeno A, Dolmans D, Spencer J, Gelula M, Prideaux D. A systematic review of faculty development initiatives designed to improve teaching effectiveness in medical education: BEME Guide No. 8. Med Teach. 2006;28(6):497–526.
3. Swanwick T. Understanding medical education evidence, theory and practice. 2nd ed. Chichester: Wiley – Blackwell (ASME); 2010.
4. Tuckman BW. Developmental sequence in small groups. Psychol Bull. 1965;63(6):384–99. https://doi.org/10.1037/h0022100. PMID 14314073.
5. Kirkpatrick D. Evaluating training programs: the four levels. San Francisco: Berrett-Koehler Publishers; 1994.

# Communication Skills for the Leaders in Health Professions Education

# 16

Santosh Salagre and Avinash Supe

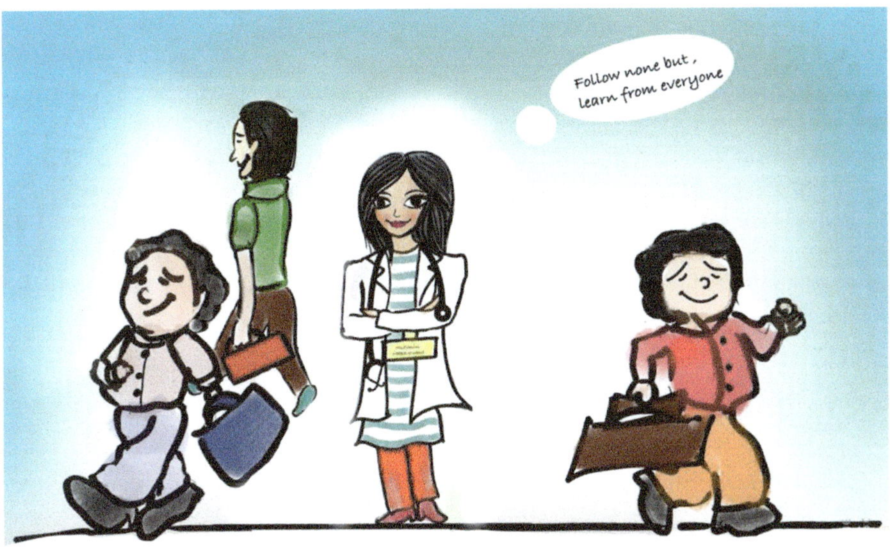


Today's leaders in health profession education need proficiency in verbal and non-verbal communication besides networking skills—Salagre and Supe

S. Salagre
Department of General Medicine, Seth G S Medical College and K E M Hospital, Mumbai, India

A. Supe (✉)
Formerly at Department of Surgical Gastroenterology, Seth GS Medical College and K E M Hospital, Mumbai, India



S. C. Parija, B. V. Adkoli (eds.), *Effective Medical Communication*,
https://doi.org/10.1007/978-981-15-3409-6_16

## 16.1 Assess the Need

Health profession educators need to assume various leadership roles throughout their professional life. These leadership roles may vary according to the future scenario of classrooms, clinical units, departments, medical colleges, or universities. In the existing undergraduate and postgraduate curricula, there is very little sensitization about playing such roles. Apart from the mandatory requirement of basic course workshops in medical education technology, medical teachers have no exposure or training in leadership.

Last two decades have witnessed a revolution in health profession education technology globally. Education Commission for Foreign Medical Graduates (ECFMG), USA has successfully implemented competency-based medical education showing a path to the developing world. Medical Council of India, in its new curriculum, has elaborated five expected roles for an Indian Medical Graduate [1]. These are clinician, leader, communicator, lifelong learner, and professional. Effective communication skills are pivotal to all these roles. Leaders in health professional education should not only develop these skills, but also transfer these skills to function effectively in the health team.

In addition to teaching skills, all leaders should be part and parcel of network among contemporaries. They also need to present or publish their experiences and innovations in medical education across the academic community. In the present era of electronic media, they should be especially proficient in harnessing newer technologies such as webinars, usage of social media as well as working with virtual platforms for effectively communicating and disseminating their thoughts to various stakeholders including learners. All these changes call for a need to equip the health professions leaders to develop strategies of effective communication.

## 16.2 Brief

An attempt has been made in this chapter to highlight:

- The need for effective communication skills for the leaders in health profession education.
- Qualities and attributes of a leader using effective communication.
- The key barriers to effective communication and steps to overcome these barriers.
- Some of the recent advances in electronic communication which the leaders need to be aware and prepared to adopt.

## 16.3 Contextualize

### 16.3.1 Scenario

Dr. Comini successfully completes 15 years as a faculty in a premier medical institute. She also undergoes an international fellowship in a medical education course and works as an active member of the medical education unit of the college. The college administration insists that she has to take up the additional responsibility of the department of medical education to revamp the activities of this department. For Dr. Comini, it is a tough decision. However, she accepts these responsibilities as a challenge. What she does is to stick on to six cardinal principles, viz. know yourself, know your audience, be specific and clear, pay attention to non-verbal communication, listen more than you speak, and finally, be positive and respectful. She takes up the challenge and comes out with flying colors!

***Exercise***: Do you think that a leader is one who turns the problems into opportunities?

## 16.4 Describe

A leader in the health profession is challenged with the issues of moving his/her organization for accomplishing its mission. This requires setting up goals, building a team, assigning and delegating tasks, organizing resources, and monitoring the progress continuously.

### 16.4.1 Effective Communication Skills

For an impactful leadership, one needs effective communication skills. The best educational leaders are also excellent communicators. They know how to reach a variety of people in many different ways. For instance, a departmental head may have a one-on-one chat with each staff member, once in every week followed by daily follow-up using email or WhatsApp. In this way, the leader engages in effective two-way communication which is needed for handling the task. With the possibility of a wide variety of tools, including social media, it is not difficult to get in touch with colleagues, students, and others, even while the leader is travelling.

### 16.4.2 Lead by Example, i.e., Walk the Talk

The best leaders lead by example, not merely by giving instruction. It is easy to issue orders and dictate from the top, but this type of leadership will not have any impact on the students or staff in implementing desirable changes. Attitudinal changes are possible only by acting as role models. Educators have a tremendous influence in molding the behavior of their students by role modeling, which is called "*hidden curriculum*." All great leaders have been influenced by their mentors. The leaders are, therefore, torch bearers to the students and the organization.

### 16.4.3 Power of Teaching and Learning

A leader in health profession should be proficient in teaching in effective utilization of both verbal and non-verbal communications. This requires continuous training and updating of skills as a learner, especially in the context of rapid obsolescence of knowledge. Fortunately, leaders today have wide access to training, continuing medical education (CME), and exposure to the latest technologies besides various avenues of learning through distance and open learning on a 24 × 7 basis.

### 16.4.4 Resourceful and Technically Competent

To be an effective leader, one needs to have learning agility. One should be resourceful and open to new ideas. The awareness and inclination to use the latest available technology is a key factor for the leaders to implement educational reforms successfully.

### 16.4.5 Self-Awareness and Confidence

A good educational leader has a proper understanding of his/her strengths and weaknesses besides the ability to receive feedback and work upon the feedback. Believing in oneself or what is called "*self-efficacy*" is a major ingredient of the motivation, next to the value attached to the goal. When a person believes in himself or herself, he or she can accomplish any task. While self-awareness is a quality of many great leaders, it can be acquired with readiness to accept feedback and reflective practice.

#### 16.4.5.1 Relevance and Importance of Effective Communication Skills

The importance of communication skills has been realized globally in achieving organizational effectiveness. The stress on teaching communication skills right from undergraduate teaching is an indicator of this trend. It is recognized as a core competency of an Indian medical graduate among other competencies, viz. to function as a clinician, health team member or leader, lifelong learner, and a professional with ethical behavior [1]. We focus on communication skills which are at the heart of effective leadership. Research conducted on leaders over long years has demonstrated that leaders spend 75–90% of their time on communication activities. This includes both verbal and non-verbal though the non-verbal assumes more importance. Albert Mehrabian proved that words have only a 7% impact on communication [2]. The tone of voice contributes to 38%, and non-verbal communication has the highest impact of 55%.

There are three main categories of communication skills which are needed for the leaders [3, 4]. However, with the beginning of a revolution in information technology, skills and strategies related to electronic communication also assume a great significance (Fig. 16.1).

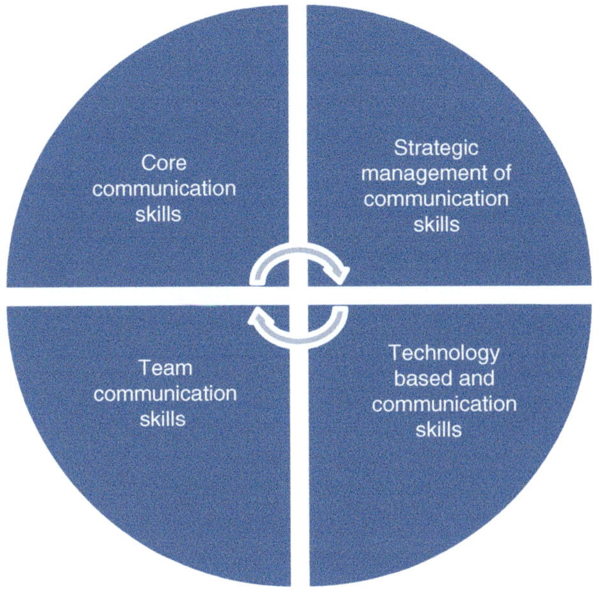


**Fig. 16.1** Communication skills needed for leaders in health professions education

a. Core communication skills.
b. Team communication skills.
c. Strategic management communication skills.
d. Technology-based communication strategies.

We will not discuss the core communication skills which are common for all, which have been adequately covered elsewhere in this book. We wish to focus on team communication skills which are of foremost importance for the leaders. With the growth of specialization and increased interdependence of job responsibilities, team work assumes the greatest significance. It is a crucial requirement both for running an educational institute or a health care service organization. In case of a health sciences university, several departments, centers, and facilities must work in cohesion which requires the free flow of communication vertically and horizontally at all point of time. The tips for effective team communication for the leaders are enlisted in Table 16.1.

### 16.4.6 Strategic Management Communication for Leaders

A strategic approach to communication is of vital importance today. Globalization has brought numerous opportunities to organizations while simultaneously increasing the potential for learning higher-level skills. These skills include (1) navigating through new and changing organizational environments, (2) focusing on the larger picture, (3) appreciating diversity of ideas in the workforce, (4) utilizing informal bases of power, (5) using communication to influence, (6) negotiating skills, (7) conflict management, and (8) listening skills.

**Table 16.1** The skills needed for effective communication in a team

| | |
|---|---|
| Adopt a humane approach | A leader succeeds when an instant connection is established with team members at the outset. Good leaders are down to earth, humble, and sensitive to others' needs and concern. |
| Avoid speaking, encourage listening | Team communication cannot be one-way traffic. Instead of self-appraisal, the leader should show a genuine interest in the team members. Active listening and body language help a lot. |
| Wait till people finish speaking<br>Do not interrupt | It is human nature to want to be heard and understood. Leaders should avoid interruptions unless it is essential<br>Encouraging team members to speak out their own opinions results in getting the best ideas. |
| Use body language that supports the words | Where words fail, body language conveys significant meaning. Posture, movement, proximity, gestures all carry more weightage than words. |
| Be there—Maintain eye contact | Eye contact can be employed to convey a lot of feelings, being one with the audience, showing empathy and a keen interest in others' opinion. The physical presence of the leader with the team is more important than an email or phone call, particularly in handling crisis situations. |
| Avoid racing to the end | There is a tendency to jump to conclusions when the leader is under extreme time pressure and surrounded by smart people. Leaders need to stop "*racing to the end*" of a conversation and be present in the moment. |
| Avoid speaking from a script, be honest and frank | Leaders who can express their views without relying on notes make a better impact as they can talk straight from their hearts. |
| Say "*we*" instead of "*I*" | Giving credit to the team is the hallmark of all leaders |
| Avoid using jargon | Jargon sometimes creates a distance between the leader and the audience. Better to avoid them and use words which are clear, concise, and easy to understand. |
| Avoid complaining and start appreciating | If a leader thinks that by criticizing the opponent, he/she becomes great, that is wrong. It may be good to start appreciating the opponent and then argue what you did better. |

Forbes emphasizes eight skills—adaptability, transparency, empathy, flexibility, humility, competent and confident communication, emotional quotient, and commitment to the vision [3]. These are general human behavioral skills but are extremely essential for a successful leader.

### 16.4.7 Technology-Based Communication Strategies

Over the years, newer technologies are invading health professions education. In fact, technology enhancement is emerging as a key issue in medical education in India. The leaders should be aware of these technologies and become proficient in using these technologies [4, 5]. Some of the technologies needed for the leaders have been listed below:

1. Face-to-face instruction using technologies: These include the followings:
   - Electronic smart-boards which can digitally capture the instructor's chalkboard drawings and make them available for review or dissemination via other online platforms.

- Audience response system for formative assessment and immediate response during quizzes.
- Power point presentations, online and offline videos, and other interactive means to deliver the content.

2. Online instruction: These include the followings:
   - E-resources hosted on a website or portal.
   - Learning management systems (LMS) to support the administration of online course delivery:
     a. MOODLE (Modular object-oriented dynamic learning environment)
     b. Blackboard learn.
     c. Massive open online courses—MOOC to support learning, providing access to learning content to a large number of learners such as Coursera and edX platforms.
     d. Medical visualization where learners get a three-dimensional view of the human anatomy.
3. Mobile and other handheld devices and apps—Use of smart phones in day to day academic and administrative activities accompanied by the use of social media has become a necessity rather than a luxury for the leaders. However, what is more, important is an effective, rational, and responsible use of these gadgets, as otherwise, it may end up in creating more problems.
4. Simulation-based instruction: Some of the examples are:
   - Mannequins with a life-like body or torso models of a human for clinical skills training
   - Simulators for developing psychomotor skills
   - Resuscitation Anne for emergency care simulation, Nursing Anne for wound care, and other patient care scenarios
   - Virtual reality environment to mirror the real-life environment in which the medical services are delivered
   - Virtual patients to imitate real patient cases, i.e., human patients.
5. Technology for assessment: These include:
   - Computer-aided assessment systems combined with quizzes for formative and summative assessments
   - Learning portfolios to facilitate the assessment and reflection of educational achievements and progress
6. Integration with clinical practice.

The examples of this are bedside clinical technologies to capture and interpret clinical data and help in patient management.

#### 16.4.7.1 Barriers to Effective Communication

Followings are the key barriers to effective communication:

- Physical—Space constraint, environment, and surroundings with noise and disturbances
- Physiological—Ill health, workplace induced stress, fatigue, poor eyesight, and hearing difficulties

- Cultural—Diversity of people in a common workplace
- Language—Expression, use of jargon, slangs, pronunciation, similar-sounding words
- Gender—Differences and ethnicity
- Interpersonal—Closeness, distance, personal values, and expectations
- Psychological—The type of personalities
- Hierarchy
- Generation gaps
- Disruptive behavior, professional rivalries

An effective leader always strives to overcome these barriers by taking the proper step. Many of the barriers can be removed by training and reorienting the staff and by resolving conflicts by appealing to super ordinate goals of the organization. The changes may also require proper reorganization of various cadres, re-defining expectations, and reallocation of resources to bridge the gaps. If for some unavoidable reasons specific barrier cannot be overcome, it is vital to communicate regarding the same. Ultimately, the relationship of trust helps in such critical situations through effective communication.

#### 16.4.7.2 Assessment of Communication Skills

Realizing the importance of communication skills, a number of tools are now available for assessing communication skills. Kalamazoo rating scale is perhaps the most popular among the various scales [6, 7]. Communication research is currently an area of interest in medical education across the globe [8]. The assessment of communication skills has been discussed elsewhere in this book.

#### 16.4.7.3 Training of Trainers

Communication skills training requires trained and dedicated teachers who are themselves, excellent communicators and role models. The suggested modalities include a variety of tools and techniques and case scenario-based strategies. It is best done in a specially designed communication skill laboratory with adequate audio-video facilities [9].

While the AETCOM module recommended by the Medical Council of India(MCI) is a good beginning, considering the huge scope of this topic and dearth of trained teachers in the field of communication skills, it is essential that each medical university and medical college develop inter-disciplinary facilities for training of trainers in communication skills using simulation and standardized patients.

Finally, the role of educational networking goes a long way in preparing the leaders for tomorrow. Mechanisms of networking need to be established across the medical colleges and the health sciences universities within the country and across the world. For this purpose, the leaders need to be open to new ideas and proficient in harnessing IT and networking skills. Health professional institutes must create infrastructure and build human resource capacity for developing these skills among all cadres and sectors of health professions education. This is the need of the hour!

### 16.4.8 Conclusion

- Verbal, non-verbal, written, and electronic communication are most vital for health professions leaders.
- Team skills are essential as leaders build teams and work in teams.
- Strategic management communications such as negotiation, adaptability, empathy, and humility are necessary for leaders.
- Electronic communication and technology have been expanding over the last two decades, and leaders must adopt newer technologies in communication by networking and sharing of ideas.

## 16.5 Evaluate

As a teacher in health profession education, you might have come across many leaders using different strategies of communication. Which of their communication components you have been impressed with and why? Substantiate your answer.

## References

1. Vision 2015. Medical Council of India. https://old.mciindia.org/tools/announcement/MCI_booklet.pdf. Accessed on 9 Sept 2019.
2. Institute of Judicious Studies. Handout 1. http://www.iojt-dc2013.org/~/media/Microsites/Files/IOJT/11042013-Albert-Mehrabian-Communication-Studies.ashx. Accessed on 9 Sept 2019.
3. Craig William. 8 Skills Leaders will need in tomorrow's workplace. https://www.forbes.com/sites/williamcraig/2019/03/26/8-skills-leaders-will-need-in-tomorrows-workplace/. Accessed9 Sept 2019.
4. Hirkani M, Supe A. Technology-enhanced learning in undergraduate health professions education: an Indian perspective. J Educ Technol Health Sci. 2018;5(2):69–79.
5. Cook DA, Triola MM. Educational technology in health professions education: current state and future directions. In: Stuart G, Triola M, editors. Enhancing health professions education through technology: building a continuously learning health system. Arlington: The Josiah Macy J Foundational; 2015. p. 71–116.
6. Novack DH, Dube C, Goldstein MG. Teaching medical interviewing: a basic course on interviewing and the physician-patient relationship. Arch Intern Med. 1992;152(9):1814–20.
7. Kurtz SM, Silverman JD. The Calgary-Cambridge referenced observation guides: an aid to defining the curriculum and organizing the teaching in communication training programmer. Med Educ. 1996;30(2):83–9.
8. Makoul G. Communication research in medical education. In: Jackson L, Duffy BK, editors. Health communication research: a guide to developments and directions. Westport: Greenwood Press; 1998. p. 17–35.
9. Jyoti Nath, Modi A, Chhatwal J, Gupta P, Singh T. Teaching and assessing communication skills in medical undergraduate training. Indian Pediatr. 2016;53(6):497–504.

# Conflict Management and Communication

17

Balachandra V. Adkoli and Swati Pawar

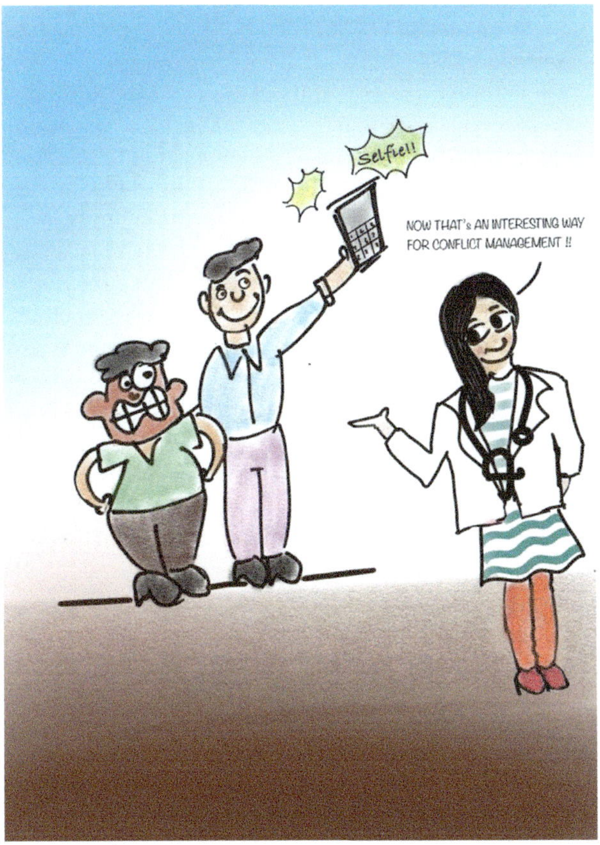


Conflicts are necessary evils in a competitive world. However, they can be resolved by effective communication—Adkoli and Pawar

B. V. Adkoli (✉)
Centre for Health Professions Education, Sri Balaji Vidyapeeth (Deemed-to-be University), Pondicherry, India
e-mail: balachandraa@mgmcri.ac.in

S. Pawar
Mahatma Gandhi Medical College and Research Institute, Pondicherry, India
e-mail: dyms@mgmcri.ac.in


S. C. Parija, B. V. Adkoli (eds.), *Effective Medical Communication*,
https://doi.org/10.1007/978-981-15-3409-6_17

## 17.1 Assess Need

Conflicts are a part and parcel of any growing society. Conflicts exist at homes. They are more common in organisations because the individuals who are different in terms of competency and motivations are put together to shoulder the jobs. In case of health care establishments the conflicts are even more frequent because the issues are often related to life and death. Refusal by the hospital to admit a patient in time may trigger a lot of anger and protest from the relatives and the public. The treating physicians may argue and fight each other on the best treatment. Even if the hospital stay is cut down or extended beyond limit, there will be disputes depending upon the positions held by the parties.

Conflicts are not limited to hospitals. They are common among those who are involved in academics. Even an action taken by a faculty member against absenting student belonging to opposite sex may be questioned and dubbed as harassment. Passing or failing such a candidate in the exam without adequate evidence may create conflicts among faculty, administration, and the student community.

An analysis of all conflicts across the board reveals that the root cause of conflict is a communication gap somewhere between the parties, sometime in the process. Had there been some effective communication, the conflict could have been avoided. This brings us to conclude that conflict resolution requires proactive communication. Unfortunately, neither the individuals nor the systems are adequately trained to handle communication.

Interestingly, research shows that conflicts per se, are not harmful to the organisation if they are handled wisely in time. In fact many of the conflicts would even lead to creative solution to the problems, thus contributing to higher productivity or higher quality of service. The trick therefore lies in understanding the dynamics of conflict management and come out with strategies that involve 'out of the box' solutions.

There is growing evidence that 65% of the performance deficits are due to strained relationship among the staff, and not due to deficiencies in skill or motivation [1]. It is, therefore, implied that medical fraternity should be aware of the strategies for resolving conflicts which would help them to increase the productivity.

## 17.2 Brief

In this chapter, we intend to:

- Discuss five styles of conflict resolution identified by management Gurus.
- Offer tips to the individuals based on their formulae.
- Offer suggestions for the organisations to prevent and manage conflicts.

## 17.3 Contextualize

### 17.3.1 Case Scenario

Extracts from Dr. Comini's diary listing the conflicts which she encountered.

Read carefully. Note the date when Dr. Comini wrote it and her position in the hierarchy.

#### 17.3.1.1 Date 24/8/1992

Today was a special day for us, the freshers of MBBS batch 1992. All of us were made to introduce ourselves about our family background, customs, traditions and hobbies etc. to the whole batch. When my turn came, I mentioned about my modest background. A young faculty member with a cynical look asked "*Miss Comini, I know that your community still follows funny kind of custom! Can you elaborate about your personal experiences?*" I was shocked and fumbled to answer this question. Luckily for me the Dean Sir came to my rescue and objected to this personal question and the session continued.

#### 17.3.1.2 Date 23/10/1997

PG training here is really exciting. Full of opportunities to learn. We were told that All India Conference on medicine is to be held in December but only one PG student will be sponsored by the department to attend this prestigious conference. I was quite keen but my competitor Dr. X. is a highly social guy, well connected too. We had a tough fight. When nothing worked I showed my voluntary project which I did during last summer vacation and explained that my abstract of the paper has been already approved by the conference! There was no option left for HOD except to sponsor my candidature. I am convinced that at times you need to fight to win the case. Sorry, Dr. X…better luck next time!!

#### 17.3.1.3 24/2/2001

Yes, of course, I am a junior faculty…but does it mean that my name is placed last among the four authors, that too for a publication in a prestigious journal? I collected data, I analysed it and I wrote the full paper, now that the paper is ready for submission, HOD Sir wants himself to be the first author, the next senior professor, the second author…the statistician, the third author. And I am the last! What a mockery of publication ethics? Any way I am happy that at least my Department will come to lime light…may be one day I will get what I deserve…

#### 17.3.1.4 Date 25/4/2019

As a senior faculty today I learnt how challenging it was to lead an institutional activity. I was assigned the responsibility of organizing a megaevent, a poster exhibition projecting the achievements of our institute. I had to first convince all departments that it was an institutional project. I appointed various committees and assigned tasks. I involved the general administration, accounts department, besides a few NGOs whom we had helped in the past. They came out with liberal sponsorships, including media coverage which helped in mobilizing huge number of visitors. The student volunteers whom we had motivated worked day and night to assist in the logistics. The exhibition was a thumping success. We celebrated the success and shared credit amongst everyone who contributed to success directly or indirectly.

***Exercise***: Review the diary pages of Dr. Comini. Under each episode think of the style adopted by Dr. Comini to resolve the conflict. Was she right or can you think of a better way?

## 17.4 Describe

### 17.4.1 What Does the Theory Say?

There are five styles of conflict resolutions adopted by the people. They are characterised by five animals, respectively (Fig. 17.1) [2, 3]:

1. Competing (Shark).
2. Avoiding (Turtle).
3. Accommodating (Teddy Bear).
4. Compromising (Fox).
5. Collaborating (Owl).

These styles are determined by a combination of two factors, viz. the extent to which a person is assertive and cooperative. Every person has a mix of these two attributes.

- Too little assertiveness and too little cooperative attitude leads to avoiding style. Turtle is the symbol. Turtle undergoes hibernation for years but still remains alive.
- Too little assertiveness and high cooperation leads to accommodating style. It is symbolic of teddy bear, who entertains others at her cost.
- Too much of assertiveness and very little cooperation leads to competing style, symbolic of shark. The shark attacks the opponent and fights to finish.

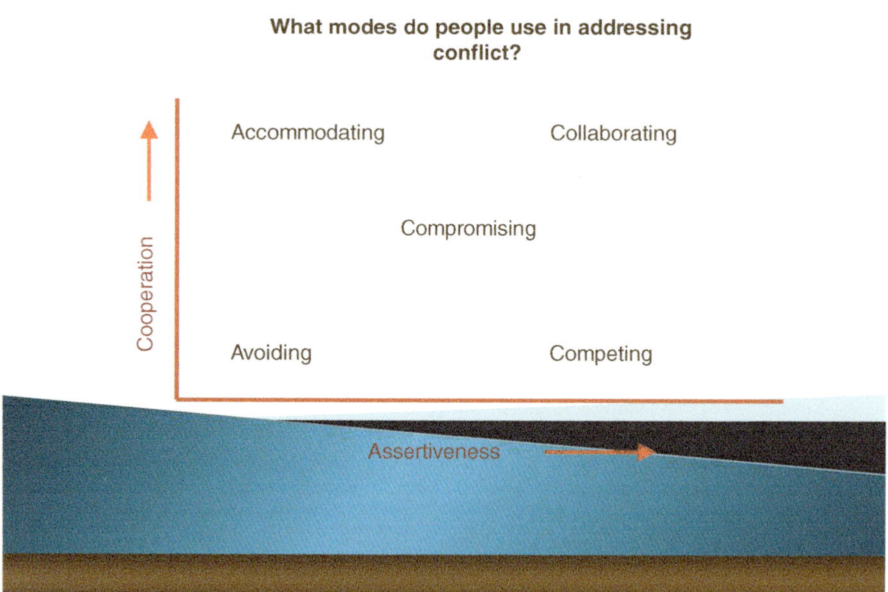


**Fig. 17.1** Five styles of conflict management

- A moderate degree of assertion and cooperation leads to compromising style. It is also called 50–50 formula. Fox is symbolic of this style.
- Lastly, high degree of assertion combined with high degree of cooperation leads to collaboration style, which is the best among the five. It is symbolic of owl, who sleeps during the day time and works at night. This is characteristic of leaders who have a long vision, who work from background, develop a strategy and accomplish the task successfully.

In order to identify the styles adopted by people, Thomas & Kilmann developed an inventory called Thomas—Kilmann Inventory (TKI), which has become popular internationally [4, 5].

It is important to note that each of the five styles prescribed by the management Gurus has its own strengths and weaknesses. A particular style may work well under a particular circumstance [6].

It is akin to the medical prescription. Every drug which is effective, has some side effect and one needs to take a call whether this side effect is acceptable or not (Table 17.1).

**Table 17.1** Table showing five styles of conflict management, tips for individuals

| Conflict resolution style | Prescribed under what circumstance? | What you need to do? | What are the side effects? |
|---|---|---|---|
| Competing (shark)<br>Example:<br>Comini's diary<br>*Date 23/10/1997* | • You are occupying higher position than your opponent<br>• You have no time as the conflict has to be resolved urgently | • Be assertive<br>• Fight!<br>• Use all your power | • You are creating an enemy<br>• Your relationship is at stake! |
| Avoiding (Turtle)<br>Example:<br>Comini's diary<br>*Date 24/8/1992* | • You are new to the situation<br>• You need to buy time<br>• There is no urgency | • Just sit back and pray for good time!<br>• Appoint a committee! | • You are only doing quick-fix job, not finding a permanent solution |
| Accommodating (Teddy Bear)<br>Example:<br>Comini's diary<br>*24/2/2001* | • You are a goodwill messenger (*Shanti-doot*)<br>• You are not bothered about your score | • Give way to your opponent to excel<br>• Do not expect return! | • Some day you may get disillusioned<br>• You are nurturing selfish souls! |
| Compromising (Fox) | • You are in conflict with an equally strong opponent<br>• You cannot wait any longer | • Bargain with the opponent and apply 50:50 formula | • It is not ideal solution for the organisation<br>• If the distribution(mediator) is not fair, this can lead to more unrest |
| Collaboration (Owl)<br>Example:<br>Comini's diary<br>*Date 25/4/2019* | • You want to produce long term result<br>• You want to build a team | • Set goal<br>• Build a team<br>• Involve *all*<br>• Recognise *all* | • It requires a lot of patience, time, and resources<br>• It may supress the ego of *pundits* because everybody is a winner here |

### 17.4.2 Ancient Indian Wisdom on Conflict Management

Kautilya's *Arthashastra* is perhaps the best known treatise on economics, politics, and governance including approaches *(Upayas)* to manage conflicts [6, 7]. According to this source, conflicts can be resolved effectively by resorting to one or more tactics in a gradual manner.

1. *Sama* is the first step in which one needs to talk to the opponent, explain the situation, the pro's and con's in a logical manner so that they resolve the conflict on the table in an amicable manner. *Sama* is a kind of collaborative style.
2. *Dana:* If *sama* does not work, you need to try with *dana,* which means offering gifts, cash or kind or honours to woo the aggrieved party. It is a kind of soft 'bribe', with good intention of resolving conflict.
3. *Bheda: Bheda* means *divide and rule* policy. You isolate the person as social boycott to build pressure on the opponent to yield. When *dana* fails, this tactics is likely to work in resolving conflict. It is like lobbying or almost threatening the opponent to face the worst consequence.
4. *Danda: Danda* is nothing but punishment, physical or mental, to force the opponent to loose and give up.

Kautilya's policy (*Neeti*) is a compendium on good governance based on sound principles. The good governance should first make a policy which is fair and transparent. A fair policy enacted by able administrators and staff can prevent so many conflicts.

### 17.4.3 A Five Point Formula for Organisations

1. *Take proactive steps* to communicate clearly the organisation's policies, expectations, job responsibilities, and compensation package in clear terms.
2. *Harness the popularity of social media* and the strengths of networks for communicating and informing the people about the policies, best practices, and redressal mechanisms which are in place to resolve conflicts.
3. *Always appeal to the superordinate goals* of the organisation, whenever two or more factions meet with a conflict.
4. *Develop a culture of giving and taking feedback* at all levels at all times. This is quite challenging as it is likely to hurt the egos of many captains and bosses who think that they run the show.
5. *Promote training programs centred around wellness* activities for the patients and staff together, to demonstrate what you wish to tell, viz. empathic listening skills, skills of honesty, humility, self-less service, and unconditional love.

Finally, individuals are equally responsible for managing their own conflicts. Besides departmental training, they can work upon changing their life-styles.

Maintaining work-life balance holds the key. Techniques practised in complementary medicine, such as Yoga, music listening, meditation, prayer, the practice of silence, can help combat work pressure and lead a stress-free life. In fact, the ultimate solution to conflict lies in the innermost layer of communication which is silence and a blissful moment!

### 17.4.4 Conclusion

- Conflict management holds the key for enhancing individual growth as well as organisational development.
- There are five styles of conflict management described in the management each symbolised by an animal—competing (shark), avoiding (turtle), accommodating (teddy bear), compromising (fox), and collaborating (owl).
- The best style depends upon the situation. Collaborating style is recommended in general.
- The ancient Indian wisdom of quadrants, *sama* (dialogue), *dana* (gift), *bheda* (isolating the problematic), and *danda* (punishment) is also worth trying.
- Conflicts can be minimised by good governance, appealing to the superordinate goals, and encouraging collaboration as against competition. Training of employees in soft skills pays rich dividends.
- Individuals can benefit by modifying their life-style changes.

## 17.5 Evaluate

After reading this chapter, recall one episode of conflict which you had faced with your colleague in your workplace. Reflecting back, what do you think, you should have done to resolve the conflict with him/her?

## References

1. Dreachslin JL, Kiddy D. From conflict to consensus: managing competing interests in your organization. Healthc Exec. 2006;21(6):9–14.
2. Callanan GA, Perri DF. Teaching conflict management using a scenario-based approach. J Educ Bus. 2006;81(3):131–9. Heldref Publications, Washington.
3. Saltman DC, O'Dea NA, Kidd MR. Conflict management: a primer for doctors in training. Postgrad Med J. 2006;82(963):9–12. https://doi.org/10.1136/pgmj.2005.034306.
4. Kilmann RH. A brief history of the Thomas-Kilmann conflict mode instrument. Available from http://www.kilmanndiagnostics.com/brief-history-thomas-kilmann-conflict-mode-instrument. Accessed on 5 Apr 2018.
5. Schaubhut NA. Technical brief for the Thomas-Kilmann conflict mode instrument description of the updated normative sample and implications for use CPP research department. 2007. Available from https://www.kilmanndiagnostics.com/sites/default/files/TKI_Technical_Brief.pdf. Accessed on 5 Apr 2018.

6. Adkoli BV, Pawar SJ. Conflict management strategies – implications for health professions education SBV journal of basic. Clin Appl Health Sci (JBCAHS). 2018;2(3):132–8. Available at https://staging.sbvu.cf/wp-content/uploads/2018/12/JBCAHS-Vol2-Issue3-July-Sept-2018.pdf.
7. Kautilya. Arthashastra. (trans: Shamasastry R). Bangalore: Government Press; 1915. Available from https://csboa.com/eBooks/Arthashastra_of_Chanakya_-_English.pdf. Accessed 16 Aug 2018.

# The Future of Communication in a Digital World

# 18

Supten Sarbadhikari

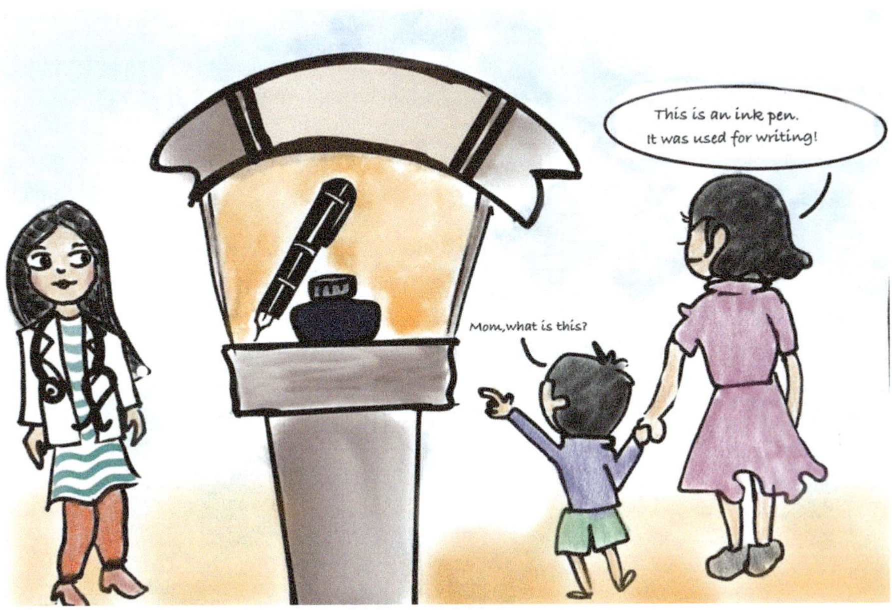


The communication patterns in a digital era are going to radically different—Supten Sarbadhikari

S. Sarbadhikari (✉)
PSG FAIMER Regional Institute, Coimbatore, India


S. C. Parija, B. V. Adkoli (eds.), *Effective Medical Communication*,
https://doi.org/10.1007/978-981-15-3409-6_18

## 18.1 Assess Need

Our global village is now becoming more and more digital, and so communication in the cyberspace or the digital world is becoming more and more important with each passing day. However, often, as in the real world, effective communication skills are lacking, and that is giving rise to misunderstandings that can become very serious.

The main reason why a different set of skills will be necessary in the online world is because there is no scope to assist through the visual interpretations from our body language that often can mitigate the actual responses in the real world.

## 18.2 Brief

Online media are becoming increasingly popular for delivering various courses. The author has been involved with such courses since 2007 [1–14]. Often students feel more comfortable in face-to-face (F2F) settings. Therefore, *blended learning*, which can have a combination of F2F and online interactions, may work better than online communications alone.

In this chapter, we will count the following prominent members of our digital world—viz. email, social media (WhatsApp, Facebook, Twitter, LinkedIn, and Instagram), and Learning Management Systems (LMS) like Moodle for the purposes of our discourse. Then we present a few scenarios to reflect upon what is acceptable and what is not. Finally, there will be a small test to ponder on your own learning and to think of ways in which you can really move further ahead.

This chapter will enable you to:

- Depict the various modalities of the digital world or cyberspace.
- Formulate a digital communication strategy.
- Value the role of communication through the digital world.

## 18.3 Contextualize

### 18.3.1 Scenario 1

Dr. Comini who is working in the Medicine department of a premier medical institute observed that patients from remote areas had to travel for about 11–24 h before they could receive specialist treatment, or meet experienced cardiologists in bigger cities [15]. She came up with an innovative idea. She developed an IT-based gateway using WhatsApp to transmit ECG images to specialists. This method harnesses the ease of communication offered by WhatsApp to connect senior cardiologists with physicians who work out of remote locations.

***Exercise***: Discuss whether such innovation is worthwhile? What are the pros and cons of using such a platform?

Clinicians around the world have started using online discussions to assess their diagnostic procedures and sharpen their skills of diagnosis and treatment. One such portal is telederm.org (http://www.telederm.org/). This portal is aimed to facilitate the discussion of diagnostic procedures, diagnosis, and therapy among dermatologists on a worldwide level. Readers may *compare this site with this Facebook community*: https://www.facebook.com/The-Community-for-Teledermatology-Dermatology-54861231844/.

Another example is the EULAR Online Course for health professionals is aimed at health professionals in rheumatology (HPRs) who play an important role in the management of rheumatic conditions: e.g., nurses, physical therapists, occupational therapists, and psychologists. The EULAR fully online course for HPRs was granted credits in the Netherlands by the accreditation committees of the following health professional disciplines: Physical therapists (60 credits), Nurses (64 credits), Nurse practitioners (50 credits), and Occupational therapists, Exercise therapists, and Podiatrists (40 credits). Further details are here: https://www.eular.org/edu_online_course_hpr.cfm?showArchive=1.

Online courses such as these mentioned offers many opportunities to a health professional for their learning activities. One of the possible answers has been summarized in this Copyleft cartoon by Giulia Forsythe [16] taken from Creative Commons [Attribution: CC0 1.0 Universal (CC0 1.0) Public Domain Dedication] (Fig. 18.1).

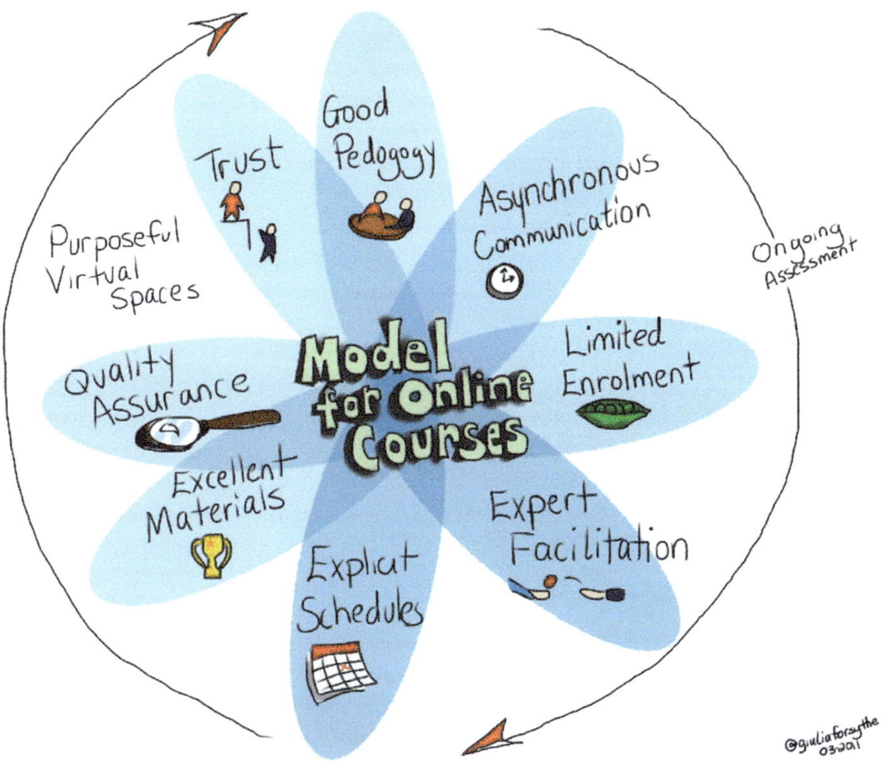


**Fig. 18.1** Components for good online courses

## 18.4 Describe

### 18.4.1 The Various Modalities of the Digital World or Cyberspace

Some of the regularly used media and platforms, for communication and teaching/learning, through the digital world, are as follows:

1. Email—Institutional or Webmail like Gmail/Yahoo/Hotmail.
2. Social Media—WhatsApp, Facebook, Twitter, LinkedIn, Instagram.
3. Learning Management System (LMS) or Course Management System (CMS) or Virtual Learning Environment (VLE)—Moodle, Sakai, D2L, Blackboard Learn, Canvas.

### 18.4.2 Digital Communication Strategy

However, for making the best use of digital media and platforms for communication, we need to have a well-defined communication strategy. Before elaborating further, let us look at two definitions.

*Netiquette* stands for Network etiquette which is a guideline for good manners in network communication and behavior [17–19]. Netiquette is derived by merging the words network and etiquette.

Some of the netiquette that the National Library of Medicine used to recommend for interacting through email lists are given below. While these were available online a few years back at http://www.nlm.nih.gov/listserv/netiquette.html now that page has become nonexistent. However, some other pages often archive content, and one such example is here: https://digital-medicine.blogspot.com/2008/09/nlm-netiquette-do-keep-postings-on_41.html?m=0.

One should not engage in harmful behavior while dealing with email or messaging. A list of 'to do's and don'ts' while handling email has been shown in Table 18.1.

One of the don't commands above says that we should not use other's materials, especially if copyrighted ones, without the owner or creator's explicit permission. One of the ways to overcome that (other than getting formal written permission from the owner/creator of copyrighted materials) is to use copyleft materials that are available freely in the public domain and can be used and reused with appropriate attributions.

*Copyleft* is a general method for making a program (or other creative work) free, and requiring all modified and extended versions of the program to be free as well [20]. The simplest way to make content free is to put it in the public domain, uncopyrighted. This allows people to share the program and their improvements if they are so minded.

Maria Pantalone says that the intersection of social media and real-life communication form two halves that can bring value and meaning to your daily interactions [21]. They are no longer separate realms, but increasingly intertwined worlds that are now both equally indispensable platforms for communication. Making the most of both of these will help to give you the best chance of success.

**Table 18.1** Netiquette for mailing, Do's and Don'ts

| | |
|---|---|
| • DO keep postings on the specified discussion topics of that particular list.<br>• DO search the list archives prior to posting a question to prevent repeat questions.<br>• DO identify yourself. Include your name and institution, if appropriate.<br>• DO use descriptive subject lines.<br>• DO send messages in plain text only as some subscriber's email systems cannot handle rich-text or HTML mail.<br>• DO keep your messages brief when posting to a list.<br>• DO quote relevant parts of the message when responding to a message, but DO NOT resend the entire original message.<br>• DO be careful when using humor in your messages. | • DO NOT "*flame*" individuals on the list. Conflict should be resolved in personal emails.<br>• DO NOT generate vacation 'auto-reply' to the list.<br>• DO NOT post-test messages to the list. Contact the list owner for assistance if you have a problem posting.<br>• DO NOT send messages with little or no meaningful content, such as "*I agree*!", to the entire list.<br>• DO NOT be critical of other's queries posted to the list. Send a private message ∗ DO NOT use all upper-case letters when writing—This is seen as shouting.<br>• DO NOT post messages containing any defamatory, abusive, profane, or offensive language, or post illegal material.<br>• DO NOT post any materials protected by copyright without the permission of the copyright owner. |

### 18.4.3 Role of Communication through the Digital World

The pros and cons of communicating through the digital world or the cyberspace are listed in Table 18.2. These are based on the opinions of various experts in this area [22–24]. Their grounding in educational principles cannot be lost sight [25]. Another important issue is that the use of digital media is actually shifting the focus in the following areas are listed in Table 18.3.These will be the determining factors while developing a robust strategy for communications in the digital world or cyberspace. Therefore, excellent teaching or course materials in the digital world must have many qualities as summarized in Table 18.4.

### 18.4.4 Medical Consultation through Digital Media

Healthcare and public health have been using digital media in diverse ways [26–29]. Whether it is Google trends or posts on Twitter and Facebook, all have been successfully utilized for tracking disease patterns, as they emerge.

Some epidemics have been tracked, almost in real-time or near real-time, through digital footprints like social media postings, of people belonging to various local or geographical communities, and trends in search phrases [30]. A digital surveillance system that uses Internet resources has enormous potential to monitor disease outbreaks in the early phase. Many studies have shown that social networking sites can be used to conduct real-time analysis for better predictions [31].

**Table 18.2** Pro's and con's of social media

| Advantages | Disadvantages |
|---|---|
| Social media is a huge step forward for humanity, as it transcends time and space barriers and can connect instantly people near and far. | They have some damaging effects on communication skills and unfortunately lasting damaging effects when social media is used in excess or obsessively. |
| Social media is a great tool when it is paired with solid in-person communication skills—Like making a face-to-face contact, listening, and being humble and patient. | The more people are invested in their online relationships, the more their face-to-face relationships suffer. |
| Facebook, Instagram, and twitter allow people to broadcast their thoughts, feelings, and milestones to their friends and the general public instantaneously. Sometimes this is a good thing. | People—Especially young people—Struggle with in-person communication because they lack practice, and they do not know the rules. How we speak, how we write, how we present ourselves influences what other people think of us. Each small, seemingly insignificant, piece of our being makes up the total of who we are. Social media has caused a complete 180° turn in how we communicate with each other. Social media often make things impersonal. Also, the abbreviated language of social media is becoming the norm for verbal communication too. One of the biggest pitfalls of the social media era is its profound impact on how we value ourselves. Ideally, validation has to come from within. |

**Table 18.3** Shifting of focus from the real to the digital World

| |
|---|
| • From audience (passive learner) to the user (active learner) |
| • From media (of instruction) to content (depth and breadth, especially through hyperlinks, most of the confusions can be clarified instantly) |
| • From mono-media (only auditory or visual) to multimedia (static to dynamic multimedia) |
| • From periodicity (only during class or clinic hours) to real-time (anytime and anywhere) |
| • From scarcity (difficult to find resources) to abundance (too many attractive resources) |
| • From editor-mediated (facilitated) to non-mediated (self-directed and self-determined or heutagogic learning) |
| • From distribution (rationed, limited) to access (whenever and wherever needed) |
| • From one way (listening or writing) to interactivity (questioning and answering through multimedia) |
| • From linear (one page or chapter after the other) to hypertext (any topic any time—whenever clarification necessary) |
| • From data (unprocessed observations) to knowledge (analysis and evaluation) |

However, for a direct healthcare professional-patient interaction, there have been various guidelines by statutory authorities and professional societies regarding communication through the digital media [32, 33]. The National Health Services (NHS), UK has specific guidelines for various categories of healthcare professionals. In India, since the medical profession has come under the ambit of the consumer protection act, litigations against doctors have risen manifold.

**Table 18.4** Ideal components of a successful online course

| | |
|---|---|
| 1. | They must be interactive, with attention to the individual students that are best suited in small groups compared to larger ones. |
| 2. | They must well-structured with clear-cut schedules that may be flexible. |
| 3. | Assignments must be analytical and not just for copying from resources retrieved by Google from the world wide web. |
| 4. | There should be ample scope for explorations by the students. |
| 5. | Discussion boards and online mailing lists (*asynchronous communication*, unlike *synchronous* communication that happens during real-time video conferencing or webinars) should be encouraged where a lot of peer to peer learning can take place. |
| 6. | Heutagogic principles [25] of self-determined learning should be kept in mind while designing the curriculum. |
| 7. | Regular formative assignments can be offered even through social media apart from the LMS. |
| 8. | The quality of the study materials must undergo both peer review, as well as pilot testing with prospective students for the courses. This can increase the trust in the facilitator(s). |
| 9. | Gamification can enhance the learning and retention experience. |
| 10. | Feedback (either way) can be instantaneously leading to quick course corrections. |

### 18.4.5 Digital Health and India's Stand

India has been one of the evolving global leaders in digital health, especially for achieving the Sustainable Development Goals (SDGs). Some of the initiatives taken in India to promote digital technologies for better health include hosting of fourth Global Digital Health Partnership Summit and the International Digital Health Symposium in 2019 [34]. "*Delhi Declaration*" was adopted to accelerate and implement the appropriate digital health interventions to improve health of the population at national and sub-national levels, as appropriate according to national context [35].

### 18.4.6 Conclusion

- The communication pattern in the digital world is going to be drastically different.
- Learning management system (LMS), course management system (CMS), and virtual learning environment (VLE) are likely to dominate the new learning society.
- The educators must be prepared to harness their capabilities in a responsible manner following the netiquettes.

## 18.5 Evaluate

Imagine about the next course or topic that you would like to teach or facilitate in the near future. Imagine the type of online resources and media that you are likely to use for delivery and assessment—both formative and summative. Write down the ground rules for communications and the expected outcomes. List as many points as possible to make your course a memorable one. Share your course planner with your trusted colleagues and find out how they feel about it.

## References


1. Sarbadhikari SN. A step-by-step primer for using the internet for medical education. Southeast Asian J Med Educ. 2007;1(1):49–51.
2. Sarbadhikari SN. Applying health care informatics to improve student learning really good stuff. Med Educ. 2008;42:1117–8.
3. Sarbadhikari SN. How to design an effective e-learning course for medical education. 2008. Available at http://www.pitt.edu/~super1/lecture/lec35331/index.htm. Accessed on 25 Mar 2019.
4. Sarbadhikari SN. Wiki and Learning Management System (LMS). 2009. Available at http://www.pitt.edu/~super1/lecture/lec43331/index.htm. Accessed on 25 Mar 2019.
5. Sarbadhikari SN. How to make healthcare delivery in India more "informed". Educ Health. 2010;23(2):456.
6. Sarbadhikari SN. A farce called the National Board of examinations. Indian J Med Ethics. 2010 Jan;7(1):20–2.
7. Sarbadhikari SN. Unlearning and relearning in online health education. (chapter 21). In: Biswas R, Martin CM, editors. User driven healthcare and narrative medicine. Hershey: IGI Global; 2011. p. 294–309.
8. Sarbadhikari SN. Web resources for assessment in medical education, chapter 23. In: Anshu ST, editor. Principles of assessment in medical education. New Delhi: JAYPEE Brothers; 2012. p. 234–42.
9. Karishma SH, Sarbadhikari SN, et al. Creating awareness for using a wiki to promote collaborative health professional education. Intl J User Driven Health. 2012;2(1):18–28.
10. Ahmed Z, Sarbadhikari SN, et al. Using online social networks for increasing health literacy on oral health. Intl. J User Driven Health. 2013;3:51–8.
11. Sarbadhikari SN. Medical informatics: a key tool to support clinical research and evidence-based medical practice (Ch 15). In: Babu AN, editor. Clinical research methodology and evidence-based medicine. 2nd ed. Tunbridge Wells: Anshan; 2015. p. 179–91.
12. Sarbadhikari SN, Srinivas M. Health informatics and health information management. In: Gyani G, Thomas A, editors. Handbook of healthcare quality and patient safety. 2nd ed. New Delhi: Jaypee; 2016. p. 206–16. Sec. 4, Ch. 17.
13. Sarbadhikari SN. E-learning. In: Mishra D, Verma D, editors. Concepts and practices in medical education: a primer. New Delhi: CBS Publishers; 2019.
14. Sarbadhikari SN, Sood JM. Gamification can act as a motivation for nurturing healthy habits. Natl Med J India. 2018;31(4):253–4.
15. Manu G. https://www.thebetterindia.com/65207/whatsapp-alleviating-poor-patient-care-himachal-pradesh/. Accessed on 25 Mar 2019.
16. Forsythe G. https://www.flickr.com/photos/gforsythe/5552385806. Accessed on 25 Mar 2019.
17. Yarmohammadian MH, Iravani H, Abzari M. Information and communications technology, culture, and medical universities; organizational culture and netiquette among academic staff. J Educ Health Promot. 2012;1:6.
18. Stach R. The knowledge board netiquette. [Online]. [cited 2004 Mar 24].
19. Harper D. How's your netiquette? Ind Distribution Syst Software. 1988;88:11–112. ABI/INFORM Global.
20. GNU. https://www.gnu.org/licenses/copyleft.en.html. Accessed on 25 Mar 2019.
21. Pantalone M. Social media and its impact on communication skills. https://infinitegrowth.com.au/social-media-and-its-impact-on-communication-skills/. Accessed on 25 Mar 2019.

22. Jacob C. How Social Media Affects Communication Skills? https://upjourney.com/how-social-media-affects-communication-skills. Accessed on 25 Mar 2019.
23. Orihuela JL. The 10 new paradigms of communication in the digital age. https://medium.com/@jlori/the-10-new-paradigms-of-communication-in-the-digital-age-7b7cc9cb4bfb. Accessed on 25 Mar 2019.
24. Clark S. Effective communication in a digital world. https://www.digitalistmag.com/future-of-work/2017/12/08/effective-communication-in-digital-world-05609824. Accessed on 25 Mar 2019.
25. Chacko TV. Emerging pedagogies for effective adult learning: from andragogy to heutagogy. Arch Med Health Sci. 2018;6(2):278–83. Available at: http://www.amhsjournal.org/article.asp?issn=2321-4848;year=2018;volume=6;issue=2;spage=278;epage=283;aulast=Chacko;type=0. Accessed on 25 Mar 2019.
26. Amelia Burke-Garcia A, Scally G. Trending now: future directions in digital media for the public health sector. J Public Health. 2014;36(4):527–34. https://doi.org/10.1093/pubmed/fdt125. Accessed on 25 Mar 2019.
27. Ventola CL. Social media and health care professionals: benefits, risks, and best practices. P T. 2014;39(7):491–520.
28. Williams V, Kovarik C. Long-range diagnosis of and support for skin conditions in field settings. Trop Med Infect Dis. 2018;3(3):84. https://doi.org/10.3390/tropicalmed3030084. Published 2018 Aug 13. Accessed on 25 Mar 2019.
29. Newberry C. How to use social media in healthcare: a guide for health professionals. https://blog.hootsuite.com/social-media-health-care/. Accessed on 25 Mar 2019.
30. Seo DW, Shin SY. Methods using social media and search queries to predict infectious disease outbreaks. Healthc Inform Res. 2017;23(4):343–8. https://doi.org/10.4258/hir.2017.23.4.343.
31. Alessa A, Faezipour M. A review of influenza detection and prediction through social networking sites. Theor Biol Med Model. 2018;15(1):2. https://doi.org/10.1186/s12976-017-0074-5. Published 2018 Feb 1.
32. NHS, UK. Social media guidelines and tools. https://www.nhsemployers.org/your-workforce/need-to-know/social-media-and-the-nhs/social-media-guidelines. Accessed on 25 Mar 2019.
33. Jagdish S. IMA asks doctors to avoid consultations on phone, Whatsapp. http://www.mymedicalmantra.com/ima-asks-doctors-to-avoid-consultations-on-phone-whatsapp/. Accessed on 25 Mar 2019.
34. Ministry of Health and Family Welfare, Government of India and World Health Organization, India. Available from: https://www.gdhpindia.org/. Accessed on 25 Mar 2019.
35. Global Digital Health Partnership, Delhi Declaration. Available from https://s3-ap-southeast-2.amazonaws.com/ehq-production-australia/25eb0facd90ee547c03071b005807288dbeac40b/documents/attachments/000/099/429/original/GDHP-Delhi_Declaration_Final.pdf?1551307009. Accessed on 25 Mar 2019.

# Part V

# Depending Upon Situations, Play Ping-Pong!

# 19 Sensitive Issues in Communication-Empowering Patients Needing Palliative Care

Gilly Burn

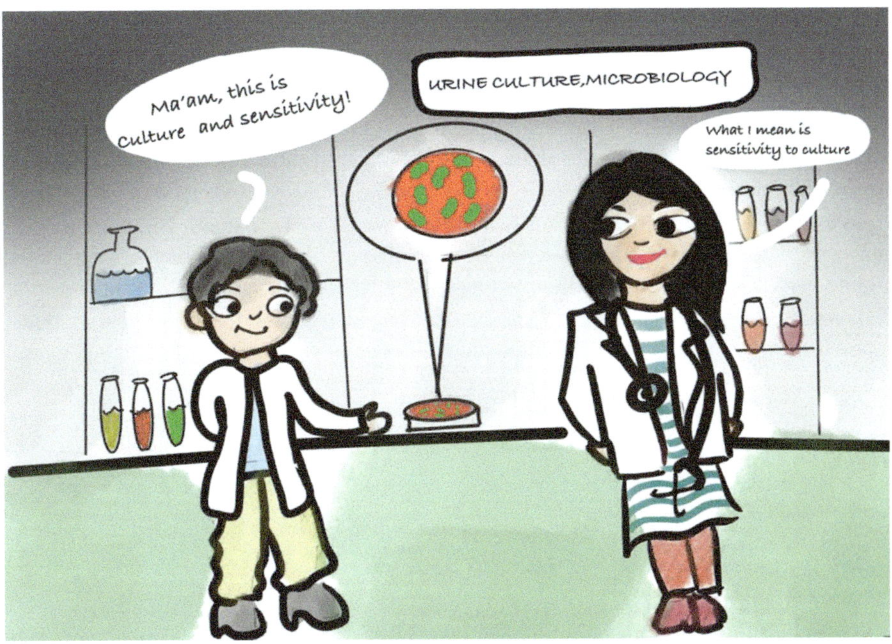


Recall the face of the poorest and the most helpless man whom you may have seen, and ask yourself if the step you contemplate is going to be of any use to them—Mahatma Gandhi.

G. Burn (✉)
Care Response International and Cancer Relief India, Durham, UK


S. C. Parija, B. V. Adkoli (eds.), *Effective Medical Communication*,
https://doi.org/10.1007/978-981-15-3409-6_19

## 19.1 Assess Need

The WHO definition of palliative care states: "*Palliative care is the active total care applicable from the time of diagnosis, aimed at improving the quality of life of patients and their families facing serious life-limiting illness, through the prevention and relief of suffering by means of early identification and impeccable assessment and treatment of pain and other physical symptoms, as well as psychological, social and spiritual distress*". Appropriately, the Indian Association of Palliative Care has adapted the WHO statement, by adding "*through socially acceptable and affordable interventions*".

Note that the WHO definition says that palliative care starts at the point of diagnosis. This is particularly relevant in the Indian context where it is estimated that 80% of patients are first diagnosed when the hope of a cure is not possible, and when palliative care is the only humane option.

### 19.1.1 What Is Empowerment?

The Oxford Dictionary defines the verb "*to empower*"—"*to give (someone) the authority or power to do something*"; to make (someone) stronger and more confident, especially in controlling their life and claiming their rights; the act of giving somebody more control over their own life or the situation they are in.

We empower patients by being respectful towards them. Robert Twycross talks of three fundamental principles in terms of relationships—a model which I have always found very helpful. He asserts that "*relationships are founded on truth, fostered by honesty and poisoned by deceit*" [1]. Without trust between a patient and the treating physician, it is impossible to have a therapeutic relationship, which will benefit the patient.

## 19.2 Brief

The objectives of this chapter are:

- To define palliative care and empowerment.
- To differentiate between different types of pain… (physical, etc.) with examples.
- To underline the role played by effective communication in palliative care.
- To describe some strategies of effective communication in the context of palliative care.

## 19.3 Contextualize

### 19.3.1 Scenario

This is a story of Mr. XY, a rickshaw puller from a metropolitan city. He had a large fungating cancer of the mandible, which had severely disfigured him. He had come to the clinic too late to be cured.

Physically he presented with unbearable, faciomaxillary pain. He was unable to eat because of the pain, and even if he got some food into his mouth, it would just come out of the hole in his cheek. He was now very weak from the lack of nourishment. The pain stopped him sleeping, and he was completely exhausted. He had stomach pains because of hunger. He had the griping pain of constipation, which added to his hunger pains. His whole body ached.

Mr. XY's disease led him to be rejected by his neighbours, friends, and even his children, because of the foul-smelling tumour, and the fact that he was constantly doubled over in pain. His trouble did not stop there. He was forced to stop pulling rickshaw as he became weak and frail. No work means no money; No money to feed or clothe his family; No money to pay for his children's education; no money for his daughter's wedding, no money to visit the doctor and pay for medication.

All these agonies added to his helplessness and made him question his God—Why me? What have I done to deserve this? What will happen to my family after my death? Who will care for them? Does anyone care? Does God care? No amount of analgesia can fix spiritual pain.

***Exercise***: Discuss various kinds of pain which Mr. XY has, as a result of different ramifications of the disease. Do you think medical care can relieve his problems? What best you can offer him as a total physician?

## 19.4 Describe

### 19.4.1 The Concept of Total Pain

Dame Cicely Saunders, a visionary and the pioneer of the modern hospice movement and palliative care, benefited millions of patients throughout the world, who have a life-threatening illness. She started her career as a nurse, then became a social worker, and finally, she qualified as a doctor at St Thomas's Hospital London. In 1967, she founded the St Christopher's Hospice in London, offering in-patient, community services, education, and research. Cicely Saunders recognised the importance of welcome and hospitality [2]. Indeed, the word *hospice*, means both guest and host—the patients and family being the guests of the caring team. This is significant in India where "*Guest is treated like a God*".

It was from here that Professor Robert Twycross did his ground-breaking research into the use of oral morphine in the 1970s. Dame Cicely understood the patient's perspective of pain, in its totality. She created the universally relevant concept of "*total pain*". This pain has physical, social, emotional, and spiritual components, which are unique to each patient's particular situation. The concept of "*total pain*" can be depicted as four overlapping circles, enabling professionals to see the patient in totality, not separating the spiritual, physical, social, and emotional components [3, 4].

The pain experienced by Mr. XY in the scenario is an example of total pain (Fig. 19.1).

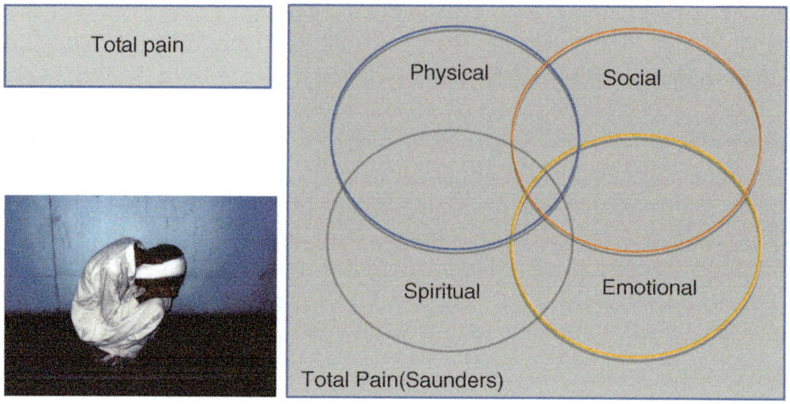


**Fig. 19.1** The concept of total pain

In order to answer the questions related to the care of patients needing palliative care, it is useful to quote the analogy of The Six Honest Serving Men, described by Rudyard Kipling way back in 1902. He said:

> "I keep Six Honest Serving Men,
> They taught me all I knew,
> Their names were Why and What and When
> and Where and How and Who."
> –Rudyard Kipling, 1902

In the context of palliative care issues, the answers can be found as follows:

- WHY?—To empower the patient/family.
- WHAT?—Does the patient WANT/NEED to know?
- WHEN?—From diagnosis until death.
- WHERE?—Clinic, ward, community.
- HOW?—With competence, compassion, sit, non-verbal communication, privacy.
- WHO?—Should tell/should be told (professional/patient/family).

***Why*** is it important to communicate the diagnosis to the patient with a life-threatening illness?

Firstly, it empowers the patient with knowledge, and begins the process of creating a relationship of trust between the professional and the patient and his family, working together with them in partnership. It enables them to make an informed choice. Do they want the treatment? Can they afford it? What are their options? It helps to reduce uncertainty, prevent unrealistic hope, and to give control to the patient and his family.

***What*** should we be communicating?

The professional needs to find out what the patient wants to know, and what the patient needs to know, about his diagnosis, in order to make informed choices. In my experience, there are some patients who want to know everything about their diagnosis, while others may say, "*I don't want to know, just talk to my relatives*". But our duty of care is, first and foremost to the patient, and only with his or her permission, should we be discussing the diagnosis with the family. Unfortunately, relatives, out of love, want to protect the patient, and will say to the doctor, "*please don't tell my wife/father/mother*". Sadly, this approach just sets up a "*conspiracy of silence*" whereby the family members know, and the patient often suspects the diagnosis, but nobody discusses it openly, and so both suffer in the silence, of keeping up a pretence, that everything is all right.

***When*** should patients be told?

In the West, patients tend to be told when all the investigations have been seen, and a diagnosis has been made. Patients should be mentally prepared, perhaps by asking, "*would you be able to tell me what's been happening to you?*" Or, "*how did all this start?*" At each visit they should be asked if they want to know what is happening, so they can maintain control of their lives. As the illness progresses towards death, some patients want to know everything, while others want limited or even, no information.

How do you know what the patient wants to know? Just ask! "*Would you like me to explain what is happening? Have you got any questions for me? Is there anyone you would like with you when I explain?*"

***Where*** should communication take place?

It may be in a clinic, the hospital ward, or the community at the patient's home affording as much privacy as possible, with both the professional and patient sitting at eye level.

***Who*** should be telling and to whom?

Ideally, it should be the treating physician: the person with all that the facts in front of them. The patient should be asked if they would like to have anyone with them when they receive significant information. There should always be a nurse present, with good communication skills, when significant news imparted so they can support and advocate for the patient.

***How?***

Invariably in India, the patients' relatives intercept and tell the doctor to inform them, and not the patient. However, the author has given questionnaires to Indian health professionals asking if they would tell the diagnosis to the patient or the relative first? Over 90% responded that they would tell the relative first and only tell the patient with the relative's permission, thus dis-empowering the patient, if the relative chooses not to allow the patient to be told the truth. However, when asked what they themselves would want, 99% of professionals wanted to be told the truth about their diagnosis, before or at the same time as their relative. When asked "*why?*", they replied that they wanted to be in control and to be able to get their affairs in order. It begs the question, "*What is the difference between a health care professional being informed of their life-threatening diagnosis, and any other patient*"?

The ways in which professionals communicate can have a positive or negative impact on a person's sense of spiritual wellbeing.

### 19.4.2 It Is All About Empathy!

Think of your patient as a VIP! Think about how would you or your nearest and dearest want to be treated? If *we* expect to be treated with respect and compassion, then surely the same goes for all our patients.

We often hear from doctors that the patient is not intelligent enough to understand their illness. But the fault is not with the patient but with the professionals because they do not have the requisite communication skills to make the information clear and understandable. After all, they have not been trained to communicate.

Think of the ways in which we can make our verbal and non-verbal communication effective. Consider how we examine and touch a patient, listen attentively, vary the tone of our voice, use the words to express, and how we welcome our patients to a strange and often frightening environment—all these things can matter in minimising their distress.

### 19.4.3 The Power of *Namaste* and Sitting

In a pilot study, patients perceived that the physician spent longer with them if they sat down, rather than standing [5]. There was a significant impact on patient satisfaction, compliance, and positive rapport. All of which added benefits of reduced lengths of stay cost-effectiveness, and improved clinical outcomes. The practical implication is that sitting beside a patient as opposed to standing is a better option.

In another study, the researcher looked at posture and communication [6]. Women who perceived the physician to be warmer, more caring, sensitive, and compassionate had less anxiety. Patients perceived doctors to be more compassionate when sitting [7].

Further research is necessary, as this could have a huge positive impact on the doctor-patient relationship.

We need to address non-verbal communication in its totality. How we use our body language, eye contact, tone of voice, the words we use, and the use of silence, all these do matter. In the age of mobile mania, it is always a good idea to turn off the mobile phone in a consultation.

The proper use of hands when examining the patient has a great potential to communicate respectful care, which can raise the person's self-esteem and feeling of comfort [8].

The use of narratives, complemented with photographs, can certainly have a positive impact on the audience.

Research has shown that using photographs helped students to develop skills in emotional recognition, cultivation of empathy, identification of narrative and awareness of multiple perspectives [9]. There is nothing like listening to the patient's story to increase the clinician's empathy and compassion [10].

**Table 19.1** Ten steps and tips for breaking bad news in the context of palliative care

| Steps to be followed | Tips and examples |
|---|---|
| 1. Preparation-very important | • Stools/chairs to sit on<br>• Know all the facts before the meeting<br>• Find out whom the patient wants to be present (e.g., relative/friend)<br>• Ensure privacy and that you will not be interrupted |
| 2. What does the patient know? | • Ask for a narrative of events by the patient. (How did it all start?) |
| 3. Is more information wanted? | • "*Test the waters*", but be aware that it can be very frightening to ask for more information<br>• *Example: "would you like me to explain a bit more*" |
| 4. Give a warning shot | *Example*<br>• "*I am afraid it looks rather serious*"<br>• Then allow a pause for the patient to respond |
| 5. Allow denial | • *Denial* is a defence mechanism and a way of coping<br>• *Allow the patient to control the amount of information* |
| 6. Explain (if requested) | • DETAIL will *NOT* be remembered but the *WAY* you explain *will* be remembered |
| 7. Listen to concerns | *Ask*<br>• "*What are your main concerns at the moment*"<br>• Allow time for the expression of feelings |
| 8. Encourage ventilation of feelings | • A KEY phase in terms of patient satisfaction<br>• It conveys *empathy* |
| 9. Summary of plan | • Summarise concerns<br>• Plan treatment<br>• Foster *realistic* hope |
| 10. Offer availability | • Most patients need further explanation (people forget the details)<br>• Adjustment takes weeks or months<br>• They may benefit from a family meeting |

These guidelines are derived from a booklet by Dr. Peter Kaye, a palliative care physician, with whom the author worked

### 19.4.4 Converting Theory into Practice

Based on the theory and practical experience in the field, the following ten steps are proposed for Breaking Bad News in the context of Palliative Care (Table 19.1).

The last word goes to Dame Cicely Saunders- a voice for the voiceless.

> Even when we feel that we can do absolutely nothing, we will still have to be prepared to stay. We should learn not only how-to free patients from pain and distress - but also how to be silent, how to listen, and how just to be there. I think if we try to remember this, we will see that the work is truly to the greater glory of God.—Saunders [2]

### 19.4.5 Conclusion

- The understanding of how to deal with the patients needing palliative care is a complex issue.
- One needs to appreciate the concept of total pain before delivering care.
- Special care should be taken to empower the patient and the family in helping themselves.
- The focus should be on providing a quality of life.
- The communication needs such greeting and welcoming the patients, active listening, genuine expression of empathy, appropriate use of body language, and posture of sitting should be considered.
- Breaking the bad news requires preparation of setting and systematic use of verbal skills and body language.

## 19.5 Evaluation

After reading this chapter, think of ways and means to address the palliative care issues in your chosen speciality. How can you acquire those skills?

Do you think the palliative care training in medical education requires interprofessional approach? If yes, how can you initiate such training?

## References

1. Twycross RG. Introducing palliative care. 4th ed. Abingdon: Radcliffe Publishing; 2003.
2. Saunders DC. Watch with me: inspiration for a life in hospice care. Lancaster: Mortal Press; 2003.
3. Saunders C. The evolution of palliative care. Patient Educ Couns. 2000;41(1):7–13.
4. Clark D. Total pain: the work of Cicely Saunders and the hospice movement. APS Bull. 2000;10(4):13–5.
5. Swayden KJ, Anderson KK, Connelly LM, Moran JS, McMahon JK, Arnold PM. Effect of sitting vs. standing on perception of provider time at bedside: a pilot study. Patient Educ Couns. 2012;86(2):166–71.
6. Bruera E, Palmer JL, Pace E, Zhang K, Willey J, Strasser F, Bennett MI. A randomized, controlled trial of physician postures when breaking bad news to cancer patients. Palliat Med. 2007;21(6):501–5.
7. Strasser F, Palmer JL, Willey J, Shen L, Shin K, Sivesind D, Beale E, Bruera E. Impact of physician sitting versus standing during inpatient oncology consultations: patients' preference and perception of compassion and duration. A randomized controlled trial. J Pain Symptom Manag. 2005;29(5):489–97.
8. Halstead LS. The power of compassion and caring in rehabilitation healing. Arch Phys Med Rehabil. 2001;82(2):149–54.
9. Shapiro J, Rucker L, Beck J. Training the clinical eye and mind: using the arts to develop medical students' observational and pattern recognition skills. Med Educ. 2006;40(3):263–8.
10. Moore RJ, Hallenbeck J. Narrative empathy and how dealing with stories helps: creating a space for empathy in culturally diverse care settings. J Pain Symptom Manag. 2010;40(3):471–6.

# The Role of Medical Humanities in the Development of Communication Skills

# 20

Upreet Dhaliwal

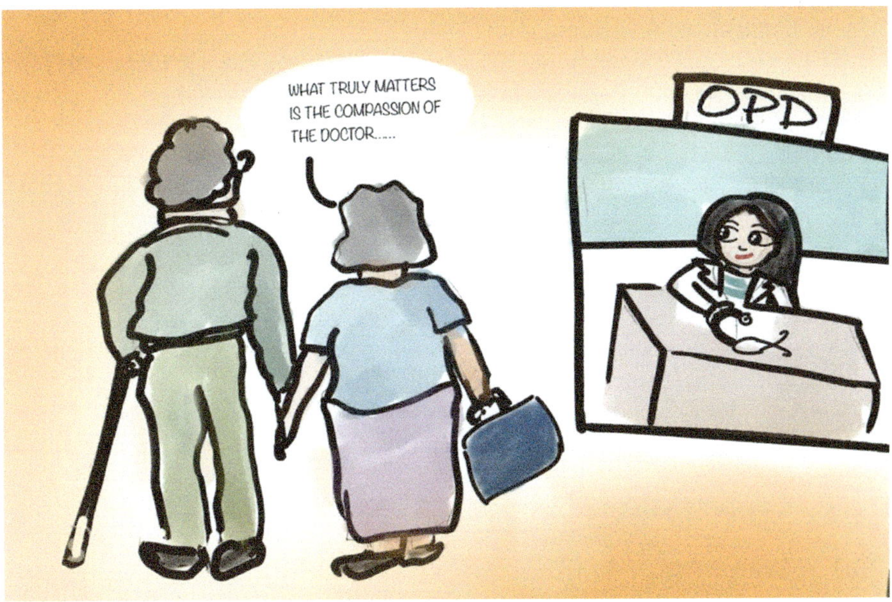


To whom shall I tell my grief?—Anton Chekhov: 'Misery', in the Schoolmistress and Other Stories, 2006

U. Dhaliwal (✉)
Medical Humanities Group, University College of Medical Sciences, University of Delhi, New Delhi, India



S. C. Parija, B. V. Adkoli (eds.), *Effective Medical Communication*,
https://doi.org/10.1007/978-981-15-3409-6_20

## 20.1 Assess Need

The therapeutic relationship begins to develop at the very first interaction between the healthcare provider and the patient. The desired outcome is the same for both stakeholders—the alleviation of suffering and the enhancement of the health of the patient. For the outcome to be achieved, both participants need to establish effective communication with each other [1].

Communication is taken for granted since we all learn to talk and write in childhood, and it is expected that our skills will improve with time and with practice; however, communication in medicine is complex and nuanced, and deserves attention [2]. For the communication to be effective, the provider must take into consideration the 'history' of the patient, the 'language' he understands, his 'cultural' and 'religious' background, and his 'human' dimensions [3, 4]. The provider, thus, has to come from a position of humanity; otherwise, the communication stands the risk of becoming meaningless and irrelevant to the patient's context, besides evoking patient dissatisfaction with care [5].

Healing is as much about science as it is about the human element of the stakeholders—this understanding is one of the reasons that humanities disciplines have begun to find a place in formal and informal medical curricula all over the globe [6, 7].

## 20.2 Brief

In this chapter, we will:

1. Demonstrate how the humanities disciplines can enhance verbal, written, and other non-verbal forms of communication.
2. Suggest ways to incorporate the humanities into the curriculum.

## 20.3 Contextualize

### 20.3.1 Scenario 1

An old man comes to the ophthalmology outpatient department (OPD) without a current OPD paper. It is not his surgical team's follow-up day, so the registration clerk does not stamp his old papers or give him a new one. You have 50 patients waiting to be seen, and it is nearly lunchtime. The registration counter has closed for the day. When you tell him this, he says 'I just want the medicines repeated'. You know he will not get his medicines if his paper is not stamped. You reach a dead end. Meanwhile, your other patients are getting restless.

Now consider this version of the same story described in a poem:

*A dogged old man blocks the entrance*<br>
*to my outpatient chamber*<br>
*with his ancient body*

*as though desperately unwilling*
*to squander what's left*
*of his fleeting time -*
*loathe to cool*
*his spent old heels*
*in the heat of what might well be*
*his last torrid summer.*
*His unspoken wish*
*to be examined at once*
*is thwarted by the person*
*manning the door:*
*Your surgeon is not here;*
*Today's not her day, and*
*Your papers aren't stamped*
*Because they're for Tuesday.*
*That's when you should visit -*
*Now stop blocking the door;*
*just...move away, please.*
*His unspoken wish*
*to be examined at once*
*is met with robust cries*
*of helpless frustration*
*from fifty others*
*who have been standing so long*
*in a serpentine queue;*
*numbing and miasmic,*
*their own pain crescendos*
*to a fidgety clamour*
*that makes them temporarily blind*
*to the old one's burden.*

***Exercise***: Think of these versions, both of which could be used to help medical students learn about the ethics of doctor–patient communication; however, the second version—the poem—adds a layer of humanity to the protagonists by giving them a three-dimensional character with thoughts and feelings. This is a strength of the humanities. It has the ability to humanize medical communication.

### 20.3.2 Scenario 2

Dr. Comini notices that students are able to take a reasonable history from patients; unfortunately, it is a bare-bones history which focuses on the illness and not on the person who is ill. Thus, the student fails to capture nuances that could impact treatment, like there may be no caregiver or the patient may be dependent on an indifferent caregiver, or there may be an underlying depression that the patient does not want to talk about.

The teacher decides to expose students to storytelling, and invites patients and their care givers to tell their stories—not necessarily stories of illness but stories of their lives—who they are, how they live, what they have achieved in their lives, and their fears and hopes.

Now consider the feedback she received from the students about storytelling. This was, indeed, delightful, for they began to see patients as humans rather than as illnesses to be cured.

## 20.4 Describe

### 20.4.1 The Provider's Role in Communication

Since the relationship is unequal, the onus is on the provider to ensure that the communication is in a language that the patient understands, and it is sensitive to the patient's needs and goals, is empathetic, is respectful of patient preferences and of the need for privacy and confidentiality, and encourages their participation in shared decision-making. The principles of effective communication also apply during communication with the patient's family, with peers, and with others in the community, and when recording patient data.

### 20.4.2 The Role of the Humanities in Communication

Several humanities disciplines are known to influence the way in which we communicate. Table 20.1 lists the disciplines and provides details of how they can help improve different aspects of communication.

**Table 20.1** Humanities disciplines and their influence on verbal, written, and other non-verbal forms of communication

| Humanities Discipline | Potential influence on communication skills |
|---|---|
| Visual art and films [8, 9] | Promote observation, reflection, critical analysis, data gathering, oral debate, and written communication |
| Various forms of theatre [10] | Promote interpersonal communication, verbal communication, appropriate and effective use of body language to build trust, presentation skills, and encourage self-expression |
| Literature, graphical literature, and poetry [11, 12] | Understand different perspectives, foster engagement with feelings and thoughts—of self and of others, and experience empathetic and effective communication |
| Newspaper incident reports and other media, including biographies and history of medicine [13, 14] | Learn ethical and professional communication, respect for diverse opinions, and truth-telling with respect and sensitivity |
| Anthropology [15] | Hone culturally competent, communication |
| Music and dance [16, 17] | Learn self-expression, non-verbal communication, culturally competent communication |
| Disability studies [18]; gender studies [19] | Hone culturally competent and respectful communication |

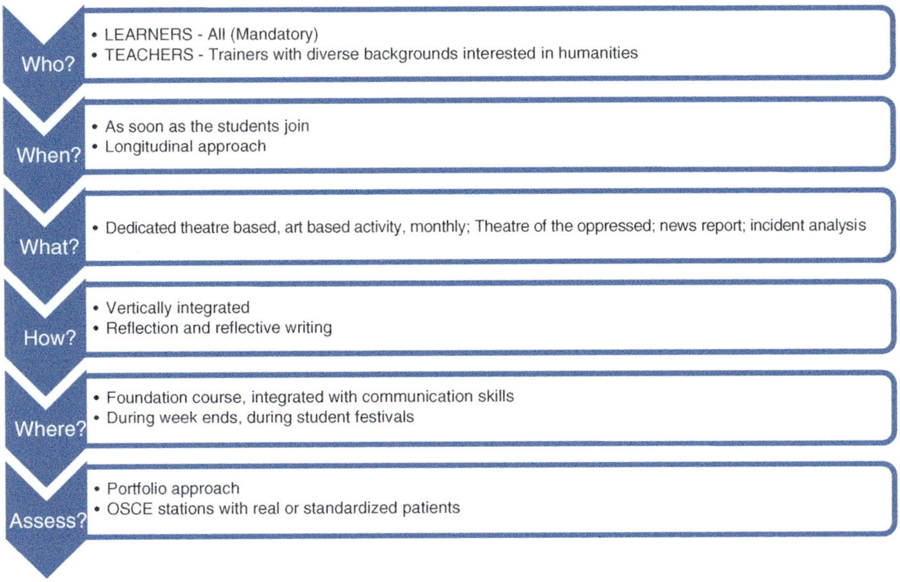


**Fig. 20.1** Points to keep in mind when devising a humanities curriculum for communication skills

### 20.4.3 Incorporating the Humanities into the Curriculum

The points to be kept in mind while incorporating the humanities into the medical curriculum have been highlighted in the following paragraphs (Fig. 20.1).

#### 20.4.3.1 Who Can be the Learners?

Communication is too important a topic to make it an elective subject. Thus, it should be mandatory for every health professions' learner to participate in the humanities initiatives.

#### 20.4.3.2 Who Can be Trainers?

The humanities are a collection of diverse tools, and teachers may or may not have an interest in using them. Health professions' teachers with a special inclination, with some experience, or with a curiosity about one or more of these tools may be encouraged to adopt them. Which humanities discipline works in a particular context will also depend on the interests of the learners. An interdisciplinary approach may ensure that a number of teachers are available; a transdisciplinary approach, with teachers being drawn in from the humanities disciplines, may be even more useful—such an eclectic mix will expose learners to the multifaceted nature of real-life communication.

#### 20.4.3.3 When Should Exposure to the Humanities Begin?

The need for communicating in an effective, contextual way begins as soon as students join a health professions course; thus, they should be exposed to communication techniques as soon as they join, i.e., during the first few months; in the case of medical students, this would be in the foundation course.

#### 20.4.3.4 What Should the Duration of Exposure to the Humanities be?

Exposure to multiple humanities modalities tabled above should continue throughout the course. A longitudinal approach could be used, with learners progressing from simpler concepts in communication (respectful communication, data gathering, presentation, communication during teamwork) to those of greater complexity (history taking, counseling, documentation, breaking bad news) commensurate with their increasing levels of competence.

#### 20.4.3.5 What Could a Humanities Curriculum Look Like?

A dedicated theatre-based, and/or art-based, and/or poetry-based activity every semester; a monthly movie chosen so that it has entertainment value, but also highlights important concepts of appropriate communication. Theatre during student festivals once annually to address areas where students, patients, caregivers, and faculty struggle because of failure in communication; news reports suggestive of breakdown of communication, and incident analysis undertaken immediately after an incident to help students make sense of the causes and consequences of poor communication; and humanities research projects for students looking to participate in intramural research.

Reflections and reflective writing should be encouraged after each humanities endeavour with feedback being provided so that the learning is internalized. Vertical integration, if it can be logistically managed, would allow a mixed class of students—from the first year through to final year—so that an opportunity is provided for peer-teaching and peer-mentoring to augment the learning of communication in a safe environment.

#### 20.4.3.6 Where Could One Find the Time?

Dedicated time should be allotted to the teaching of humanities. It would be ideal to devote about 3–4 h a week during the foundation course or in the first 2 weeks after joining a health professions course. Later on, dedicated slots should be set aside by all disciplines for training in communication skill, with additional opportunities provided after classes and during weekends, and at the time of student festivals.

#### 20.4.3.7 Ways to Assess the Humanities Curriculum for the Achievement of Communication Goals

Humanities learning can be best assessed by means of student portfolios that include written reflections, poems, narratives, and oral presentations. Assessment can also be done in the form of OSCE stations, assessed by observers using rubrics. Standardized patients can be used effectively for assessing a humane attitude. It is more feasible to assess the development of humanities by internal assessment rather than external assessment.

#### 20.4.3.8 The Role of Institutions and Universities

Encourage faculty and students to be creative so that institutional culture evolves to one where humanistic communication is the norm. Humanities interventions in health professions education are engaging, enriching experiences that achieve more than just the stated goals. Student acceptance is often high since didactic teaching is replaced by activities that stimulate imagination and creativity (Fig. 20.1).

### 20.4.4 Conclusion

- Several humanities disciplines are known to influence verbal, written, and other non-verbal forms of communication.
- The humanities highlight the human element of the stakeholders—patients, care providers, and caregivers.
- Through a study of the humanities, learners can approach communication through an understanding of the patient's context.
- Exposure to multiple humanities modalities should begin early in the medical course, and should continue throughout the course, starting with simpler concepts in communication, and progressing to more complex concepts as learner competency increases.

## 20.5 Evaluate

If you have decided to read this chapter, then you are already convinced of the role of the medical humanities in medical education. Figure out what humanities discipline appeals to you and begin to use it in your endeavours with students. Imagine that there are no rules except mutual respect and safety, then, through cooperation with your learners, evolve a paradigm that works in your context.

## References

1. Jones J, Willis D. Doctors' communication of trust, care, and respect: it takes two to make therapeutic relationship work. BMJ. 2004;328(7451):1318. author reply 1319.
2. Pun JK, Matthiessen CM, Murray KA, Slade D. Factors affecting communication in emergency departments: doctors and nurses' perceptions of communication in a trilingual ED in Hong Kong. Int J Emerg Med. 2015;8(1):48. https://doi.org/10.1186/s12245-015-0095-y.
3. Craxì L, Giardina S, Spagnolo AG. A return to humane medicine: Osler's legacy. Infez Med. 2017;25(3):292–7.
4. Bittner-Fagan H, Davis J, Savoy M. Improving patient safety: improving communication. FP Essent. 2017;463:27–33.
5. Nguyen TV, Hong J, Prose NS. Compassionate care: enhancing physician-patient communication and education in dermatology: part I: patient-centered communication. J Am Acad Dermatol. 2013;68(3):353.e1–8. https://doi.org/10.1016/j.jaad.2012.10.059.
6. Kelly M, Dornan T. Mapping the landscape or exploring the terrain? Progressing humanism in medical education. Med Educ. 2016;50(3):273–5. https://doi.org/10.1111/medu.12967.

7. Dhaliwal U, Singh S, Singh N. Promoting competence in undergraduate medical students through the humanities: the ABCDE paradigm. RhiME. 2015;2:28–36.
8. Boisaubin EV, Winkler MG. Seeing patients and life contexts: the visual arts in medical education. Am J Med Sci. 2000;319(5):292–6.
9. Wellbery C, McAteer RA. The art of observation: a pedagogical framework. Acad Med. 2015;90(12):1624–30. https://doi.org/10.1097/ACM.0000000000000801.
10. Hoffmann-Longtin K, Loue S, Love LM, Liu HY, Power CM, et al. Active learning on center stage: theater as a tool for medical education. MedEdPORTAL. 2019;15:10801. Available from https://www.ncbi.nlm.nih.gov/pmc/articles/PMC6476526/.
11. Davies EA. Why we need more poetry in palliative care. BMJ support palliat Care. 2018;8(3):266–70. https://doi.org/10.1136/bmjspcare-2017-001477.
12. Charon R, Hermann N, Devlin MJ. Close reading and creative writing in clinical education: teaching attention, representation, and affiliation. Acad Med. 2016;91(3):345–50. https://doi.org/10.1097/ACM.0000000000000827.
13. Vachon B, LeBlanc J. Effectiveness of past and current critical incident analysis on reflective learning and practice change. Med Educ. 2011;45(9):894–904. https://doi.org/10.1111/j.1365-2923.2011.04042.x.
14. Bryan CS, Longo LD. Perspective: teaching and mentoring the history of medicine: an Oslerian perspective. Acad Med. 2013;88(1):97–101. https://doi.org/10.1097/ACM.0b013e31827653f5.
15. Davenport BA. Witnessing and the medical gaze: how medical students learn to see at a free clinic for the homeless. Med Anthropol Q. 2000;14(3):310–27.
16. Wilson C, Bungay H, Munn-Giddings C, Boyce M. Healthcare professionals' perceptions of the value and impact of the arts in healthcare settings: a critical review of the literature. Int J Nurs Stud. 2016;56:90–101. https://doi.org/10.1016/j.ijnurstu.2015.11.003.
17. Newell A, Kleinman P. Doctors can dance. Lond Rev Educ. 2012;10(2):133–44.
18. Coret A, Boyd K, Hobbs K, Zazulak J, McConnell M. Patient narratives as a teaching tool: a pilot study of first-year medical students and patient educators affected by intellectual/developmental disabilities. Teach Learn Med. 2018;30(3):317–27. https://doi.org/10.1080/10401334.2017.1398653.
19. Luz C, Hall D, Gardner P, Hennessey CW, Lammers L. Transformative theatre: a promising educational tool for improving health encounters with LGBT older adults. Gerontol Geriatr Educ. 2016;37(3):292–306. https://doi.org/10.1080/02701960.2015.1127812.

# 21 Communication Skills for Medical Professionals: Perspectives from the Middle East

Mona Hmoud Al-Sheikh and Muhammad Zafar Iqbal

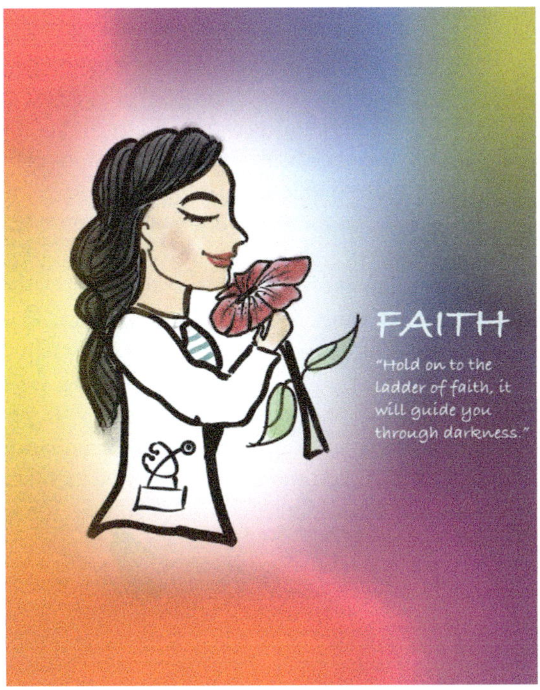


Communication should be simple, effective and culturally appropriate—Mona and Zafar

M. H. Al-Sheikh (✉) · M. Z. Iqbal
Medical Education Department, College of Medicine, Imam Abdulrahman Bin Faisal University, Dammam, Saudi Arabia
e-mail: zafar@iau.edu.sa



S. C. Parija, B. V. Adkoli (eds.), *Effective Medical Communication*,
https://doi.org/10.1007/978-981-15-3409-6_21

## 21.1 Assess Need

Communication is defined as *a two-way process involving speech, writing, or non-verbal means that aim to create shared interpretation for those involved* [1]. Effective communication between health professionals and patients is the key ingredient to a safe and quality healthcare system [2]. It is also responsible for building a satisfactory and conducive relationship between all stakeholders. Between doctor and patients, it helps in building rapport, improving patient satisfaction, coping with prescriptions, and ensuring desired positive outcomes. On the other hand, effective communication between health professionals (doctors, undergraduate and post-graduate trainees, nurses, auxiliary medical staff) helps in building safe, trustworthy, supportive, and professional working environment [3].

Effective communication is among the most fundamental skills which are essential for health professionals. Its value increases further in a multicultural and multilingual culture where many factors affect the interaction between the stakeholders. Some of the most commonly recognized factors include language, ethnicity, literacy level, health awareness, religious, and/or social beliefs [2]. Most of these factors are directly related to the different communities which are living and working in the Gulf region (Saudi Arabia, United Arab Emirates, Bahrain, Oman, Qatar, and Kuwait). Although some studies conducted in Middle East reported nationality and language diversity to be an insignificant barrier, however, more literature is inclined otherwise [2, 4, 5].

Despite the huge significance of effective communication in the literature, unfortunately, it remains the most underrated skill in the gulf region. One wonders if there is a system available to assess the level of communication gap and its fallouts in healthcare services. Another intriguing question is that do we really realize the value of communication skills in our professional training? If yes, then what measures have we taken so far to ensure successful achievement and demonstration of effective communication? It is about time that we focus on incorporating and assessing communication skills in our health professionals so that safe and quality healthcare services can be ensured.

## 21.2 Brief

This chapter highlights the significance of effective communication in the healthcare system of the Middle Eastern region, which is largely populated by the multicultural and multilingual communities. In this chapter, we have tried to:

- Discuss the cultural and lingual issues that can become a barrier in providing quality healthcare.

- Explain a detailed rationale on why teaching communication skills to healthcare providers is essential.
- Offer practical tips on how effective communication skills can be learned, and practised by the health professionals working in the Middle East.

## 21.3 Contextualize

### 21.3.1 Scenario 1

An expatriate, Gyne/Obs specialist, working in a teaching hospital in the Middle East, performed an internal examination on a middle-aged woman belonging to a tribal area. During the examination, he was unable to feel the cervix. Using the speculum to view the cervix, he discovered a white round tumour covering the cervix. After finding the tumour, he immediately consulted his senior, and they decided to take a biopsy. Upon inquiry by the local consultant, the patient reluctantly disclosed that she had placed an onion in her vagina (a normal practice in her village) to induce labour. Somehow, the patient hesitated in sharing this information with the doctor thinking that the doctor may not be able to comprehend or appreciate the use of the home remedy. Surely, it was a unique experience for the expatriate doctor.

***Exercise***: Now imagine yourself in a similar kind of situation and reflect on how would you cater such kind of cultural barriers?

### 21.3.2 Scenario 2

This is the story of Ms. SSN, who has been working as a senior staff nurse in a tertiary care hospital of Saudi Arabia for the past 4 years. When she was newly recruited, she was a very hardworking and professional worker, but she did not have any command on the local (Arabic) language. From time to time, she used to seek help from her fellow colleagues to communicate with Arabic speaking patients. One day, she was working in the in-patient surgery ward on a night shift. During the night shift, an old patient, who was in his post-operative care, called Ms. SSN and said '*jib futa*'. At first, she was taken by surprise, and she thought to herself that she might have misheard it. To clarify her understanding, she asked the patient politely '*aish*' meaning '*what?*'. He then repeated the same word '*jib futa*' again but with a bit firm tone. This time, she was in shock because this word holds bad meaning (prostitute) in her native language. Dismayed in her thoughts, she returned to the nursing counter, and started crying. Seeing her crying, one of the native colleagues approached her and inquired about the matter. Ms. SSN told her reluctantly that the old man in bed number so and so had abused her and called her '*futa*'. At first, her colleague looked surprised and asked, "*what is the problem in that?*" Then Ms. SSN told her the meaning of this word in her native language. After listening to the issue, her colleague smiled and explained to Ms. SSN that in Arabic, '*gib*' means '*bring*', and '*futa*' means '*towel*'. By putting her hand on Ms. SSN's shoulder, she politely said, '*My dear, all he is asking for is a towel and nothing else*'. After listening to this, Ms. SSN felt relieved, but this incidence made her realize the value of learning the local language for effective communication with patients and for her own professional growth.

***Exercise***: Deliberate how Ms. SSN can overcome her language barriers in both the short and long term?

## 21.4 Describe

The communities within the Gulf region are a unique blend of Arabs and expatriates which differ in traditions, cultural backgrounds, and spoken languages [6]. Therefore, the two most commonly known barriers to effective communication in gulf countries are cultural and linguistic barriers. In this section, we will explain in detail how cultural and linguistic diversities affect communication between stakeholders (doctors, nurses, other health professionals, patients, and their families) of the local healthcare system.

### 21.4.1 Cultural Barriers

The local Arabs are predominantly Muslims, and they strictly follow Islamic values and beliefs which are deeply rooted in their lifestyles. Locals strongly believe in modesty, evil eye, family values, modest female clothing, and spirituality [4]. Some of the most common cultural norms of the local Arab community are as follows:

1. *Extended family structure:* Big families consisting of parents, grandparents, unmarried brothers and sisters, married sons with their wives and children all live together under one roof.
2. *Shame and honour:* The feeling of kinship '*hammula*' is prominent in the Arab world. Any insult to the tribal origin is considered a felony.
3. *Mental and physical disabilities:* Mental illness and physical disabilities are a stigma in most Arab communities and are usually kept hidden from the society. People feel ashamed of admitting these disabilities because society might perceive them as hereditary; thus, the reputation of the whole family is considered at stake.
4. *Infertility:* Infertility is perceived as a shame rather than a disease, and many times it leads to divorces.
5. *Physical contact:* Physical social contact such as hand-shaking and hugging between males and females is strongly discouraged and is prohibited in Arab culture.

6. *Doctor–family communication instead of doctor–patient communication:* The information related to the disease is expected to be given to the entire family and not to the patient alone. Family presence is highly valued and their opinion matters in the choice of treatment and later on in treatment compliance.
7. *Gender bias:* Most of the times, patients and families expect a female obstetrician to attend the gynaecological issues, whereas the male staff is not preferred to be present in the delivery room.

On the other hand, the expatriates living in this region belong to various ethnicities; they follow different religions and customs based on their backgrounds. In Saudi Arabia alone, expatriates constitute almost 30% of the total population [2], whereas in UAE, the total population of locals is under 10% [4]. Considering the complex multicultural norms in Arab countries, it is inevitable to expect a healthcare worker to possess both medical and cultural competence [7]. The cultural competence is an essential requirement to interact effectively with people of different cultures and beliefs. The know-how of the professional staff about the regional and cultural norms helps in reducing diagnostic errors, drug complications, misunderstandings among doctors/patients, co-workers, and families [8]. Despite the fact that cultural competence is an important pre-requisite, the literature suggests that many times, health professionals struggle in accommodating patients' customs and beliefs, especially those who belong to the non-Muslim world. Many studies [9–12] have highlighted this issue where health professionals face difficulties in coping with the spiritual and religious needs while ensuring high standards of medical care. The religious and cultural discordance may create a serious communication gap between patients and health professionals which not only affects healthcare quality but also causes patient dissatisfaction and cultural conflicts (Fig. 21.1).

### 21.4.2 Linguistic Barriers

In the healthcare system of gulf countries, most health professionals are expatriates which majorly belong to India, Pakistan, Indonesia, Philippines, America, Canada, and the United Kingdom [4, 13, 14]. All of these countries have their own mother languages which fairly differ from the Arabic language. Although the official mode of communication in teaching institutes and hospitals in the Gulf is English, still, Arabic language remains the primary spoken tongue within the community. This language barrier may not be considered as an emergency challenge between healthcare providers as most of the local and expatriate health professionals communicate in English. Yet, it remains an overarching issue when it comes to local patients who are not fluent in English, and they use Arabic as their principal language for communication [15]. This linguistic barrier may cause misinterpretation of patient needs and medical issues, resulting in patient demotivation, poor treatment compliance, and sub-standard patient care [4]. On the other hand, miscommunication between

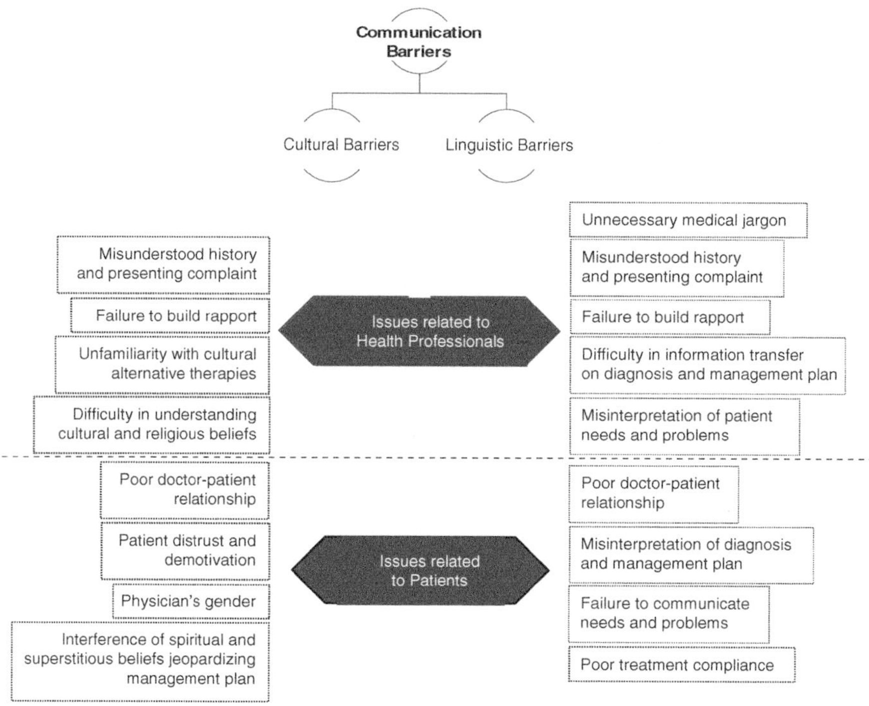


**Fig. 21.1** Communication barriers and their potential outcomes in the Middle East

health professionals can cause malpractice, medicolegal errors, misinterpretation of clinical findings, procedural errors, and poor healthcare outcomes [16] (Fig. 21.1).

### 21.4.3 Teaching and Learning Communication Skills

Many scholars [17–20] stress upon improving communication between health professionals and patients in order to achieve high-quality healthcare. In these studies, a structured training on communication skills has been advocated as an integral component of undergraduate, postgraduate, and continuing professional development of healthcare, providers to prevent communication-related issues.

It has now become a necessity rather than a luxury to train health professionals on how to communicate effectively in healthcare settings. Many health professional programs [1] and national bodies [21] have already incorporated communication skill in their competency-based training frameworks. Some programs have also introduced communication skills courses at entry-level of medical and other allied health sciences degree programs. Despite its recognition as a key competency, it has not been conceived by many health sciences curricula in the Gulf region, especially outside medicine [22]. In literature, many guides and frameworks exit on developing communication skills, some of them are local [12], while others are international [23–25]. These models can be used as guides to develop a training framework which can fulfil the contextual needs of the regional community.

Usually, individuals have their own pre-developed communication styles and preferences prior to health professional education and training [26]. However, in the context of healthcare practices, effective communication is highly technical and may require structured training, practice, and constructive feedback to develop the skill further [27]. The training should ideally be based on the principles of patient-centred approach where patient-oriented clinical evidence guide the learning outcomes, clinical scenarios, and problem statements of the training courses [12]. These dedicated courses on communication skills should be an integral part of undergraduate as well as postgraduate pedagogy [17, 28, 29].

To make these courses more effective, especially in undergraduate education, early patient exposure starting from year one of medical/health sciences training can play a key role [30]. This approach can help the students in understanding patient needs and medical humanities in addition to improving their communication skills. Communicating directly with patients can also help students improve their scientific perspective and awareness regarding social traditions [31]. At the same time, teachers should catalyse the learning process by acting as role models and guiding students on how to communicate effectively with patients. Ahmed [32] suggested that patient exposure in the early years of health professional training should be primary care and family centres oriented rather than tertiary care hospitals to augment doctor–patient communication training.

In certain cases, there are not enough opportunities to train health professional students via direct patient exposure due to the lack of patients in some healthcare domains or simply due to the lack of patient consent. In this scenario, simulation-based training through mannequins and simulated patients can be the best possible alternative [33]. It allows learners to develop their communication skills by practising in a safe and controlled environment in which they are free from the fear of harming the patients or getting penalized [34]. Simulation is a student-centred, experiential learning method in which learners are exposed to various complex medical problems which mimic real-life clinical scenarios. In this controlled environment, multiple opportunities for rehearsal and constructive feedback are provided to optimize student learning [35]. The potential benefits of simulation-based training are well known in health professions education. Jay et al. [36] reported a higher quality of counselling skills in trainees who attended simulation course as compared to those who did not. Similar findings were reported by Kaplonyi et al. [34], who observed significant attitudinal changes in students with respect to their communication skills.

At the level of practising physicians and healthcare workers, much work is required to develop their communication skills. These qualified doctors, nurses, and other health professionals can be trained through continuous professional development programs such as workshops, seminars, conferences, and certification courses [18, 37]. Although continuous professional development is an integral part of licensure extensions and promotions in almost all gulf countries, most of these activities are clinical skills-oriented. Less attention has been given on conducting

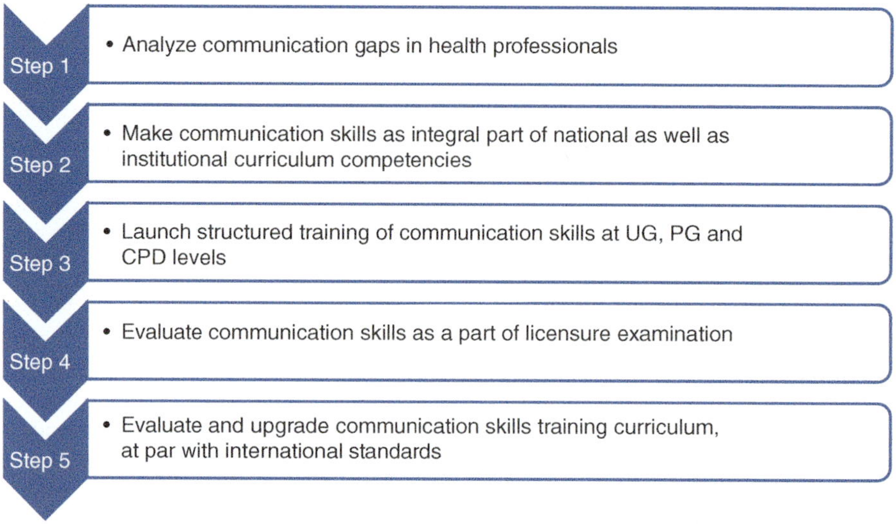


**Fig. 21.2** Steps in incorporating communication skills into the curriculum

professional development activities on communication skills [38]. The training courses on communication skills should be a norm in which the health professionals are exposed to communication sensitive issues such as breaking bad news to patients, dealing with gynaecological, sexual, or oncological issues and counselling patients suffering from terminal illness or chronic disease etc. [32].

In addition to the training of health professionals at an institutional level, a dedicated assessment component on the Arabic language can be incorporated in the official licensure examination of the gulf countries. This will help in assessing the lingual and cultural competence of potential candidates in addition to their medical knowledge and skillset. This practice is already well established in many countries such as USA, UK, Canada, and Australia, where the health professional applicant has to demonstrate effective communication skills through IELTS, TOEFL, and aptitude tests. A brief summary of the essential steps required for incorporating effective communication skills among health professionals is given in Fig. 21.2.

### 21.4.4 Conclusion

- Effective communication skills can help in overcoming cultural and linguistic barriers in the gulf region.
- Health professionals with polished communication skills can address patient issues more efficiently, and can help in bringing down healthcare costs inflicted by medical errors and legal penalties.
- A thorough analysis of cultural, verbal, and non-verbal communication issues through the lens of various stakeholders; patients, healthcare workers, adminis-

trative bodies is required. This systematic evaluation will provide the groundwork for commencing structured training of health professionals on intercultural communication skills.
- The health professional institutes should provide the necessary support to their healthcare staff by offering language training services.
- In addition to the training of health professionals, it has been suggested that a dedicated assessment section on the Arabic language can be incorporated in the official licensure examination of the gulf countries.

## 21.5 Evaluate

From this chapter, you had an overview of how essential effective communication skills are in the Middle Eastern healthcare system. Being a health professional, imagine a position is vacant in a primary care hospital situated in the tribal area of a gulf country. Take a few minutes to reflect on the following:

- How will you cater to the cultural and lingual communication gap if you get a job offer?
- What will be your short- and long-term approaches?

## References

1. Denniston C, Molloy E, Nestel D, Woodward-Kron R, Keating JL. Learning outcomes for communication skills across the health professions: a systematic literature review and qualitative synthesis. BMJ Open. 2017;7(4):e014570.
2. Almutairi KM. Culture and language differences as a barrier to provision of quality care by the health workforce in Saudi Arabia. Saudi Med J. 2015;36(4):425–31.
3. Schyve PM. Language differences as a barrier to quality and safety in health care: the joint commission perspective. J Gen Intern Med. 2007;22(2):360–1.
4. Albahri AH, Abushibs AS, Abushibs NS. Barriers to effective communication between family physicians and patients in walk-in Centre setting in Dubai: a cross-sectional survey. BMC Health Serv Res. 2018;18(1):1–14.
5. Khalifah AM, Celenza A. Teaching and assessment of dentist-patient communication skills: a systematic review to identify best-evidence methods. J Dent Educ. 2019;83(1):16–31.
6. Almutairi A, McCarthy AL. A multicultural nursing workforce and cultural perspectives in Saudi Arabia: an overview. The Health. 2012;3(3):71–4.
7. Shen Z. Cultural competence models and cultural competence assessment instruments in nursing: a literature review. J Transcult Nurs. 2015;26(3):308–21.
8. Delphin-Rittmon ME, Andres-Hyman R, Flanagan EH, Davidson L. Seven essential strategies for promoting and sustaining systemic cultural competence. Psychiatry Q. 2013;84(1):53–64.
9. Al-Yateem N, AlYateem S, Rossiter R. Cultural and religious educational needs of overseas nurses working in the Kingdom of Saudi Arabia and the United Arab Emirates. Holist Nurs Pract. 2015;29(4):205–15.
10. Sidumo EM, Ehlers VJ, Hattingh SP. Cultural knowledge of non-Muslim nurses working in Saudi Arabian obstetric units. Curationis. 2010;33(3):48–55.

11. Halligan P. Caring for patients of Islamic denomination: critical care nurses' experiences in Saudi Arabia. J Clin Nurs. 2006;15(12):1565–73.
12. Alsaad SM, Alshammari SA, Almogbel TA. Appraisal of the communication skills of residents in the family medicine program in Central Saudi Arabia. Saudi Med J. 2016;37(7):804–8.
13. Aldossary A, While A, Barriball L. Health care and nursing in Saudi Arabia. Int Nurs Rev. 2008;55(1):125–8.
14. Aboul-Enein FH. Personal contemporary observations of nursing care in Saudi Arabia. Int J Nurs Pract. 2002;8(4):228–30.
15. Al-Khathami AM, Kojan SW, Aljumah MA, Alqahtani H, Alrwaili H. The effect of nurse-patient language barrier on patients' satisfaction. Saudi Med J. 2010;31(12):1355–8.
16. Rehim SA, DeMoor S, Olmsted R, Dent DL, Parker-Raley J. Tools for assessment of communication skills of hospital action teams: a systematic review. J Surg Educ. 2017;74(2):341–51.
17. Carey JA, Madill A, Manogue M. Communications skills in dental education: a systematic research review. Eur J Dent Educ. 2010;14(2):69–78.
18. Bylund CL, Brown RF, di Ciccone BL, Levin TT, Gueguen JA, Hill C, et al. Training faculty to facilitate communication skills training: development and evaluation of a workshop. Patient Educ Couns. 2008;70(3):430–6.
19. Hobgood C, Sawning S, Bowen J, Savage K. Teaching culturally appropriate care: a review of educational models and methods. Acad Emerg Med. 2006;13(12):1288–95.
20. Werner A, Holderried F, Schäffeler N, Weyrich P, Riessen R, Zipfel S, et al. Communication training for advanced medical students improves information recall of medical laypersons in simulated informed consent talks–a randomized controlled trial. BMC Med Educ. 2013;13(1):15.
21. Zaini RG, Bin Abdulrahman KA, Al-Khotani AA, Al-Hayani AMA, Al-Alwan IA, Jastaniah SD. Saudi Meds: a competence specification for Saudi medical graduates. Med Teach. 2011;33(7):582–4.
22. Bachmann C, Abramovitch H, Barbu CG, Cavaco AM, Elorza RD, Haak R, et al. A European consensus on learning objectives for a core communication curriculum in health care professions. Patient Educ Couns. 2013;93(1):18–26.
23. Makoul G. The SEGUE framework for teaching and assessing communication skills. Patient Educ Couns. 2001;45(1):23–34.
24. Rider EA, Hinrichs MM, Lown BA. A model for communication skills assessment across the undergraduate curriculum. Med Teach. 2006;28(5):e127–34.
25. Salmon P, Young B. Creativity in clinical communication: from communication skills to skilled communication. Med Educ. 2011;45(3):217–26.
26. Salmon P, Young B. The validity of education and guidance for clinical communication in cancer care: evidence-based practice will depend on practice-based evidence. Patient Educ Couns. 2013;90(2):193–9.
27. Wouda JC, van de Wiel HBM. Education in patient–physician communication: how to improve effectiveness? Patient Educ Couns. 2013;90(1):46–53.
28. Vogel D, Meyer M, Harendza S. Verbal and non-verbal communication skills including empathy during history taking of undergraduate medical students. BMC Med Educ. 2018;18(1):1–8.
29. Kelly M, Nixon L, Broadfoot K, Hofmeister M, Dornan T. Drama to promote non-verbal communication skills. Clin Teach. 2019;16(2):108–13.
30. Cade J. An evaluation of early patient contact for medical students. Med Educ. 1993;27(3):205–10.
31. Bensing J. Bridging the gap.: the separate worlds of evidence-based medicine and patient-centered medicine. Patient Educ Couns. 2000;39(1):17–25.
32. Elzubier AG. Doctor-patient communication: a skill needed in Saudi Arabia. J Family Community Med. 2002;9(1):51–6.
33. Bremner MN, Aduddell K, Bennett DN, VanGeest JB. The use of human patient simulators. Nurse Educ. 2006;31(4):170–4.
34. Kaplonyi J, Bowles KA, Nestel D, Kiegaldie D, Maloney S, Haines T, et al. Understanding the impact of simulated patients on health care learners' communication skills: a systematic review. Med Educ. 2017;51(12):1209–19.

35. Bakogiannis A, Darling JC, Dimitrova V, Roberts TE. Simulation for communication skills training in medical students: protocol for a systematic scoping review. Int J Educ Res. 2019;93:243–9.
36. Jay M, Schlair S, Caldwell R, Kalet A, Sherman S, Gillespie C. From the patient's perspective: the impact of training on resident physician's obesity counseling. J Gen Intern Med. 2010;25(5):415–22.
37. Alofisan T, Al-Alaiyan S, Al-Abdulsalam M, Siddiqui K, Hussain I, Al-Qahtani M. Communication skills in pediatric training program: national-based survey of residents' perspectives in Saudi Arabia. J Fam Community Med. 2015;23(1):43.
38. Berkhof M, van Rijssen HJ, Schellart AJM, Anema JR, van der Beek AJ. Effective training strategies for teaching communication skills to physicians: an overview of systematic reviews. Patient Educ Couns. 2011;84(2):152–62.

# Cultural Sensitivities in Communication: A Southeast Asian Countries Perspective

# 22

Muzaherul Huq and Shegufta Mohammad

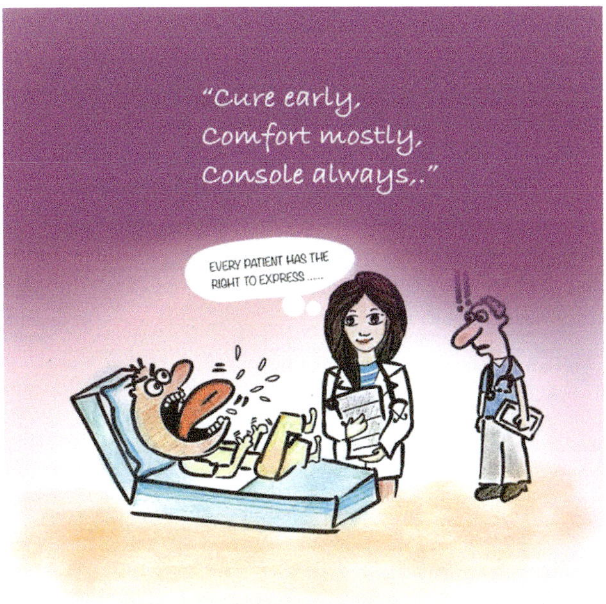


Do not ignore the cultural sensitivities in honing your communication skills—Muzaherul Huq and Shegufta Mohammad

M. Huq (✉)
Formerly at WHO, SEARO, Dhaka, Bangladesh

S. Mohammad
Update Dental College and Hospital, Dhaka, Bangladesh



S. C. Parija, B. V. Adkoli (eds.), *Effective Medical Communication*,
https://doi.org/10.1007/978-981-15-3409-6_22

## 22.1 Assess Need

Cultural sensitivity means being aware that cultural differences and similarities exist and have an effect on values, learning, and behaviour [1]. The twenty-first century belongs to the era of global communication. Widespread migration of people of various types of culture for various reasons is an issue of concern in communication. In order to successfully communicate with a wide variety of people in a migrating world, we need to be aware of cultural sensitivity in communication [2].

It is a well-known fact that a common gesture which is highly appreciated in one cultural context can be very offending in a different culture. We all read Gulliver's travels. The problems of such communication gaps are sometimes magnified beyond proportion, especially in a technology-driven, fast-paced global village. People do not have time for deep understanding by discussing such an issue over a cup of tea. Before you have time to correct the mistake, it is already viral. A strange feature of modern living is a tendency of the people to put everything in a negative perspective. Even if a comment or a remark is made in passing, it is twisted by the media resulting in a controversy. This problem is often vitiated by the hyperactive social media in a digital world.

Unfortunately, during conventional medical education, there is no scope for training the medicos to appreciate the cultural sensitivities around the world. When the graduates go abroad for a job, they will be surprised or even shocked to see and accept the cultural differences, thereby leading to moments of embarrassment. Preparing the medicos for appreciating cultural diversities during medical education is, therefore, the need of the hour.

## 22.2 Brief

In this chapter, an attempt has been made to:

- Explain the meaning of cultural sensitivity in communication.
- Discuss the importance of cultural sensitivity.
- Suggest a strategy to apply and incorporate knowledge and attitude needed for effective communication to handle cultural sensitivity in the context of the Southeast Asian.

## 22.3 Contextualize

### 22.3.1 Scenario 1

As a part of the activities of medical education unit, Dr. Comini organized a three day international seminar on quality assurance. The participants for this seminar came from different background including medical officers, staff nurses, and technical staff. The resource person travelled from USA. The seminar was held in a meticulous manner. At the concluding day of the seminar, a farewell function was arranged for all participants including the resource person. During the farewell function, the resource person was about to hug a lady participant to express his thanks and appreciation. However, this behaviour though quite normal in the home country of the resource person creates a big furore and embarrassing moments for the lady participant and the whole group.

***Exercise***: Reflect on this episode and comment on the situation. Was the resource person right or the audience created unnecessary panic? Think of how the cultural sensitivities play important role.

## 22.4 Describe

Southeast Asia (SEA) provides a unique picture of diversity of landscape, religions, languages, and culture. The region has 11 countries, viz., Brunei, Burma (Myanmar), Cambodia, Timor-Leste, Indonesia, Laos, Philippines, Singapore, Thailand, and Vietnam. However, according to WHO network, SEA Region includes countries such as India, Sri Lanka, Nepal, Bangladesh, DPR Korea, and Maldives. SEA has a population of over 642 million, consisting of 8.5% of world's population. Some of the countries in this region have hundreds of languages spoken by the people. The major religions practiced are Buddhism, Hinduism, Christianity, and Islam. It is logical to expect that the region presents wide cultural diversities, variations in food habits and cultural norms.

There are three main areas wherein knowledge of cultural sensitivity can play an important role. They are related to:

- Workplace communication.
- Communication during health care delivery.
- Educational—student–teacher interaction.

### 22.4.1 Workplace Communication

According to the United Nations Organization, 232 million people are now living in a country that they were not born [3]. The forces of the free-market economy coupled with globalization is now a major trend in health care establishments. This is how we face much cultural diversity every day. In a workplace full of multicultural people a person, therefore, requires special management skills. After all, good teamwork is needed to bring out success in any organization. It is, therefore, necessary to address cultural sensitivities involved in a workplace.

### 22.4.2 Communication During Health Care Delivery

Health care is a vital industry. A lot of countries are now focusing on health care tourism in a big way [4]. It is reported that Malaysia received 360,000 foreign patients from the Association of Southeast Asian Nations (ASEAN) region in 2007. In Thailand, the number of foreign patients more than doubled in 5 years, from around 630,000 in 2002 to 1,373,000 in 2007. It is estimated that during 2007, approximately 750,000 Americans travelled to other countries for health care. This trend makes it difficult for physicians and caregivers to communicate effectively with patients, especially if they lack cultural sensitivity. When *culturally sensitive communication* is used, the patients are likely to experience a more positive and beneficial relationship with clinicians. For instance, in certain states, in India, the rural women shy away from being examined by male doctors. The caregivers should, therefore, take necessary precaution to face such challenges.

### 22.4.3 Educational Student–Teacher Interaction

Research and experience demonstrate that students who are fully immersed in cultures abroad and who learn another language are better-equipped to function in the global workforce [5]. They become strategic thinkers and problem-solvers, and excellent communicators using more than one language.

Students are also beginning to recognize their own benefits by learning and appreciating other cultures for professional reasons and career advancement. According to the International Organisation for Economic Co-operation and Development, the number of international students worldwide rose from 0.8 million in 1975 to 3.7 million in 2009. In addition, UNESCO's Institute for Statistics found that the number has been increasing by about 12% each year [5]. Another area of training where cultural affinity plays an important role is the practice of mentoring, which is a potential instrument for the benefit of both mentors and mentees. Experience shows that mentoring is more effective when the mentor and the mentee share the same cultural background.

#### 22.4.3.1 Jehova's Witness

The sensitivities surrounding medical treatment for Jehovah's witnesses can place doctors in difficult medico-legal dilemmas [6]. The Jehovah's Witness religion is a Christian affiliation with millions of members in more than 200 countries worldwide. Jehovah's witnesses are well-known for their refusal to receive blood transfusions, which may lead to various challenges for medical practitioners involved in the treatment and management of Jehovah's witness patients. Jehovah's witnesses believe that it is against God's will to receive blood and, therefore, they refuse blood transfusions, even if it is their own blood. The acceptance of blood transfusions by Jehovah's Witnesses has, in some cases, led to expulsion from and ostracization by their religious community. This type of scenario requires careful communication skills with proper knowledge regarding religious culture.

Culture is nothing but the social behaviour and norms evolved by human societies. It includes ideas, customs, and social behaviour of a particular people or society. Every human being grows in a particular cultural environment. A person's lifestyle and point of view are always shaped according to his/her cultural perspective. For example, in Japan, people have a strong sense of the history of culture. From outside, we can see the rich history but if we want to live, work, or study there, then, we need to find out the subtle cultural uniqueness which is still embroidered in their day-to-day life. They have a strong sense of obligation and gratitude, a sense of compassion and sympathy for others, and a strong sense of WE versus THEY. It is like a submerged iceberg from the top; only a little bit is visible (Fig. 22.1). Southeast Asian countries like Nepal and Bhutan have very special cultural practices which should be understood by the expatriates for successful living there.

Each country has its own

- Historical culture.
- Religious culture.
- Ethnic culture.
- Language culture.
- Food culture.
- Lifestyle culture.

Cultural differences are due to landscape and extreme weather condition. They are also due to varied economic condition and the possibility of relocation.

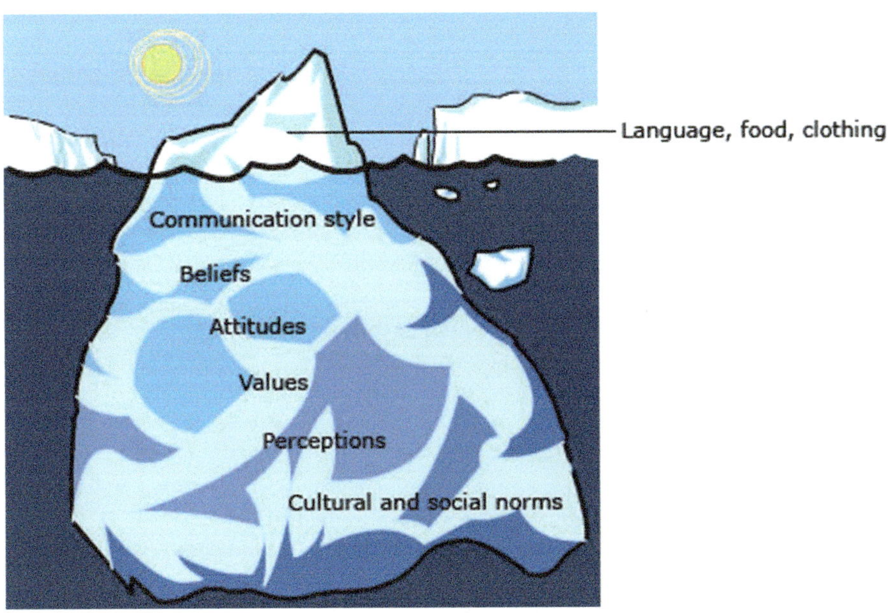


**Fig. 22.1** Different aspects of cultural sensitivity (Iceberg)

#### 22.4.3.2 Southeast Asian Countries Context of Cultural Sensitivity

Southeast Asian countries have long enriched heritage and culture. The people here are very diverse in culture. They belong to different religions and speak different languages. The countries have remote places and villages where people are living an isolated life in their own community nurturing own culture. Whether it is a remote village in Nepal or an island in the Maldives, they have their unique cultural identity. In order to help them and to communicate with them, one needs to be aware of their culture.

### 22.4.4 Strategies to Promote Cultural Sensitivity

In order to promote cultural sensitivity, we need to have a knowledge of language, food and clothing first, which is the most visible part of the culture. Then we need to understand their communication patterns, beliefs, attitudes, values, perceptions, besides cultural and social norms (Fig. 22.1).

#### 22.4.4.1 Cross-Cultural Communication Barriers

There are several barriers to cross-cultural communication:

- *Ethnocentrism cultural imposition*: The emotional attitude that one's own culture is superior to all others.
- *Stereotyping*: Generalizing about a person while ignoring the presence of individual differences.
- *Discrimination*: Differential treatment of an individual due to minority status; actual and perceived.
- *Tone difference*: Formal tone change becomes embarrassing and off-putting in some cultures.

If the cross-cultural differences are understood, it will be easy for working in a different land. The best way to inculcate cultural sensitivity is to address this issue during early childhood upbringing. However, the schools and medical colleges have the responsibility of nurturing the cultural growth by arranging talks, discussions, and debates on this topic, and more importantly by organizing cultural exchange programs between two institutes belonging to different countries.

### 22.4.5 Conclusion

- Cultural sensitivities assume a great significance in working with a health team.
- It becomes all the more important in a migrating world.
- An attitude of tolerance and accepting the differences holds the key.
- Training in cultural sensitivity should start from early childhood, duly nurtured during undergraduate medical education and reinforced periodically.

## 22.5 Evaluate

Having read this chapter, now you are in a position to take small homework. Eliciting your peers' help, you can role-play a different scenario at the workplace or educational institute involving multicultural participants, how they respond to a particular issue like population explosion.

## References

1. Mohan J. Dutta, communicating about culture and health: theorizing culture-centered and cultural sensitivity approaches. Commun Theory. 2007;17(3):304–28. https://doi.org/10.1111/j.1468-2885.2007.00297.x.
2. Brooks LA, Manias E, Bloomer MJ. Culturally sensitive communication in healthcare: a concept analysis. Collegian. 2018;26(3):383–91. https://doi.org/10.1016/j.colegn.2018.09.007. Available online 12 October 2018.
3. Helble M. The movement of patients across borders: challenges and opportunities for public health. Bull World Health Organ. 2011;89:68–72. https://doi.org/10.2471/BLT.10.076612.
4. Dalen JE, Alpert JS. Medical tourists: incoming and outgoing. Am J Med. 2019;132(1):9–10. https://doi.org/10.1016/j.amjmed.2018.06.022.
5. Williams TR. Exploring the impact of study abroad on students' intercultural communication skills: adaptability and sensitivity. J Stud Int Educ. 2005;9(4):356–71. https://doi.org/10.1177/1028315305277681.
6. JEHOVA'S witnesses, Wikipedia. Available at https://en.wikipedia.org/wiki/Jehovah%27s_Witnesses. Accessed on 25 Aug 2019.

# 23 Salutogenesis Approach to Communication

Ananda Balayogi Bhavanani

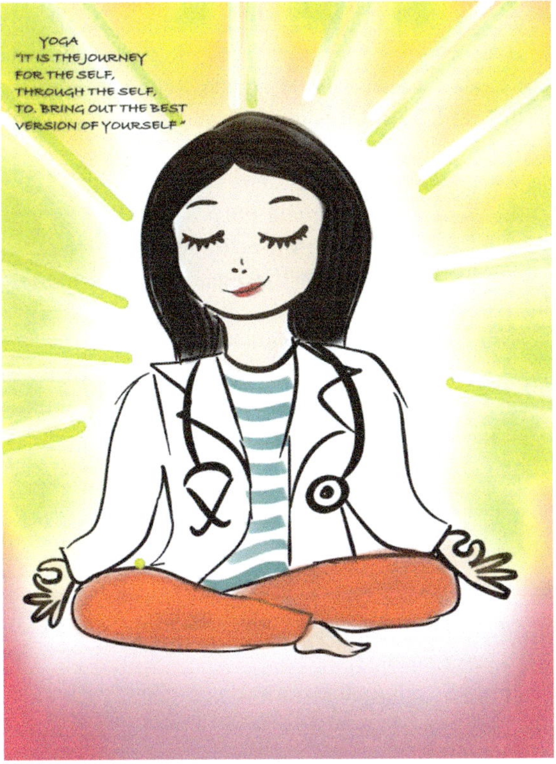


Compassion becomes real when we recognize our shared humanity.—Pema Chödrön

A. B. Bhavanani (✉)
Centre for Yoga Therapy Education and Research (CYTER), Sri Balaji Vidyapeeth (Deemed-to-be University), Pondicherry, India
e-mail: yoga@mgmcri.ac.in


S. C. Parija, B. V. Adkoli (eds.), *Effective Medical Communication*,
https://doi.org/10.1007/978-981-15-3409-6_23

## 23.1 Assess Need

In modern times, medical doctors are being increasingly targeted by the general public for lacking apparently a "*humanistic*" approach to their patients. One of the possible reasons is perhaps our overemphasis on the role of disease (pathogenesis) as against the overall human well-being, termed Salutogenesis. A time has come to shift the emphasis.

As healthcare providers, our role is to provide "*care*" in a compassionate and competent manner. This is the humanistic angle that makes medicine an art. "*You treat a disease, you win, or you lose. If you treat a person, I guarantee you'll win, no matter what the outcome*" [1]. Healing in a holistic sense has faded away from medical attention and is rarely discussed in modern medicine, especially in therapeutics.

The Indian tradition of healing understands health and well-being as a dynamic continuum of human nature and not a mere "*state*" to be attained and maintained. The lowest point on the continuum may be understood as having the lowest speed of vibration, and manifests as death, whereas the highest point with the highest vibration is that of health, well-being, and even a conceptual awareness of immortality. In between the extremes of this continuum lie the states of normal health and disease.

This is in tune with the concept of eudemonia described by Aristotle as a "*well-lived*" life that fulfils a person's ultimate purpose, and gives them meaning. This may also be related to the concepts of self-actualization of Abraham Maslow and to the meaning/purpose of life known in the Japanese culture as *Ikigai* and as self-responsibility (*swadharma*) in Indian tradition that enables the individual to attain a sense of coherence that is essential for well-being [2–5].

The shift in the emphasis is also called for in view of an increase in the burden of diseases often arising from rapid changes in the lifestyle, mounting pressure from the pharmaceutical industries, diagnostic technologies which have escalated the medical costs beyond the reach of the common man.

## 23.2 Brief

In this chapter an attempt will be made to:

- Explain the meaning of salutogenesis, and contrast it with the pathogenesis.
- Be aware of the plethora of medically unexplained symptoms (MUS).
- Suggest a holistic approach to various dimensions of the human being, and how they impact human life in health and disease.
- Outline the influences of an optimal healing environment (OHE).
- Identify methods through which clinicians can communicate, and address all dimensions of well-being.

## 23.3 Contextualize

### 23.3.1 Scenario 1

Mr. A, a young man of 24, was complaining of abdominal pain for many months, and after an extensive battery of investigations, was finally recommended to have surgery. Despite his condition, no one found time to talk to him in detail, and enable him to be at ease. Everyone was busy filling out forms and writing reports. Day-by-day he became more and more withdrawn and depressed. He was referred to psychiatry, and got a few more medications to add to his list. When the "*D*" day came, he was wheeled into the OT, and as his parents and family members waited outside, there was no one to provide the strength and support at their time of need. To everyone's dismay, despite all the efforts by the team of excellent surgeons, he did not survive the 6-h surgery.

As the bereaved parents and other family members broke down outside the OT, there was not a soul in sight to support them with a shoulder to cry on. "*What about those who are left behind, still alive?*" asked a new intern. "*If you want to face their wrath, go there, if not, mind your business*," said his friend as he rushed to another case.

***Exercise***: Step into the shoes of the patient and the bereaved family. Is the manner in which "*we dispose of our cases*" acceptable?

### 23.3.2 Scenario 2

Some years ago, a patient with terminal cancer was referred to Dr. HK, for an intensive healing retreat, which was helpful for the individuals to try self-healing. The patient showed great physical, mental, and emotional improvement during the retreat but unfortunately died of his cancer-related complications 4 weeks after the retreat. When the therapist called up the wife to console her, she said, "*Doctor, you have given him the best possible option which he could get at the end of his life. You have enabled him to leave his body in a much better state of mind and spirit than would have happened if he had not attended your retreat*." Her daughter piped in, "*Therapy is not just about curing people of their illnesses, but in such terminal illnesses is more importantly about helping them endure it and die with peace, courage, and dignity*."

***Exercise***: Comment on the response given by the daughter of the patient.

## 23.4 Describe

### 23.4.1 Meaning of Salutogenesis

Salutogenesis may be defined as all the factors involved in manifesting and sustaining a sense of well-being and wholesome wellness. It is derived from the Latin *Salus* meaning "*health*" and the Greek *genesis* meaning "*source*." Hence in combination, it implies, "*Sources of health*."

A study by Levinson and colleagues found that the doctors who had never been sued spent more than 3 min longer with each patient than those who had been sued did [6]. Acharya *Sushrut*, an ancient Indian Surgeon (~600 BC) defined health as "*a dynamic balance of the elements and humor, normal metabolic activity, and efficient elimination coupled with a tranquil mind, senses, and contented soul*" [7].

When we consider such a comprehensive approach to the well-being, we must take into consideration all aspects of their life, including diet, lifestyle modifications, attitude reconditioning, as well as the appropriate therapeutic and medical recipes.

All of these are integral components of holistic, or rather, wholesome therapeutic process. When such an approach is adopted, the quality of life improves drastically, and in many cases, so does the quantity.

### 23.4.2 Mind-Body Connection

Indian traditional systems of healing describe the influence of the psyche (*Mind-body)*, on the body, thus creating disease (*vyadhi)*. This is the basis of psychosomatics and mind-body medicine, and is termed *adhijavyadhi*. This is in tune with psycho-neuro-immunology (PNI) which realizes that how we think and feel can both positively and negatively influence our nervous, endocrine, and immune responses. One path leads to health, while the other to disease and suffering. Virtually every health problem that we face today either has its origin in psychosomatics, or is worsened by the psychosomatic aspect of the disease. The mind and the body seem to be continuously fighting each other. What the mind wants, the body will not do, and what the body wants, the mind will not do. This creates a dichotomy, a disharmony, in other words, a disease. By paying careful attention to personal history, one can nearly always trace origins of psychosomatic disease back to patterns of mental and emotional pressures (Box 23.1).

**Box 23.1 Stress-Related Disorders: Four Distinct Phases**

Psychosomatic, stress-related disorders appear to progress through four distinct phases [1].

1. Psychic Phase: During this phase a person will have stress. This will be seen in the form of irritability or disturbed sleep.
2. Psychosomatic Phase: Here, some physiological symptoms will appear. There can be high blood pressure.
3. Somatic Phase: This phase is marked by a disturbed function of organs, particularly the target, or involved organ.
4. Organic Phase: During this phase, there will be full manifestation of the diseased state. One needs to focus on palliative care and quality of life.

Even though the bio-psychosocial model is gaining popularity, there exist major barriers to the integration of mind-body principles and modern clinical practices. A report by Astin and colleagues attributed this to inadequate attention to such methods in medical training as well as the lack of time, insufficient monetary incentives, and a larger cultural ethos that favor the "*quick-fix*" over the more difficult task of examining the role of such factors [8]. They identified various adverse factors, such as:

- Lack of knowledge of evidence base.
- Inadequate attention paid to the mind-body area in training.
- Perceived lack of competence to use mind-body methods.
- Inadequate time, lack of economic incentive.
- The perception that psychosocial factors are beyond their capacity to control.
- The perception that patients do not want to address psychosocial/lifestyle issues.
- Cultural beliefs that addressing the psychosocial domain is not within the purview of physicians.

### 23.4.3 Salutogenesis and the Sense of Coherence (SOC)

According to Aaron Antonovsky, SOC can be understood as a "*pervasive, long-lasting, and dynamic feeling of confidence that one's internal and external environments are predictable and that there is a high probability that things will work out as well as can be expected*" [9]. More the person has SOC, the better he has chances of well-being and quality of life [10].

The three components of SOC are based on the notion that:

1. One's life is comprehensible.
2. It is manageable.
3. It is meaningful.

The sense of life being comprehensible is a cognitive process where the individual has the sense "*My world is understandable*." The coping skill in the second component enables the individual feel, "*My world is manageable*," while the motivational aspect of life having a sense of meaningfulness manifests in the individual feeling, "*My world has meaning*." The comprehension, meaningfulness, and manageability (SOC approach) in chronic diseases keep them "*well*" despite any limitations, and is similar to "*physically disabled*" becoming "*differently abled*." When an individual has these three aspects manifesting in their life, they have a sense of health, wellness, well-being, and wholesomeness.

Through our words and actions, can we learn to communicate with our patients in such a way that these three aspects come alive? It is only then that the health-promoting aspects of healing start to manifest in them. We need to help them comprehend their life better. This is only possible if we truly "*know*" them. This takes

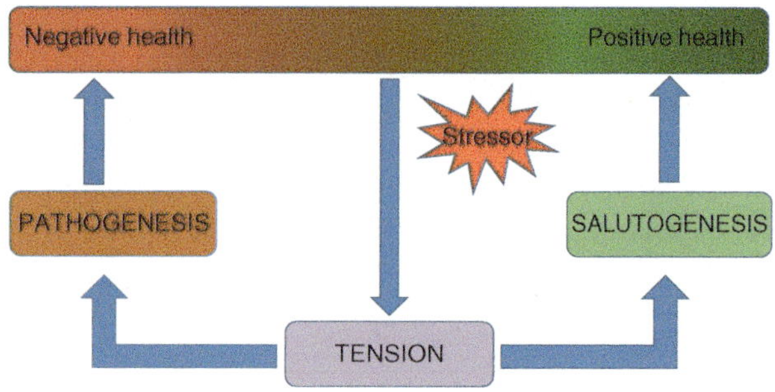


**Fig. 23.1** Antonovsky's own way of explaining the health continuum and the salutogenic direction

time and patience. Often people are not aware of their inherent capacities and potential. We need to help our patients move from "*impossible*" to "*I Am Possible!*" (Fig. 23.1).

Sometimes, just "*being there*" for the person may be all that is required. It is useful to ask them openly in a caring manner, "*Can I help you in anyway?*" Another way we can help them is through compasionate statements like, "*I am there for you*," or "*We will get through this together*". Helping them to see the bigger picture can help overcome emotional reaction. Spirituality, religion, and personal beliefs have been shown to correlate highly with all WHO-QOL domains in a cross-cultural study conducted by the WHO-QOLSRPB covering 18 countries with 5087 respondents [11]. After all it is your perspective which really matters. The following quote has been tried successfully to elevate the morale of a diseased person. "*To an ant, every wave is a tsunami, while to the giant even the tsunami is just another wave…do you want to be an ant or a giant?*" A comparative account of pathogenesis versus salutogenesis approach has been given in the Table 23.1.

### 23.4.4 Medically Unexplained Symptoms

Patients usually come to the healthcare provider because they experience bodily symptoms. However, often, we find in a large majority that the clinical picture does not meet any existing diagnostic criteria for known diseases or disorders [12]. In some cases, this may happen because symptoms are recent and evolving. But in a large majority, symptoms are persistent but, either by their character or the negative results of the clinical investigation, they cannot be attributed to any known disease. This, so-called "*medically unexplained symptoms*" (MUS) can be very frustrating. It is estimated that MUS account for up to 45% of all general practice consultations, while a study based in secondary care indicated that about 50% of patients had no clear diagnosis at 3 months [13].

Emphasis should be laid on early intervention, and on services that are accessible and acceptable to patients. The commissioning guidance emphasizes the need for care pathways that integrate physical and mental healthcare, and join primary, secondary, and tertiary services seamlessly.

**Table 23.1** Comparisons between pathogenic and salutogenic approaches to patient care

| Quality | Pathogenic approach | Salutogenic approach |
|---|---|---|
| Goal | Trying to give the patient better medical interventions | Trying to improve the external and internal environment |
| Key question | What causes diseases? | What promotes health? |
| Efforts | Attempts to avoid the problems | Attempts to manifest potential |
| Focus | Trying to cure the medical condition | Enabling manifestation of health in all its dimensions |
| Attitude | The healthcare provider is the master doing it for the patient | There is equal responsibility on both sides as a team |
| Methodology | Always trying to fix that part of the system that is not working and set it right | Developing the individual's health assets, thus enabling them to function at optimal health |
| Philosophy | Save the life of the individual and prolong it as much as possible | Enable the individual to have a life worth living by discovering how to live fully |
| Theological | Reactive against pain or loss | Proactive towards gain or growth |
| Who heals? | The healthcare provider; paternalism; dependence | The patient themselves; culture of active health |
| Empowerment | To the provider and system | Patient empowers to "*take charge*" of their own life |
| Role of provider | The expert who cures | Facilitates self-healing |
| Endpoint | Symptom relief | Ever-evolving life journey... an ongoing process |

### 23.4.5 Creating an Optimal Healing Environment

The term Optimal Healing Environment (OHE) was coined by the Samueli Institute in 2004 with a focus on "*the processes of recovery, repair, renewal, and reintegration that contribute to a person's physical, mental, social, and spiritual health and well-being*" [14]. We should not forget that healing and cure are mutually complementary, and both are essential.

The concept of OHE can be understood through four domains:

1. Internal domain: This domain deals with the development of healing intention and the experience of a sense of personal wholesomeness. Expectation, hope, understanding, and belief can foster the healing intention.
2. Interpersonal domain: This domain deals with the cultivation of healing relationships through communication, compassion, social support, and empathy. It also deals with the creation of healing organizations through capable leadership, healthy teamwork, and optimal use of modern technology.
3. Behavioral domain: This consists of the adoption and practice of healthy lifestyles by the individual. It means the application of integrative, collaborative medicine that is person-centered, family centered, and sensitive to cultural

differences in the patient population. A healthy lifestyle is an individual choice with regards to diet, physical activity, exercise, relaxation as well as cultivation of positive thought and overcoming the negative thoughts and habits that otherwise lead to addiction and debilitation.

4. External domain: The environment affects the way we heal. It is vital to build healing spaces taking into consideration the color, light, art and architecture, smells, and air movements as well as the utilization of music and reduction of unnecessary jarring sounds. All healthcare institutions need to foster ecological sustainability as make sure their structures are eco-friendly, green, energy-efficient, and in tune with nature as much as possible.

### 23.4.6 Adopting an Holistic Approach

#### 23.4.6.1 Lifestyle Choices

Adopting a healthy lifestyle is a key factor in promoting wellness. Healthy food, exercise, positive thinking, and service beyond self are ideal formula. In fact, the traditional Indian lifestyle encompasses a wholesome approach (Box 23.2).

**Box 23.2 Traditional Indian Lifestyle Approach**

- Healthy physical activities and exercise (*achar*).
- Healthy mental patterns and attitudes towards life (*vichar*).
- A healthy, nourishing diet with adequate intake of water and balanced intake of fresh food (*ahar*).
- Healthy recreational activities to relax body and mind (*vihar*).
- Healthy interpersonal and intrapersonal relationships (*vyavahar*).

Helping the patient move from incoherence to coherence:

There are four steps in helping the patients move from incoherence to coherence, viz., denial, anger, depression, and acceptance, with an acronym—DADA [15].

- Denial: The person denies the condition. "*It cannot be true, especially not for me*." They check and double-check the reports, and take umpteen opinions with many consultants. It is here that we need to be supportive of them. Compassionate listening and calm demeanor are vital to handle patients in this stage.
- Anger: When the diagnosis is confirmed, they get angry with everyone, and even the creator has no escape from his wrath. "*Why me?*" "*Why only me?*" Again, empathy is a vital quality to communicate with them at this point of time, and giving them some personal space which often helps them to let the steam off.

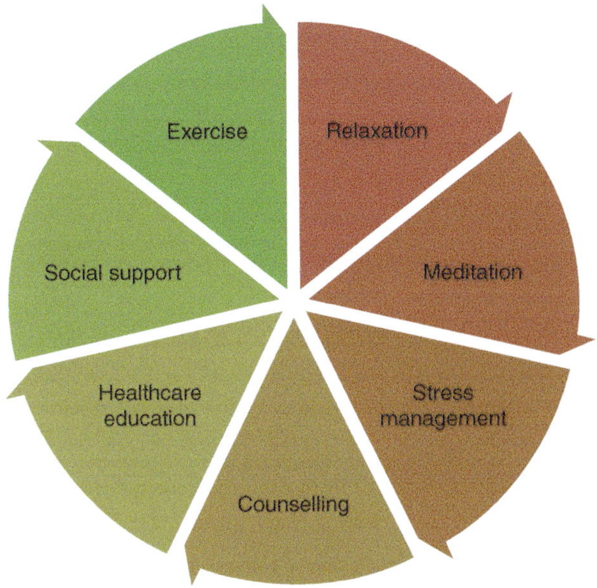


**Fig. 23.2** Suggested approaches for coping with psychological stresses

- Depression: Subsequently, when the psychic clutter settles down, they begin to think that there is no escape, and sink into a state of depression followed by the withdrawal from society and friends. We need to be with them during this phase, and give a helping hand to overcome depression. Giving them a sense of purpose and meaning is vital at this point. Spiritual practice can be highly useful.
- Acceptance: When they finally decide to accept the problem, and face it with courage, healing happens. This acceptance is not in the form of passive resignation, but in the form of the undertaking of a dynamic resolute decision to progress and make the best efforts towards health. Once we get them here, our job becomes much easier henceforth. The patients with terminal illnesses can be best served by effective communication more than anything else to overcome their depression and anxiety (Fig. 23.2).

The great Austrian psychiatrist and Holocaust survivor *Viktor Frankl* (1905–1997) is best-known for his indispensable 1946 psychological memoir Meaning which describes the primary purpose of life: the quest for meaning, which sustained those who survived [16]. He declares "*Everything can be taken from a man but one thing: the last of the human freedoms—to choose one's attitude in any given set of circumstances, to choose one's own way.*" For those engaged in communication with fellow suffering human beings, he says, "*Love is the only way to grasp another human being in the innermost core of his personality….*" This is where empathy and compassion come into our medical profession as the guiding lights.

### 23.4.7 Conclusion

- Salutogenesis is a holistic concept. It deals with all the factors involved in manifesting and sustaining a sense of well-being and wholesome wellness.
- The heart of salutogenesis is the sense of coherence whose three components are based on a sense that one's life is comprehensible, manageable, and meaningful.
- An optimal healing environment (OHE), a healthcare system designed to stimulate and support the inherent healing capacity of patients, families, and their care providers.
- The concept of OHE can be understood through four domains that are: internal domain, interpersonal domain, behavioral domain, and external domain.
- A holistic approach to health includes healthy physical activities (*achar*), healthy mental patterns (*vichar*), nourishing diet (*ahar*), healthy recreation (*vihar*), and healthy relationships (*vyavahar*).

## 23.5 Evaluate

Imagine about the next patient whom you meet in the ward. How would you like to understand them as a "*wholesome being*"? What are the key elements you would bring to the conversation?

What would you avoid? What would you do to make sure you are communicating salutogenesis and empowering the individual?

How would you go about creating an optimal healing environment in your workplace? What are the changes you would make with regard each of the domains?

## References

1. En.wikiquote.org. Patch Adams (film) - Wikiquote [online]. Available at: https://en.wikiquote.org/wiki/Patch_Adams_(film). (2019). Accessed 5 Sept 2019.
2. The Theory of Self-Actualization [Internet]. Psychology Today. 2019. [cited 6 September 2019]. Available from: https://www.psychologytoday.com/intl/blog/theory-and-psychopathology/201308/the-theory-self-actualization.
3. Ikigai [Internet]. En.wikipedia.org. 2019. [cited 6 September 2019]. Available from: https://en.wikipedia.org/wiki/Ikigai.
4. Bhavanani AB. The yoga of responsibility. Yoga Life. 2011;42(9):3–10.
5. Vaandrager L, Kennedy L. The application of Salutogenesis in communities and neighborhoods. 2016 Sep 3. In: Mittelmark MB, Sagy S, Eriksson M, et al., editors. The handbook of Salutogenesis [Internet]. Cham: Springer; 2017. Chapter 17.
6. Levinson W, Roter DL, Mullooly JP, Dull VT, Frankel RM. Physician-patient communication: the relationship with malpractice claims among primary care physicians and surgeons. JAMA. 1997;277(7):553–9.
7. Bhavanani AB. Yoga Chikitsa: the application of yoga as a therapy. Dhivyananda Creations: Pondicherry; 2013.
8. Astin JA, Goddard TG, Forys K. Barriers to the integration of mind-body medicine: perceptions of physicians, residents, and medical students. Explore (NY). 2005;1(4):278–83.

9. Antonovsky A. Health, stress, and coping. San Francisco: Jossey-Bass Publishers; 1979.
10. Antonovsky A. The salutogenic model as a theory to guide health promotion. Health Promot Int. 1996;11:11–8.
11. World Health Organization-Quality of Life – Spirituality, Religion and Personal Beliefs Group (WHO-QOL SRPB) Group. A cross-cultural study of spirituality, religion, and personal beliefs as components of quality of life. Soc Sci Med. 2006;62(6):1486–97.
12. Rosendal M, Olde Hartman TC, Aamland A, et al. "Medically unexplained" symptoms and symptom disorders in primary care: prognosis-based recognition and classification. BMC Fam Pract. 2017;18(1):18.
13. Chew-Graham CA, Heyland S, Kingstone T, Shepherd T, Buszewicz M, Burroughs H, et al. Medically unexplained symptoms: continuing challenges for primary care. Br J Gen Pract. 2017;67(656):106–7.
14. Sakallaris BR, MacAllister L, Voss M, Smith K, Jonas WB. Optimal healing environments. Glob Adv Health Med. 2015;4(3):40–5.
15. Bhavanani AB, Ramanathan M. Yoga therapy for chronic diseases: psychosomatic aspects. In: Souvenir of International Day of Yoga celebrations 2k17 at SBVU, Puducherry. 19–23, June 2017. p. 57–63.
16. Viktor E. Frankl Quotes (Author of Man's Search for Meaning) [Internet]. Goodreads.com. 2019 [cited 6 September 2019]. Available from: https://www.goodreads.com/author/quotes/2782.Viktor_E_Frankl

# Role of Music in Therapeutic Communication

# 24

Sumathy Sundar

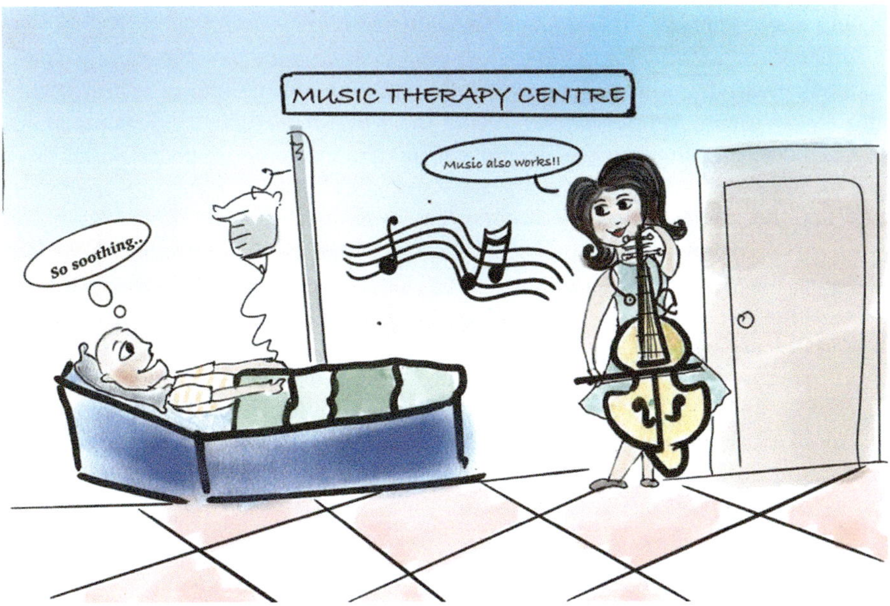


Music as a mind and body therapy complements medical care—Sumathy Sundar

S. Sundar (✉)
Center for Music Therapy Education and Research, Sri Balaji Vidyapeeth (Deemed-to-be University), Pondicherry, India


S. C. Parija, B. V. Adkoli (eds.), *Effective Medical Communication*,
https://doi.org/10.1007/978-981-15-3409-6_24

## 24.1 Assess Need

The earliest form of communication even before man learned to use language has been regarded to be music. Even now in modern times, music is one of the fewest ways that people can connect with each other without the need for any common language. It is an integral part of our lives as it is all-pervasive. Music is considered to be a universal language for social interactions, even though it lacks a semantic system, and does not convey a definitive meaning as it provides a framework for effective communication with its power to impact our feelings, thoughts, and emotions.

In the clinical context, on one side, the importance of effective communication of clinicians with patients and also within the healthcare team is known to impact the patient care outcomes. Poor communication skills affect the functional outcome and satisfaction levels of patients [1]. There is constantly a need in the healthcare delivery system to revisit ways and means to improve communication skills which have a direct impact on the clinical outcomes.

Recent research by brain hyper-scanning method indicates that there is simultaneous positive brain activity in both the patient and the therapist during their musical therapeutic interactions paving the way for positive clinical outcomes. Also, both music and speech processing share common neural circuits in the brain.

The field of music therapy as complementary medical care is being explored only recently under the ambit of integrative medicine in hospitals and medical schools. Most of the hospitals are not yet equipped with an optimum healing environment to treat patients with a salutogenic approach focused on health and wellness. Music as a mind-body therapy is said to act on the brain to induce positive emotions, cognition, reduce stress, and through the mind-body information systems translate into health-related behaviors, and enhance physical, psychological, social, and spiritual well-being of patients visiting the hospital. This holistic approach of treating the patients is garnering attention worldwide [2].

## 24.2 Brief

The chapter addresses the followings:

- What does musical communication entail in interpersonal communication?
- What is therapeutic communication with music?
- How can therapeutic communication be applied in (a) clinical communication among the interdisciplinary team, and (b) patient care setting?
- Tips for therapists to use music as a primary medium of communication to heal the patients.

## 24.3 Contextualize

### 24.3.1 Scenario

Dr. Comini, a newly joined faculty in the department of medicine, experienced difficulty in adjusting to a new environment and multi-cultural setting of the institute and the hospital. She was a bright but very shy and inexperienced girl. However, she had a high aptitude for music and to some extent, skilled too, in music. She was finding it very difficult to adapt to the institutional culture, and her shyness restricted her from communicating effectively with her colleagues and students. Her ineffective communication resulted in the other senior faculty members in the department underestimating her academic abilities. She also could not connect well with her students in the classes, and the students performed poorly in the subjects that she handled. She was depressed and had mood swings. Singing and playing the violin was the only way that she could regulate her emotions, and improve her moods outside the college hours.

At this point in time, her roommate, who was a music therapist in the same medical school invited Dr. Comini to observe the music therapy sessions whenever she had free time. She was very excited to find that her music therapist roommate had the innate ability to connect with her colleagues and the patients very well with her musical communication. She got an opportunity to observe music therapy sessions with a female patient who had a stroke and lost her communication, and had a diagnosis of aphasia. She was awestruck to see how communicating through musical experiences made the female patient regain her speech to a considerable extent which made her move forward in her day-to-day activities, and express her needs verbally. This unique experience was an eye-opener for Dr. Comini to explore music therapy as a part of her career profile.

On the founder's day of the medical school, the Chancellor announced a few fellowship programs for internal faculty. Dr. Comini bagged a 1-year fellowship in "*Music therapy as a complementary medicine with a salutogenic approach*"

***Exercise***: What was the turning point in the career experience of Dr. Comini?

## 24.4 Describe

### 24.4.1 Leveraging Musical Elements in Interpersonal Communication

Interpersonal communication is an important aspect of teamwork, leading to satisfactory patient outcomes. Interdependence is an important aspect of treatment requiring a good understanding within the interdisciplinary team treating the patient.

The success of the treatment depends on the good understanding among treating team, which mainly depends upon the communication.

The role of music has been recognized globally since ancient time. However, the therapeutic effects of music are of recent interest. Nevertheless, pieces of evidence are now available around the world to highlight the role of music therapy not only in enhancing the healing process in patients, but also contribute to the optimum performance of treating team [1–6].

Use of musical leverages like pitch, rhythm, tempo, timbre, and intensity convey the communicative intent effectively in speeches [3]. Therapists use melodious voice and variations in pitch to communicate their intentions. The suitable inflexion in voice creates interest and eagerness in the listeners. The rhythm in the voice expresses appropriate emotions and urgent needs. The use of pauses, while speaking, provides enough time for the listener to process the information, and respond effectively (Fig. 24.1).

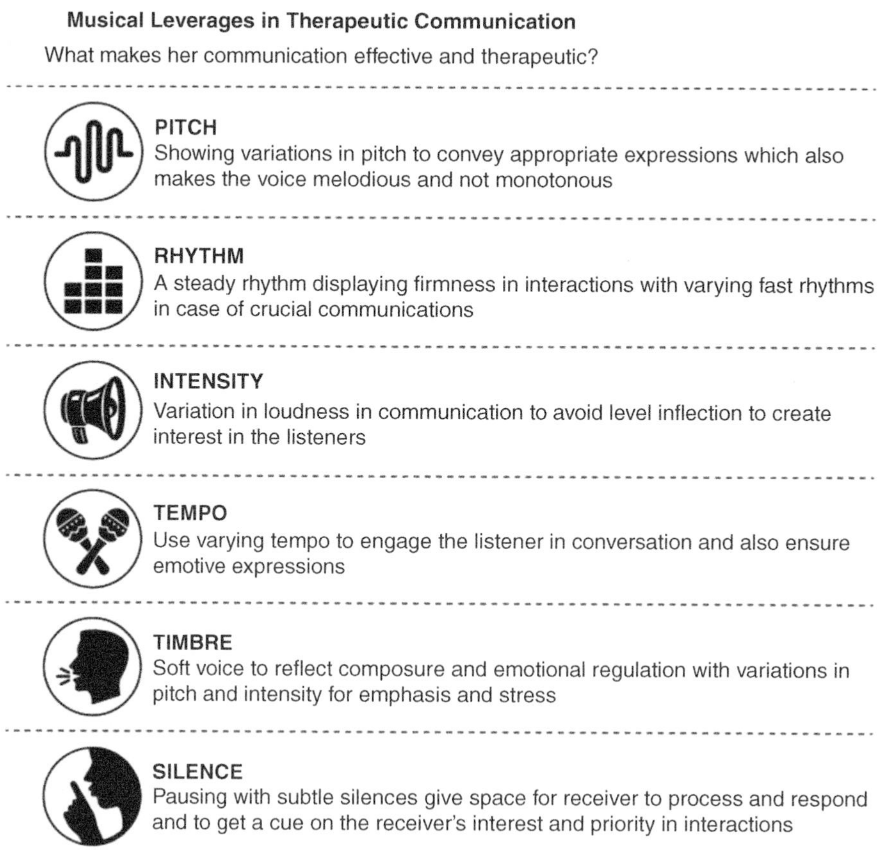


**Fig. 24.1** Therapeutic clinical communication using music

### 24.4.2 Therapeutic Communication Using Music

The hospital journey for a patient involves many psycho-physiological stressors like pain, emotional disturbances, financial stress, sleep disturbances, anxiety, depressive feelings, and irritable moods. These result in a decline in the Quality of Life (QOL) and dissatisfaction in social relationships within the family and community. The stressors may relate to the process of diagnosis, the diagnostic or interventional procedures that one has to undergo, the side effects of the medication or the treatment, and the prognosis of the treatment. These can be overcome by effective clinical communication among the interdisciplinary treating team during this time. The focus should be on treating the patient as a whole and not just the disease. Bringing a balance between the mind, body, and the soul of the patient requires a caring approach which entails an empathetic and therapeutic communication with the patient (Fig. 24.2).

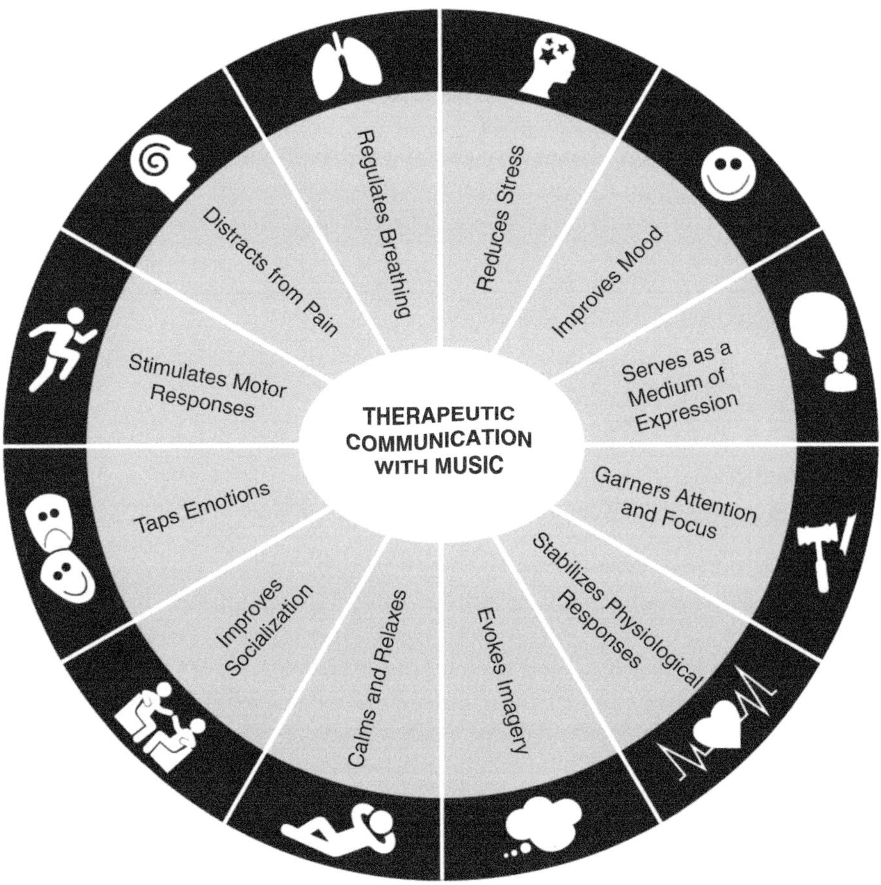


**Fig. 24.2** The list of beneficial effects of music therapy

Therapeutic communication using music entails presenting musical experiences to patients with a focus to improve, sustain, or restore their health emphasizing an integrative approach using the principles of mind and body medicine. When patients engage themselves in musical experiences provided by the music therapist, music acts on the brain. It evokes positive emotions, reduces negative emotions, and reduces stress. These changes are mediated through the brain information transfer systems including autonomic, endocrine, and immune pathways, that reduce stress, resulting in health benefits.

Presenting therapeutic musical experiences is also an effective way of communicating with interdisciplinary team members. It helps to reduce their own stress, cope with their work pressures, and perform optimally in care giving.

### 24.4.3 Therapeutic Communication Through Music

Varied applications of music therapy in key areas of hospital services are highlighted as follows:

#### 24.4.3.1 Department of Obstetrics and Gynecology: How to Calm and Relax the Patients

Musical experiences like chanting and singing can be used to evoke "*Shanta Rasa*" (stands for peace, calm, and tranquil experience) a relaxation response evoked by a music therapist in the anxious pregnant women undergoing labor [4].

During the course of labor, the use of deep breathing and chanting experiences as a rhythmic cue with laboring women is to:

- induce relaxation.
- reduce anxiety.
- cope with the laboring pain.
- reduce behavioral symptoms of pain.
- support during regular contractions.

One can effectively communicate the impact of music on fetal health, and appreciate how musical experiences can reduce fetal distress during labor.

#### 24.4.3.2 Department of Pediatrics: How to Distract from Pain

The parents of neonates and infants coming for immunization programs in the pediatric department suffer from moderate to high levels of anxiety among the parents holding the babies and the infants crying a lot. As a music therapist one can do wonders to distract the infants from pain, and reduce the behavioral symptoms of pain, while also reducing the distress levels of such parents.

- Keep your music therapy kit ready, including a hand puppet and finger puppets.
- Approach the infants and the parents even in the waiting area before the immunization procedure.
- Maneuver movement of puppet, singing lullabies, and playing keyboard in a synchronized manner.

One can realize that the babies who were crying and restless are distracted in no time with this simple technique. You can further train and coach the parents about what they can do at their homes using music with their infants.

Initiation of lactation and breast milk secretion is a complex process and studies have indicated that if mothers are stressed during and after delivery, breast milk secretion and feeding process may be delayed. To de-stress mothers who have just delivered.

- Teach them to sing lullabies to their babies.
- Write a welcome song for the newborn baby and sing.
- Sing along with the mother to create a bonding between the mother and the newborn.
- Allow the baby to listen to music to improve suckling during breastfeeding.

Record some lullabies to give it to the mothers for use at home. You can communicate to them on how mother-infant bonding develops through music.

#### 24.4.3.3 Department of Pulmonary Medicine: How to Regulate Breathing?

Patients diagnosed with chronic obstructive pulmonary diseases (COPD) have difficulty in breathing, have high levels of anxiety, and have stress in coping with their day-to-day life activities. As a music therapist, one can relax the patient, and regularize their breathing patterns by following these simple procedures.

- Talk to the patients about the benefits of singing on breathing.
- Be ready to use chants along with the breathing exercises.
- Use all the seven notes of Indian classical music for oral, respiratory exercises.
- Facilitate playing simple wind instruments by the patients to reduce symptoms of dispend.
- Sing favorite music of the patients as positive reinforcement.

You can communicate to the patients how to integrate music in their daily lives to regularize their breathing and improve their quality of life with daily use of music in the form of singing along with the breathing exercises.

#### 24.4.3.4 Department of Cardiology: How to Stabilize Physiological Responses?

Patients undergoing catheterization and cardiac procedures often experience high levels of anxiety and physiological disturbances. Music therapy has been found to be effective in bringing down the anxiety and reducing the physiological disturbances for these patients [6].

- Remember to take your diary for a list of relaxing ragas in consonance to time theory.
- Use soothing raga improvisations to turn them on to the para-sympathetic mode.
- Modulate your voice and amplitude by observing the patient's facial expressions and other non-verbal responses.
- Maintain slow tempo, and repeat short melodic key phrases of the raga softly.
- Administer a full relaxation session for about 15 min.
- Note to entrain the internal biological rhythms to your music.

The patients can be calmed down, and their physiological disturbances can be regularized, and breathing becomes even.

#### 24.4.3.5 Department of Neurology: How to Improve Communicative Abilities in Dysarthria?

Music can be a strong source of motivation and hope for treating patents having neurological problems such as dysarthria. The steps to be followed are as follows:

- Administer chants as breathing exercises.
- Plan oral motor exercises.
- Use *sapthaswaras* (Seven notes) for oral motor exercises for activating the articulators responsible for speech production.
- Sing their favorite music to motivate them.
- Do not be judgmental on how they sing. The singing process is important.
- Write songs of hope, and sing along with the patients.
- Be patient and be available to them psychologically supporting them during their emotional vent.

#### 24.4.3.6 Community Outreach to Transgender Community: How to Improve Self-Esteem and Socialization

The problem faced by the transgender community often relates to their low self-esteem. Music plays positive role in boosting the self-esteem. In fact group singing is highly recommended in such cases.

- Carry percussion instruments with you for drumming activities that engages the participants.
- Write and compose a song to express their feelings and emotions.

- Plan a group singing activity.
- Encourage emotional expression through their singing the preferred music.

#### 24.4.3.7 Faculty and Staff of Interdisciplinary Team: How to Reduce Stress?

Faculty and staff in medical schools often experience multiple stressful situations, and find difficulty in coping with these situations. Periodical stress management programs (SMP) using music as a lifestyle management strategy helps them to cope better with stressful situations.

- Schedule periodic SMPs for all staff and faculty in rotation.
- Plan activities for generating positive emotions through music.
- Facilitate group singing.
- Conduct drumming activities.
- Facilitate rhythmic movements using music.

Communicate to all the faculty and the staff, the power of music to induce positive emotions and cognition to have a positive impact on their body and mind, and how attending music-based SMPs could improve their mood and interpersonal relationships, and help them in cope with stressful situations.

Music therapy is an emerging area of interest in biomedical sciences. There is a need for further research on which particular music (*raga* or tala) works best with which patient and under what circumstances. More and more centers of music therapy are being opened, and it is likely that music therapy can one day occupy a prominent place as a complement to mainstream medicine. The emphasis on body-mind medicine and salutogenesis will push music therapy to a new level (Table 24.1).

**Table 24.1** The challenges in music therapy and possible solutions

| The challenges in music therapy | Solutions and way forward |
|---|---|
| Lack of awareness about music therapy among clinicians and administrators | Sensitization programs; providing evidence base; involvement of clinicians |
| Lack of facilities and infrastructure | Setting up of an optimal healing environment in hospitals and medical schools, and focus on mind-body therapies such as music therapy |
| Lack of trained personnel | More training programs have to be augmented |
| The challenges of bringing an interdisciplinary approach | Maintaining the right balance between science and humanities |

### 24.4.4 Conclusion

- Music therapy has gained a lot of interest and attention.
- Use of physical, psychological, social, cognitive, and spiritual facets of music and engaging patients, medical faculty, and students to improve their health.
- Using music as a primary medium of communication has a therapeutic influence.
- Using musical leverages in verbal communication improves interpersonal communication among interdisciplinary healthcare professionals.

## 24.5 Evaluate

After reading this chapter think about the way in which music therapy can be complemented in your department/discipline.

## References

1. Institute for Health Care Communication. Impact of communication in Health Care. 2011. Available from https://healthcarecomm.org/about-us/impact-of-communication-in-healthcare/. Accessed 26 Sept 2019.
2. Sundar S. Understanding music therapy: clearing misconceptions. Ann SBV. 2014;3:8–11.
3. Cohen SD, Wei TE, Defraia DC, Drury CJ. The music of speech: layering musical elements to deliver powerful messages. Relevant Rhetoric. 2016;2:1–24. Available from https://www.researchgate.net/publication/228835122. Accessed 26 Sept 2019.
4. Ramesh B, Sundar S, Jayapreetha R, Samal S, Ghose S. Effects of culture-based chants on labor pain during the latent stage of labor in primigravidae mothers: a randomized controlled trial. J Basic Clin Appl Health Sci. 2018;2(1):16–9.
5. Ajmera S, Sundar S, Amirtha Ganesh B, Bhavanani AB, Dayanidy G, Ezhumalai G. A comparative study on the effect of music therapy alone and a combination of music and yoga therapies on the psycho-physiological parameters of cardiac patients posted for angiography. J Basic Clin Appl Health Sci. 2018;2(4):163–8.
6. Sundar S, Ramesh B, Dixit PD, Venkatesh S, Das P, Dhandapany G. Live music therapy as an active focus of attention for pain and behavioral symptoms of distress during pediatric immunization. Clin Pediatr. 2016;55(8):745–8.

# Take-Home: Communication Skills Can Be Taught

# 25

Indika Karunathilake and Chamindri Witharana

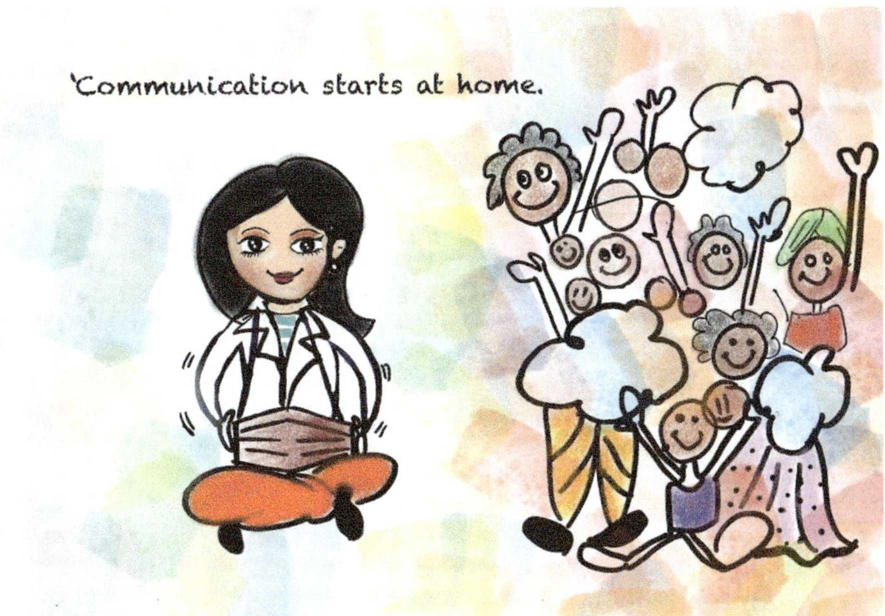


The good physician treats the disease; the great physician treats the patient who has the disease—William Osler.

I. Karunathilake (✉)
Department of Medical Education, Faculty of Medicine, University of Colombo, Colombo, Sri Lanka
e-mail: indika@medarc.cmb.ac.lk

C. Witharana
Faculty of Medicine, University of Colombo, Colombo, Sri Lanka
e-mail: chamindri@bmb.cmb.ac.lk



S. C. Parija, B. V. Adkoli (eds.), *Effective Medical Communication*,
https://doi.org/10.1007/978-981-15-3409-6_25

## 25.1 Assess Need

Effective communication is a key essential in clinical practice. The practice of good communication skills is of utmost importance for the development of a trustworthy relationship between the doctor and the patient. It also results in benefits such as reduction in errors and better compliance leading to cost effectiveness. Since many litigation cases occur due to medical errors, communication plays key role in preventing such cases. While patients will derive better care, the health professionals are likely to have better job satisfaction [1, 2]. On the other hand, ineffective communication has been one of the main reasons for growing dissatisfaction among patients and the general public.

Patients expect better doctor–patient communication. With economic growth and increasing education, patients are becoming more and more aware of their rights, and many of them want to play a more pro-active role in their treatment. The need for effective communication between the doctor and the patient, and increasing patient demands for autonomy and self-determination are the two major challenges before healthcare organizations.

Effective communication is not an inborn quality. It can be acquired by systematic training. However, the present curricula of medical education do not lay adequate emphasis on training in communication skills.

## 25.2 Brief

In this chapter, we shall:

- Revisit the process of doctor–patient communication.
- Summarize methods of teaching and assessing communication skills in medical education.
- Discuss how communication skills can be taught in Southeast Asian countries.

## 25.3 Contextualize

### 25.3.1 Scenario

Dr. Comini's journey in medicine began with her image as a shy and low profile medical student hailing from a remote area. She was subjected to constant challenges in terms of learning in a new environment, participating in seminar and journal clubs, teaching large classes, handling clinical responsibilities, pursuing research, and finally, serving as a leader in medical education. Her journey saw ups and downs, hopes and expectations, success and failure all through which she handled effectively. She believed in teamwork. She converted problems into opportunities. Dr. Comini is now Head of the Department, a seasoned educator, and a leader in the health profession with a combination of pedagogical skills, communication and networking skills to provide leadership at a national and international level.

***Exercise***: Ponder over the various issues related to the communication skills, which Dr. Comini had to learn. List a few points what you could learn from Dr. Comini's experience and make a plan for applying these principles in your workplace.

## 25.4 Describe

The overall picture emerging from the South-east Asian countries regarding communication skills is mixed with positive and negative findings. A research conducted in a teaching hospital in Sri Lanka revealed that majority of the patients expect social niceties like greeting, social smile, offering a seat, avoiding jargon, adequate time, paraphrasing, and empathy [2]. However, only 50% of doctors identified the need for the patient's involvement in decision-making, and a significant proportion of patients (29%) feel that doctors do not entertain patient's point of view.

A study conducted in Indonesia found that doctor–patient communication is more of one-way style with little input from the patients. The patients were generally dissatisfied with doctors' communication style. Doctor–patient communication appeared to be affected by cultural characteristics related to "*social distance*" and "*closeness of relationships*" [3]. A large-scale study conducted in two Medical Schools in Pakistan showed that medical students still believe in doctor-centered approach in communication [4]. In Bangladesh, there is increasing public dissatisfaction with the medical profession due to problems of communication. A qualitative survey indicated that intern were very poor in communicating with their patients. The major deficiencies observed in history-taking were: lack of efforts in exploring patients' psychosocial concerns, providing empathy, discussing patients' personal issues, beginning and ending interviews. Other deficit areas identified were lack of warmth towards the patient, failure to listen to the patients and poor use of questioning during history-taking [5]. In Nepal, it was found that the attitudes of medical students towards communication skills training were not favorable among Nepalese medical schools [6]. Formal training in communication skills in many South-east Asian medical schools is yet to start.

### 25.4.1 Some Initiatives and Good Practices

#### 25.4.1.1 AETCOM Modules in Indian Medical Universities

In order to make the existing MBBS curricula more effective in tune with the healthcare needs of the country, Medical Council of India (MCI) has taken a bold step by proposing new teaching–learning approaches including a structured longitudinal program on attitude, ethics, and communication, which is named as the Attitude, Ethics, and Communication Module (AETCOM) [7, 8]. This model offers a framework of competencies that students must achieve. It also offers approaches to teaching–learning methods and assessment of communication skills.

#### 25.4.1.2 Sri Lankan Initiatives

One of the early initiatives taken by the Faculty of Medicine, University of Colombo was to introduce behavioral science components in to medical curriculum. This stream included communication skills and ethics. Following the Colombo initiative, all State Faculties of Medicine have modified their curricula with an increased emphasis on teaching communication skills. However, the overall response was mixed as the attendance was not uniform [9, 10].

Communication is a two-way process of giving and receiving information through any number of channels [11]. The communication process is influenced by many factors such as knowledge, self-concept, ethical, and cultural factors.
Listening to patients, empathy, and paying attention to verbal, non-verbal, and para-verbal commands are vital for effective communication. On the other hand, excessive use of technical jargon, hurried interaction, showing arrogance are not liked by the patients. Patients want doctors to be supportive and empathetic. In this process body language rather than verbal communication assumes a great role [12, 13].

### 25.4.2 An Empathetic Approach to Doctor–Patient Communication

Empathy is an essential attribute for healthcare professionals. Empathy involves intellectual, thoughtful as well as the emotional behavior of a person with altruism and commitment to serve and care for the patient [14].

### 25.4.3 The Process of Doctor–Patient Communication

An expert panel of the Association of American Medical Colleges (AAMC) identified seven tips which are fundamental to all encounters between clinician and patient (Table 25.1).

**Table 25.1** Seven tips for encounters between clinician and patient: Identified by Association of American Medical Colleges (AAMC)

| No. | Tips for doctors |
|---|---|
| 1 | Build the relationship |
| 2 | Open the discussion |
| 3 | Gather information |
| 4 | Understand the patient's perspective |
| 5 | Share information |
| 6 | Reach agreement on problems and plans |
| 7 | Provide closure |

These can be taught to the students during the communication-training programme using the framework of the Calgary–Cambridge patient interview model which is popular globally [15].

Ideally, as the patient comes in, he/she should be greeted, and a seat should be offered verbally or by the gesture. Active-empathic listening is an important component of effective doctor–patient communication. It includes both verbal and non-verbal communication.

For effective doctor–patient communication, it is important to understand the expectations of patients. An increasing number of patients now expect social niceties such as greeting, social smile, offering a seat, and expression of empathy. Most of the doctors have correctly perceived these expectations. However, the hospital set up in the South Asian region is still hierarchical, and most patients accept doctor-centered approaches such as, giving instructions rather than explanations, and asking specific questions rather than open-ended questions. Patients appreciate allowing them to express an opinion.

### 25.4.4 Challenging Situations Encountered During Doctor–Patient Communication

Communicating with special categories of patients such as terminally ill patients, small children, those who are affected by war or disasters, marginalized social groups, victims of domestic or sexual violence can be challenging, and call for a unique set of skills mix. Doctors need to be trained in those special skills and techniques.

The current advances of information and communication technology open up both advantages and well as unforeseen challenges for doctor–patient communication. The impact of social media on privacy and confidentiality can be profound.

There are several barriers to effective communication. Language is one of the barriers in a multi-cultural context. Intervening of a translator sometimes creates a communication gap between the doctor and the patient. Overcrowded clinical set-ups, which are common in South Asia, pose problems for the doctors to listen to the patients (Fig. 25.1). Some doctors try to keep distance from the patients. Either they talk less or sometimes even belittle patients [16]. The excess use of mobile phone by the doctors has become another major barrier in paying full attention to the patients.

### 25.4.5 The Teaching of Communication Skills in Medical Education

Teaching why and how of doctor–patient communication has then become a pivotal goal in medical education, gradually included in undergraduate curricula as a means to enhance the ability to collect relevant information, build strong therapeutic relationships and foster patient care. Innovative approaches are needed to teach medical students, effective and compassionate communication [17]. Role-plays, case

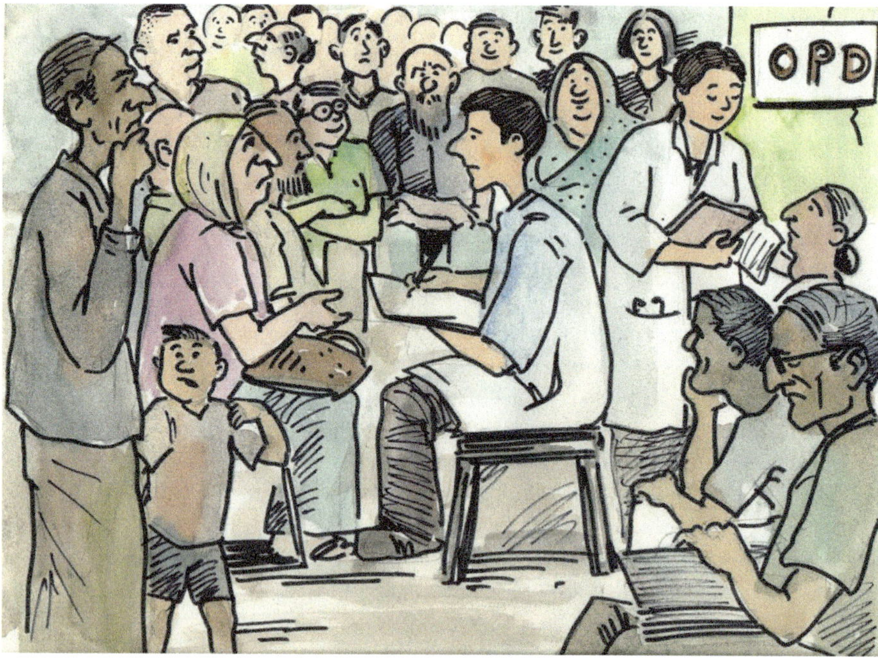


**Fig. 25.1** Learning communication skills in a crowded clinic setup can be challenging

scenarios, videos, and simulated patients are effective ways to teach communication skills. Role modeling by clinical teachers has been recognized as the most powerful tool for teaching empathy (Fig. 25.2).

Simulation is now considered as a valuable educational tool in undergraduate medical education because of its capability to practice and obtain feedback any number of times as required for achieving mastery. A simulated patient is a hired person who acts like a patient but is trained well to behave like a real patient [18].

The role of technology in communication is now widespread. Online social media (Twitter, Facebook, WhatsApp, YouTube, Flickr, Google+, LinkedIn, etc.) are now being increasingly used by doctors and medical students. Appropriate use of technology in communication can be a challenge for medical students and health professionals. Therefore, an awareness of the implications on ethics, professionalism, relationships, and profession need to be highlighted.

### 25.4.6 When to Teach Communication Skills?

The most suitable and effective time during the medical course to learn doctor–patient communication is still a matter of debate, with some researchers stating that a longitudinal design covering several years could be more effective. According to sound educational principle, periodical reinforcement is essential for effective

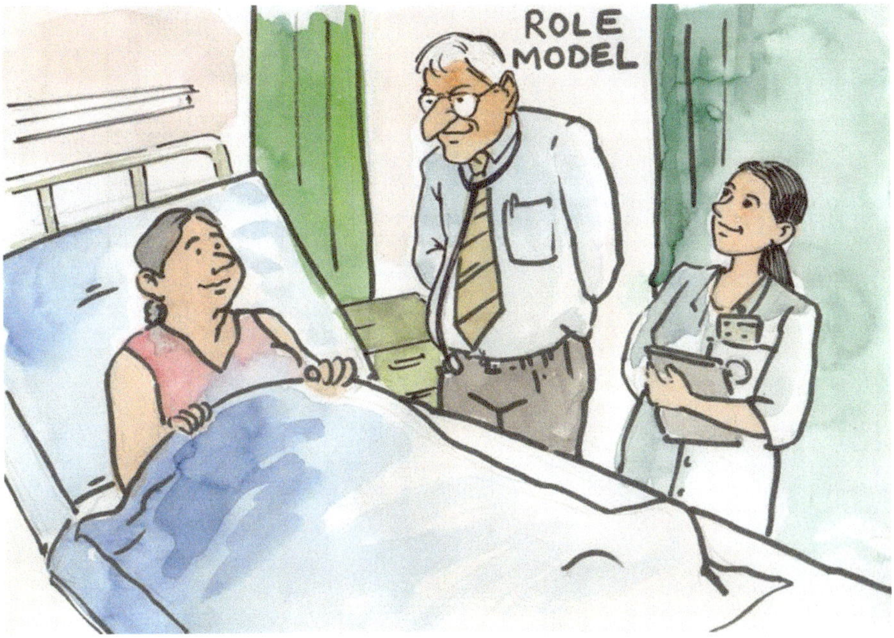


**Fig. 25.2** Role-modeling by clinical teachers

learning. In the pre-clinical years, students are not adequately prepared to develop these skills as they would not have exposure to seriously ill patients. While on the wards during clinical clerkships, students will have some exposure. However, the mentors in the wards may not be able to serve as optimal role models.

A decline of communication skills during clerkships in undergraduate medical students has been reported, namely in empathy, patient-centered attitudes, and attitudes toward the doctor–patient relationship. Communication skills learned in the first year of undergraduate medical education can, in fact, be challenged during clinical practice when students are confronted with time constraints, demanding contexts, role models with different communication styles, and real patients [19]. The use of standardized patients and communication skill labs are much desired facilities for enriching communication training. The use of case scenarios, video-movies followed by reflective exercises, role modeling and role play, engagement in community activities such as village or school health camps, village festivals, and social service activities give ample opportunity.

### 25.4.7 How to Assess Clinical Communication Skills?

Periodic assessment of retention and application of communication skills is of utmost importance to assess the progress of learning and final outcome. The assessment should, therefore, have both formative assessment and summative assessment.

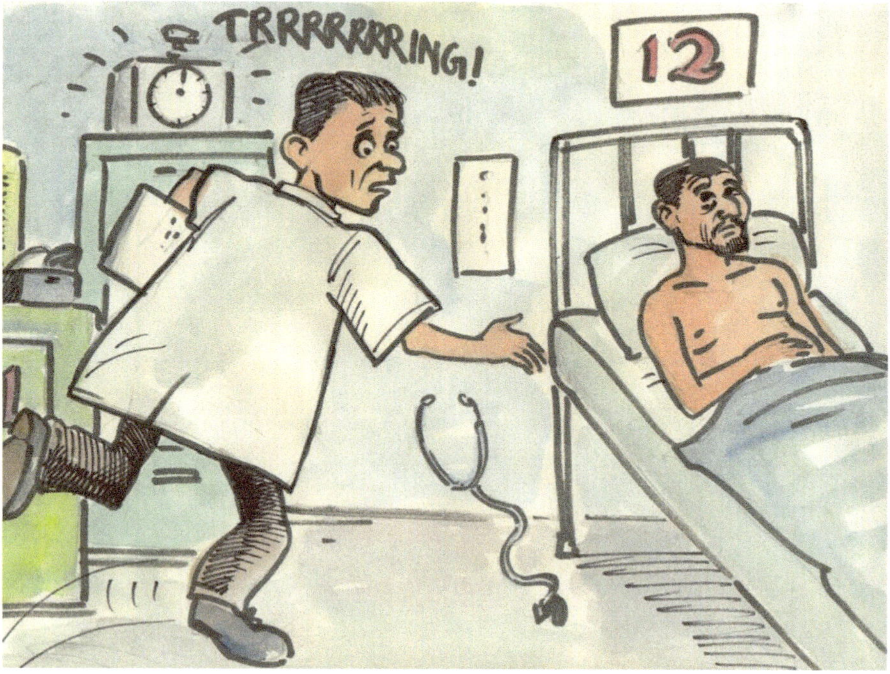


**Fig. 25.3** Assessment of communication skills in OSCE setting

The written assessments alone cannot effectively assess students' performance in communication skills. This calls for using a variety of assessment tools, such as Objective Structured Clinical Examinations (OSCE), self-rating scales, direct observations, video observations, patients' perceptions, and the number of patient recoveries [20]. OSCE can be successfully used in the assessment as it helps in giving specific feedback on what was done well and what could be improved. However, OSCE requires meticulous planning of logistics and resources in terms of real or simulated patients, besides standardized checklists to be filled by trained observers (Fig. 25.3).

Successful communication skills assessment can be done at three levels:

1. Subjective perception about knowledge can be assessed by a written test or a self-evaluation.
2. Objective assessment of communication skills, e.g. with OSCE; and
3. Assessing an output aspect of the communication process, e.g. simulated patient's perception.

The assessment of communication skills, therefore, falls in line with the current trend of assessment utilizing both objective and subjective tools including Multiple Source Feedback (MSF) in the setting of workplace-based assessment [21].

One of the practical models for teaching and assessing communication skills is called "*SEGUE model to denote: Set the stage, Elicit information, Give information, Understand the patient's perspective, End the encounter*" [22].

### 25.4.8 Conclusion

- Communication skills are of vital importance for medical graduates in a competency based medical education.
- It is necessary to identify the barriers to effective communication and make efforts to remove these barriers.
- Most effective methods consist of role modeling, role play, case scenario-based teaching in small groups, use of video followed by reflection.
- Teaching communication skills in workplaces is highly effective.
- The training should start early but continue longitudinally throughout the medical curriculum rather than taught as a single module.
- The approach to assessment should be comprehensive, including a variety of tools and techniques for providing Multiple Source Feedback.

## 25.5 Evaluate

After reading this chapter, prepare a concept map or flow chart of steps showing how you would like to propose effective communication skill training program in your institute.

## References

1. Madsen PL, Pedersen BD, Aspegren K. Communication skills training for medical students: from the simple to the complex. Ugeskr Laeger. 2005;167(38):3581–3.
2. Perera HJM. Effective communication skills for medical practice. J Postgrad Inst Med. 2015;2:20:1–7.
3. Claramita M, Van Dalen J, Van Der Vleuten CP. Doctors in a Southeast Asian country communicate sub-optimally regardless of patients' educational background. Patient Educ Couns. 2011;85(3):e169–74.
4. Ahmad W, Krupat E, Asmaa Y, Attique R, Mahmood U. Attitudes of medical students in Pakistan toward the doctor-patient relationship. PeerJ. 2015;3:e1050.
5. Khanom M, Ata M, Khair R, Ghose A, Faiz MA. Introducing training on doctor-patient communication skill among the pre-intern physicians: a suggested model. Bangladesh J Med Educ. 2018;9(2):32–6.
6. Shankar RP, Dubey AK, Mishra P, Deshpande VY, Chandrasekhar TS, Shivananda PG. Student attitudes towards communication skills training in a medical college in Western Nepal. Educ Health. 2006;19(1):71. Abingdon-Carfax Publishing Limited.
7. Medical Council of India. Attitude, Ethics and Communication (AETCOM) Competencies for the Indian Medical Graduate. 2018. Available at https://old.mciindia.org/UG-Curriculum/AETCOM_book.pdf. Accessed 1 July 2019.

8. Zayapragassarazan Z, Kumar S, Kadambari D. Record review of feedback of participants on Attitude, Ethics and Communication Module (AETCOM) proposed by Medical Council of India (MCI). Online Submission. 2019;11(1):43–8.
9. Jayasinghe S. A new curriculum: a shift for innovation, reforming medical curriculum, lessons from an established medical school in Sri Lanka. Colombo: Jayasinghe; 2002. p. 21–2.
10. Galappatthy P, Abdulla AA, Goonesekera DT, Hanwella DR, Fernando SSD, Seneviratne RA, et al. The impact of behavioral science inputs relevant to clinical work during professorial clinical rotations: perceptions of final year medical students of the University of Colombo. In: Presented at International Conference on Curriculum Change in Medical Schools, Faculty of Medicine, Colombo, Sri Lanka. 2002.
11. Olupeliyawa A, Gooneratne K, Tillakaratne S, Wickramasinghe K, Karunathilake I, Samarasekera D. Graduates' perceptions regarding their final year training. Southeast Asian J Med Educ. 2007;1:25–9.
12. Ha JF, Longnecker N. Doctor-patient communication: a review. Ochsner J. 2010;10(1):38–43.
13. Brahmbhatt K, Lodhiya K. Teaching and assessment of basic clinical communication skills among undergraduate third year medical students in Gujarat. Int J Commun Med Public Health. 2019;6(4):1461–6.
14. Mudiyanse RM. Doctor patient communication for effective healthcare. SLMA news. 2018;11(3):10–3.
15. Burt J, Abel G, Elmore N, Campbell J, Roland M, Benson J, et al. Assessing communication quality of consultations in primary care: initial reliability of the global consultation rating scale, based on the Calgary-Cambridge guide to the medical interview. BMJ Open. 2014;4(3):e004339.
16. Stovall EL. Barriers for the doctor and the patient. In: NCCS - National Coalition for Cancer Survivorship. 2016. Available at: https://www.canceradvocacy.org/resources/communicating-with-your-doctor/barriers-for-the-doctor-and-the-patient/. Accessed on 8 July 2019.
17. Ellman MS, Fortin AH. Benefits of teaching medical students how to communicate with patients having serious illness: comparison of two approaches to experiential, skill-based, and self-reflective learning. Yale J Biol Med. 2012;85(2):261.
18. Weller JM, Nestel D, Marshall SD, Brooks PM, Conn JJ. Simulation in clinical teaching and learning. Med J Aust. 2012;196(9):594.
19. Taveira-Gomes I, Mota-Cardoso R, Figueiredo-Braga M. Communication skills in medical students–an exploratory study before and after clerkships. Porto Biomed. J. 2016;1(5):173–80.
20. Sari SM, Rahayu GR, Prabandari Y. The correlation between written and practical assessments of communication skills among the first year medical students. Southeast Asian J Med Educ. 2014;8(2):49.
21. Karunathilake I. The importance of teaching and assessing communication skills in medical education. Southeast Asian J Med Educ. 2014;8(2):1.
22. Modi JN, Chhatwal J, Gupta P, Singh T. Teaching and assessing communication skills in medical undergraduate training. Indian Pediatr. 2016;53(6):497–504.

Printed by Printforce, United Kingdom